Perioperative Addiction

Ethan O. Bryson · Elizabeth A.M. Frost
Editors

Perioperative Addiction

Clinical Management of the Addicted Patient

Foreword by David L. Reich

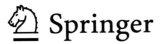 Springer

Editors
Ethan O. Bryson, MD
Associate Professor
Department of Anesthesiology
Department of Psychiatry
Mount Sinai School of Medicine
New York, NY, USA

Elizabeth A.M. Frost, MBChB, DRCOG
Professor
Department of Anesthesiology
Mount Sinai School of Medicine
New York, NY, USA

ISBN 978-1-4614-0169-8   e-ISBN 978-1-4614-0170-4
DOI 10.1007/978-1-4614-0170-4
Springer New York Dordrecht Heidelberg London

Library of Congress Control Number: 2011939085

Printed on acid-free paper

Springer is part of Springer Science+Business Media (www.springer.com)

Foreword

One of the greatest clinical challenges for any anesthesia trainee or practitioner is his/her first experience with a patient with a substance use disorder, whether it be acute, chronic, or iatrogenic. With the ready availability of drugs (over the counter, prescription, and illicitly obtained), complex pharmacology is already present prior to introducing anesthetic drugs. Tolerance and untoward drug interactions set the stage for unpredictable and adverse outcomes.

It is extremely difficult for us to accept the fact that some of our colleagues may also have substance use disorder – a sometimes-fatal disease that harms patients and destroys lives and careers. We often respond with the classic Kübler-Ross grief cycle and then forget quickly when a colleague suddenly disappears to undergo inpatient treatment, is quietly dismissed, or worse still, is found dead. With few forums to discuss addiction and an obligation to protect confidentiality, we create a collective amnesia. We take little or no action to prevent the next occurrence.

Even leaders of national societies, large healthcare institutions, academic departments, and group practices find it agonizing to develop strategies and policies for education, prevention, detection, discipline, treatment, and rehabilitation of the addicted professional. Our own departmental experience over my 26-year tenure has included deaths, careers cut short, and rehabilitations – both successful and failed. The strategy of selective rehabilitation is opposed by many who argue that the risks outweigh the benefits. There are few data to refute that position, despite notable successes.

However, we are gathering information regarding the causes and thus possible treatment or reversal of drug abuse. While much of the information is incomplete, the framework is being developed for a better understanding of the complex nature of addiction. The announcement this year (2011) that a vaccine to treat abuse is available for trial is encouraging.

Drs. Bryson and Frost have assembled a superb group of authors to address these difficult situations. They are to be commended for exploring the existing literature and bringing the experts together to create a cohesive text.

Shortly prior to becoming a United States Supreme Court Justice, Louis Brandeis wrote, "Publicity is justly commended as a remedy for social and industrial diseases. Sunlight is said to be the best of disinfectants; electric light the most efficient policeman."[1] It is my hope that this text will spur us to deal openly and more effectively with the challenges of anesthesia professionals caring for all sufferers from substance use disorder.

New York, NY   David L. Reich

---

[1] Brandeis LD: "Other People's Money" (Chap. 5: What Publicity Can Do), 1914, Public Domain. http://www.law.louisville.edu/library/collections/brandeis/node/196 (accessed January 3, 2011).

Preface

Almost since the beginning of time, man has been intrigued and often overcome by the consumption of substances that alter the perception of everyday life. Well-intended groups, religious organizations, and governments, among others, have struggled with means to legislate and control the ensuing problems with varying success. Yet, drug abuse has continued to escalate, albeit in an ever-changing form, and battle lines have been drawn. This year (2010) the size of one American tobacco company's annual sales has topped $66 billion, which is twice the gross domestic profit of a country such as Uruguay. The company is suing Uruguay (and Brazil) for unspecified damages from lost profit, as these countries have increased warning labels on cigarette packages. Indonesia depends on tobacco jobs and tax revenue as well as payment from tobacco companies for survival and thus has not joined the other 171 countries in the WHO Tobacco Free Initiative. In other words, companies can hold entire countries hostage. However, not only taxes from tobacco sustain governments but also taxes from alcohol, which have fueled more than one war, and with the newly expanded licensing of medical marihuana, undoubtedly even more revenue will flow into government pockets and quickly become essential for running diverse programs.

Anesthesiologists are not immune from addiction but may even be subjected to an environmental hazard from ingestion of trace amounts of substances that later lead to addiction. Alternatively, as has been considered, the ready availability and access to controlled substances may make anesthesia an attractive profession for some individuals and thus foster their addiction. Certainly, it is only recently (last 100 years or so) that overindulgence in narcotics and alcohol has been considered an unworthy trait in physicians. Prior to that, addiction was romanticized by authors and poets and readily adopted by many famous practitioners of medicine. Indeed, several of our most important discoveries in anesthesia evolved from playful experimentation with drugs.

Of course, as anesthesiologists, we often encounter patients who are acutely or chronically abusing drugs, sometimes of multiple origins. These agents not only alter the physiology of the body but also interact with anesthetic agents to cause several, often unpredictable, changes in systemic parameters.

In this text, we have gathered together practitioners with a special interest in the effects of abused substances in all the various manifestations. We realize that this is a rapidly changing and emerging topic, and one that is unlikely to disappear in the near future (the history is too long). We still have much to learn and a long road to travel.

New York, NY   Ethan O. Bryson
                                                                    Elizabeth A.M. Frost

Contents

Contributors

Amy S. Aloysi, MD Department of Psychiatry, Mount Sinai School of Medicine, New York, NY, USA

Ethan O. Bryson, MD Department of Anesthesiology and Department of Psychiatry, Mount Sinai School of Medicine, New York, NY, USA

R. Lyle Cooper, PhD, LCSW College of Social Work, University of Tennessee, Nashville, TN, USA

Sherry Cummings, MSW, PhD College of Social Work, University of Tennessee, Nashville, TN, USA

Samuel DeMaria, Jr., MD Department of Anesthesiology, Mount Sinai School of Medicine, New York, NY, USA

Chad Epps, MD Department of Anesthesiology, University of Alabama at Birmingham, Birmingham, AL, USA

Department of Clinical and Diagnostic Sciences, University of Alabama at Birmingham, Birmingham, AL, USA

Jonathan N. Epstein, MD College of Physicians and Surgeons, Columbia University, New York, NY, USA

Department of Anesthesiology, St. Luke's Roosevelt Hospital, New York, NY, USA

Elizabeth A.M. Frost, MBChB, DRCOG Department of Anesthesiology, Mount Sinai School of Medicine, New York, NY, USA

Clifford Gevirtz, MD, MPH Somnia Pain Management, New Rochelle, NY, USA

Heather Hamza, MS, CRNA Department of Anesthesiology, Los Angeles County Medical Center, University of Southern California, Los Angeles, CA, USA

Michelle M. Jacobs, PhD Department of Psychiatry, Mount Sinai School
of Medicine, New York, NY, USA

Department of Pharmacology and Systems Therapeutics, Mount Sinai School
of Medicine, New York, NY, USA

Alan D. Kaye, MD, PhD Department of Anesthesiology, LSU School
of Medicine, Louisiana State University, New Orleans, LA, USA

David Knez, DO Pittsburgh, PA, USA

Michael Lewis, MD Department of Anesthesiology, University of Miami
Miller School of Medicine, Miami, FL, USA

Migdalia Saloum, MD Department of Anesthesiology, St. Luke's Roosevelt
Hospital, New York, NY, USA

Corey Scher, MD New York University School of Medicine, New York, NY, USA

Andrew Schwartz, MD Department of Anesthesiology, Mount Sinai School
of Medicine, New York, NY, USA

Fouad Souki, MD Department of Anesthesiology, Jackson Memorial Hospital,
Miami, FL, USA

Dirk Wales Wearing Masks Series, Rainbow Productions, Chicago, IL, USA

Julia L. Weinkauf, MD Department of Anesthesiology, Mount Sinai School
of Medicine, New York, NY, USA

Elizabeth Laura Wright, PhDc, MNA, CRNA Department of Clinical and
Diagnostic Sciences, University of Alabama at Birmingham, Birmingham, AL,
USA

Part I
Background

Chapter 1
A History of Addiction in Medical Personnel

Elizabeth A.M. Frost

The passage of time and the changing perception of societal mores have blurred the lines between legality and the nonprescription ingestion of many drugs. The human race has long sought several goals in life: relief of pain, dominance over others, and discovery of a state distinguished by supreme emotional and intellectual elevation. Under the guise of seeking means to alleviate pain, many health care workers have liberally partaken of drugs in an attempt to determine which agents would be most efficacious. Physicians, especially in the military, found that strength and endurance came from cocaine ingestion and liberally gave it to themselves and to the soldiers. Others found that prescribing narcotics freely for all types of conditions ensured a stable and satisfied clientele. Of course, along the way, there were numerous accounts of the wonders and enhanced states that were to be achieved by using these substances. But, on the other hand, there were doctors who fought hard against universal access to narcotics, alcohol, and tobacco and who advocated strongly for the recognition of addiction as a disease.

Ancient Civilizations

Opium may have been first used in Sumeria about 5000 BC as suggested by an ideogram for opium, which has been translated as HUL or "joy" [1]. The Sumerians occupied a region in southern Mesopotamia, modern-day Iraq. As the earliest known civilization, they developed agricultural techniques that allowed the people to grow and store abundant food, making migration after crops and grazing land unnecessary. Undoubtedly, the poppy was one of the crops, cultivated not only to relieve pain but also to induce pleasure and sleep (Fig. 1.1). From the countries of

E.A.M. Frost (✉)
Department of Anesthesiology, Mount Sinai School of Medicine, New York, NY, USA
e-mail: elzfrost@aol.com

E.O. Bryson and E.A.M. Frost (eds.), *Perioperative Addiction:*
Clinical Management of the Addicted Patient, DOI 10.1007/978-1-4614-0170-4_1,
© Springer Science+Business Media, LLC 2012

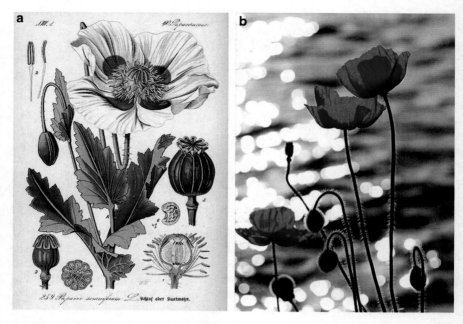

Fig. 1.1 The poppy plant as depicted in an old manuscript and as it appears in the field. Opium is derived from the pods and two crops can be grown annually. (**a**) Left side from: http://en.wikipedia.org/wiki/Opium_poppy. (**b**) Right side from: http://en.wikipedia.org/wiki/poppy

Asia Minor, the poppy was brought to Egypt during the 18th dynasty (c. 1550–c. 1292 BC), when the most successful pharaohs ruled (Thutmosis I–IV, Hatshestut, Tutankamun, and Akhenaten among others) [2]. Two varieties of the poppy, *Papaver somniferum* and *P. rhoeas* are described, the last reported to have been grown in the gardens of the pharaohs, represented in their ornaments and depicted in ancient paintings. In Greco–Roman times, Thebes (Luxor) was a famous center for growing poppies and exporting opium to the Greek islands and throughout the Mediterranean [3]. Use of poppy (nepenthe in Greek) to assuage grief (Demeter in despair over the seizure of Persephone by Pluto) and to forget sorrows (Helen to Telemachus and his comrades) is described in Homer's *Iliad* and *Odyssey*. Greek physicians also widely described the use of the poppy. Theophrastus (373–287 BC), the successor to Aristotle, wrote nearly nine books on an *Enquiry into Plants*, carefully describing the hypnotic and narcotic properties of the poppy as well as its therapeutic effects in curing sorrow and passion and creating a state of indifference to ills [4]. Three physicians in particular influenced the widespread use of poppies and opium: Discorides of Anazarba (Asia Minor 1–2^{MD}c A.D), Galen of Pergamon (129 AD–161 AD) (Fig. 1.2), and Paulus of Aeginata, a Greek physician who lived in Rome in the seventh century and complied seven books on all medical and pharmaceutical knowledge [4, 5] (Fig. 1.3). Paulus described five species of poppies, each differing in effects and potency. Although opium was widely available, physicians around the

Fig. 1.2 Aelius Galen
of Pergamon, now Bergama
in Turkey, was a famous
Greek physician of the
second century AD.
From: http://en.wikipedia.
org/wiki/Galen

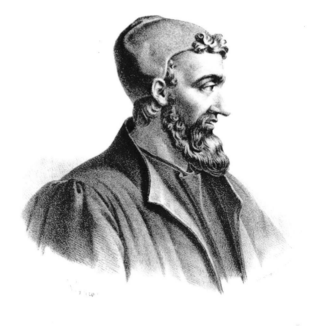

ninth to eleventh century in the Arabic world prescribed opium in moderation for
therapeutic uses. Practitioners considered the poppy and hemp plants as potent
medicines to be used with caution [4]. An eleventh century guide to the pharmacist
in the Adudi Hospital in Baghdad included 200 good, white, and fat poppies in
many pharmaceutical forms to be used for colds, coughs, urinary tract ailments,
gout, and headaches and as a general antidote [4].

By the tenth century, the Arab world expanded east to India and the borders of
China, west to the Iberian Peninsula, and north to Morocco. A new religious faith
took hold and several dissident and radical groups sprang up. The use of drugs was
introduced in many of these cells to help members endure long hours of meditation
and fasting [6]. One of these groups, *the Assassins* developed in the eleventh
century. Its members were drugged with opium and cannabis and were committed
to annihilation of the Arab state in general and the Crusaders in particular.

The thirteenth century saw the rapid cultivation of a shrub, the qat, imported
from Ethiopia to Yemen. The chewing of the fresh leaves and twigs "for spiritual
satisfaction and bodily repose" became an integral part of the life of the Yemenis and
has stayed so until today [4]. The active ingredients include cathine and cathinone,
chemicals related to amphetamines and norepinephrine.

The British had been trading with China since 1635 with informal relations.
There was a high demand for Chinese goods such as silk and tea but little use for
European fare in China. Also, the Chinese insisted in trading in hard currency

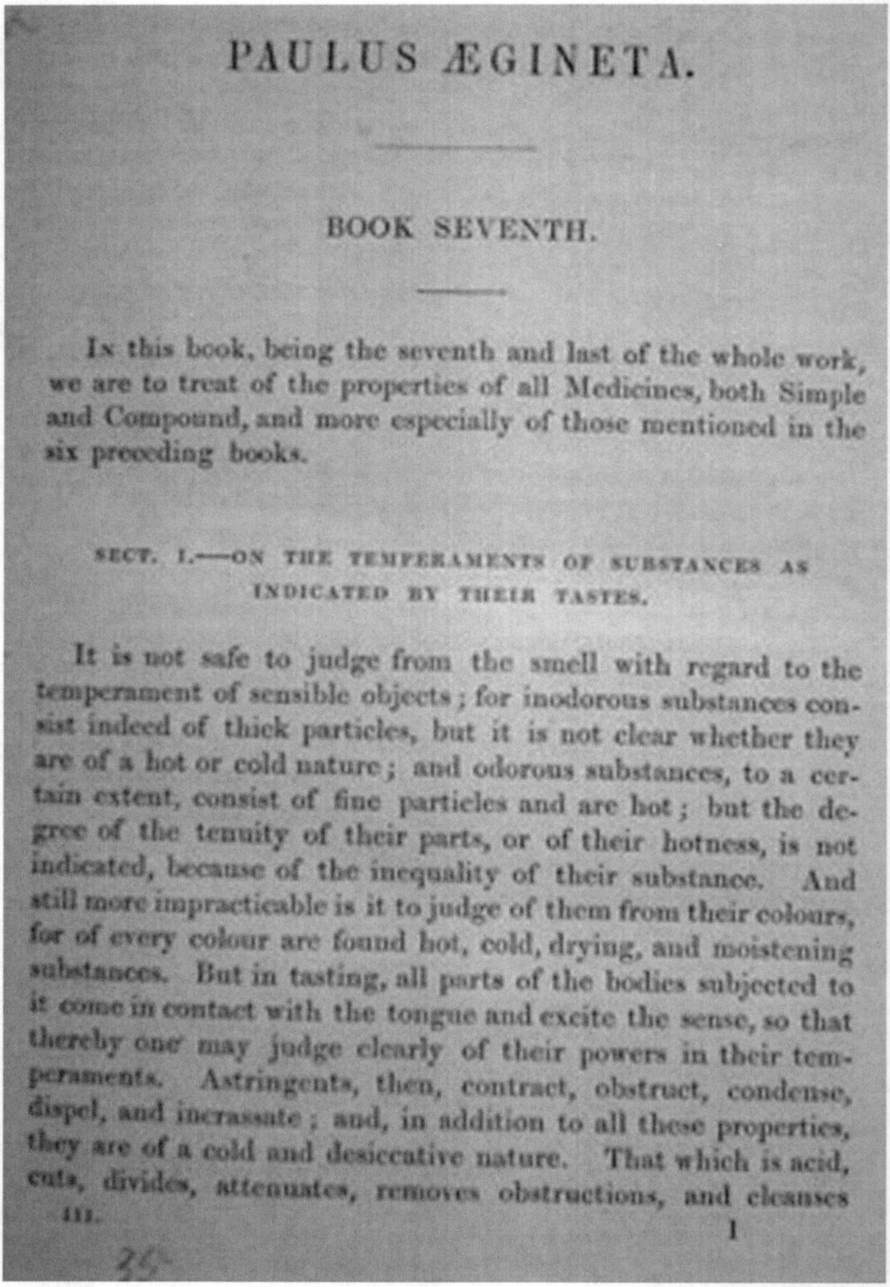

PAULUS ÆGINETA.

BOOK SEVENTH.

In this book, being the seventh and last of the whole work, we are to treat of the properties of all Medicines, both Simple and Compound, and more especially of those mentioned in the six preceding books.

SECT. I.—ON THE TEMPERAMENTS OF SUBSTANCES AS INDICATED BY THEIR TASTES.

It is not safe to judge from the smell with regard to the temperament of sensible objects; for inodorous substances consist indeed of thick particles, but it is not clear whether they are of a hot or cold nature; and odorous substances, to a certain extent, consist of fine particles and are hot; but the degree of the tenuity of their parts, or of their hotness, is not indicated, because of the inequality of their substance. And still more impracticable is it to judge of them from their colours, for of every colour are found hot, cold, drying, and moistening substances. But in tasting, all parts of the bodies subjected to it come in contact with the tongue and excite the sense, so that thereby one may judge clearly of their powers in their temperaments. Astringents, then, contract, obstruct, condense, dispel, and incrassate; and, in addition to all these properties, they are of a cold and desiccative nature. That which is acid, cuts, divides, attenuates, removes obstructions, and cleanses

III.

I

Fig. 1.3 Paulus Aeginata was a Greek physician who lived in Rome. He condensed all the knowledge of medicine from several civilizations into seven books that were translated by F Adams into English in the nineteenth century. Book 7 is devoted to pharmaceuticals, mainly herbs of which opium is one

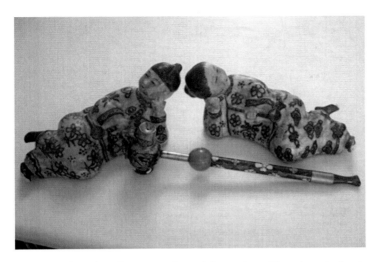

Fig. 1.4 Two porcelain opium figures are shown lying and smoking. An actual opium pipe is between them

such as silver and gold. In the eighteenth century, despite ardent protests from the Qing government, British traders began to import opium from India. An instant consumer market grew up because of the highly addictive nature of opium. The Yongzheng Emperor prohibited the sale and smoking of opium in 1729 and only allowed a small amount to be imported for medicinal purposes. The British East India Company had gained a monopoly in trade by 1773 and established an elaborate trading scheme relying on legal markets and partial leverage of illegal ones through Canton, Calcutta, and the Chinese coast line from British ships to native merchants. By the 1820s, China was importing 900 tons of Bengali opium annually. Chinese troops boarded British ships in international waters and destroyed cargo in 1839 and the British retaliated. The First Opium War lasted from 1839 to 1842 and the Chinese were defeated. Trade escalated despite considerable conflict within the British Government (Gladstone in particular). Tensions mounted and the Second Opium War was waged from 1856 to 1860. Again, the Chinese were defeated and the country fell victim to the widespread use of opium paraphernalia used in depicted is Figs. 1.4–1.7. Opium dens sprang up throughout the country and survive even until today (Fig. 1.8).

Wine has been used at least from the times of the ancient Egyptians. A papyrus dating from around 3500 BC depicts a brewery [7]. But approximately 1,000 years later, one of the first prohibitionist teachings (authored by an Egyptian priest) to a pupil warned, "I, thy superior, forbid thee to go to the taverns. Thou art degraded like beasts" [8]. There are many references to the benefits of wine in the Bible. For example, Proverbs, 31:6–7 (350 BC), exhorts "Give strong drink to him who is perishing and wine to those in bitter distress; let them drink and forget their poverty, and remember their misery no more." And in Ecclesiastics chapter 31, verse 27,

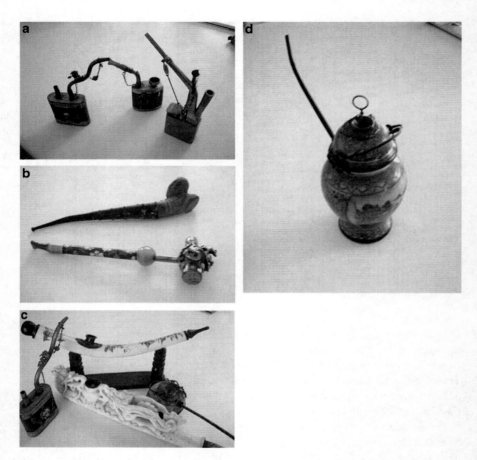

Fig. 1.5 Several opium pipes from South East Asia are demonstrated

"Wine is as good as life to a man, if it be drunk moderately; what life is then to a man that is without wine? For it is made to make men glad." Many wines were produced and distributed widely in the Roman Empire (Fig. 1.9). Hippocrates, as did many other physicians after him, advocated strong wine for many acute diseases (Fig. 1.10) [9]. Wine was the main anesthetic for centuries, both on the battlefield and for the public.

Tobacco was introduced into Europe by Columbus and his crew returning from America in 1493 and quickly became popular. By the seventeenth century, farmers in Virginia were growing tobacco, which was then exported to England. At the same time, Czar Michael Federovitch in Russia ruled that smoking tobacco was punishable by death. The death penalty was also decreed in the Ottoman Empire but the passion for smoking persisted [10].

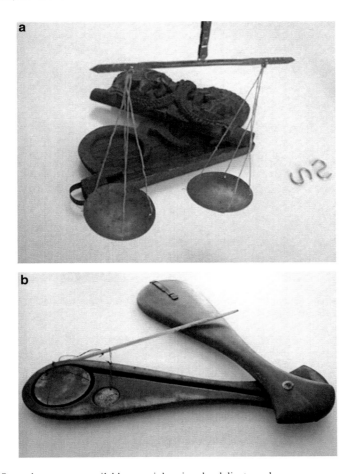

Fig. 1.6 Several means are available to weigh opium by delicate scales

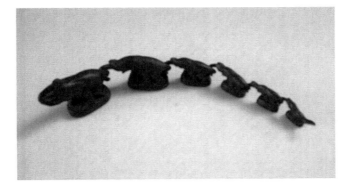

Fig. 1.7 These graded elephants are used to determine the weight and thus the amount of opium sold

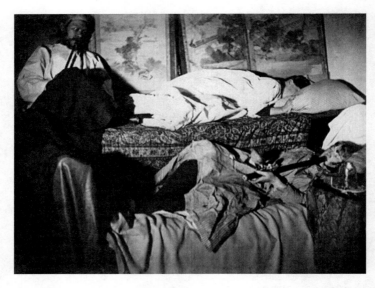

Fig. 1.8 An opium den is shown with one man and two women lying and smoking pipes. From: http://en.wikipedia.org/wiki/Opium_den

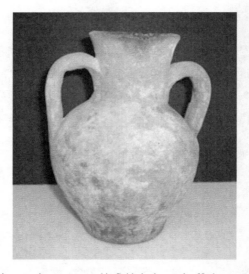

Fig. 1.9 This Roman wine vessel was excavated in Saida in the south of Lebanon and dates to about 50 BC

Physician Influence

From the Middle Ages until the twentieth century, many prominent physicians advocated the use of drugs. Thomas Sydenham (1624–1689), known as the English Hippocrates and the undisputed master of the English medical world, wrote "Among the remedies which it has pleased the Almighty God to give to man to relieve his

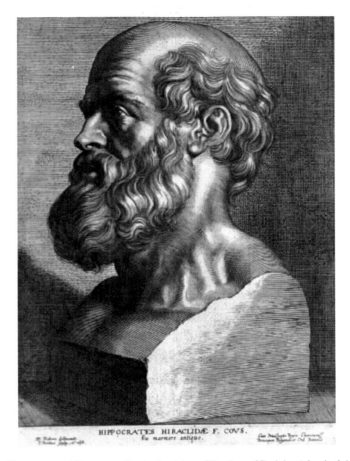

Fig. 1.10 Hippocrates of Kos was a Greek physician of the Age of Pericles (classical Athens) and is generally claimed to be the Father of Western Medicine. From: http://en.wikipedia.org/wiki/Hippocrates

sufferings, none is so universal and efficacious as opium" (Fig. 1.11) [11]. Dr. Sydenham originated the formula for laudanum, an alcoholic tincture of opium (also suggested by Paracelsus in 1525). One of his apprentices, Dr. Thomas Dover (1662–1742), introduced a cure-all prescription, Dover's Powder in 1732. It consisted of a mixture of opium, ipecacuanha, and potassium sulfate [12–14]. This formula produced a relatively reliable and consistent potion in an era when there was no regulation of medications and little standardization in preparation. Medications could be purchased at apothecary shops with or without doctors' prescriptions or at backstreet stores that sold drugs along with food, clothing, and other necessities of life. The major issue at the time in the use of opiate-based medications was not that they contained a narcotic, but whether the consistency of the formula or the misuse by the patient caused overdose. Dover's Powder provided a stable product that, because of the ipecacuanha caused vomiting at higher doses and thus could not be taken in

Fig. 1.11 Thomas Sydenham (1624–1689) was an English physician, known as the English Hippocrates. The Sydenham Society is named after him. From: http://en.wikipedia.org/wiki/Thomas_Sydenham

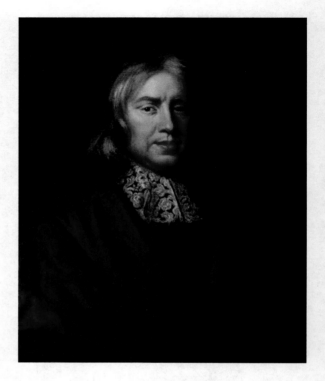

excess at any one time. The powder came to be trusted by the general public and widely prescribed by physicians for over 200 years. It was considered such a safe remedy that it was even prescribed for children. Although the powder was originated as treatment for gout, it was advocated for a wide variety of disorders, including insomnia, diarrhea, bronchitis, tuberculosis, chronic headache, insanity, menstrual disorders, pain, malaria, syphilis, and smallpox. Physicians used it throughout the eighteenth and nineteenth centuries along with many other opium-based patent and official preparations. Often both physicians and patients mistook its narcotic properties, which relieved pain and created a sense of well-being, as curative rather than palliative, and little was understood of the destructive nature of addiction until well into the nineteenth century. Dr George Wood, a professor of medicine at the University of Pennsylvania and president of the American Philosophical Society, authored a treatise on therapeutics in 1868. He described the pharmacologic effects of opium: "A sensation of fullness is felt in the head, soon to be followed by a universal feeling of delicious ease and comfort, with an elevation and expansion of the whole moral and intellectual nature, which is, I think, the most characteristic of its effects… It seems to make the individual, for the time, a better and greater man… The hallucinations, the delirious imaginations of alcoholic intoxication, are, in general, quite wanting. Along with this emotional and intellectual elevation there is also increased muscular energy; and the capacity to act and to bear fatigue is greatly augmented" [15]. Following such recommendations, it was common

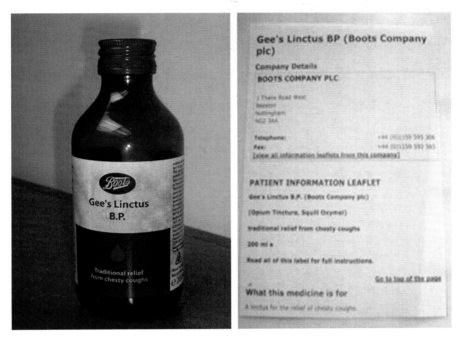

Fig. 1.12 Gee's Linctus was marketed in the United Kingdom over the counter as a cure for respiratory conditions for people of all ages. It contains tincture of opium and the advertisement was accessed on the Internet on October 21st 2010

for middle- and upper-class people, especially women and those with chronic diseases, to be addicted to opiates that were frequently seen in innocuous health elixirs or in remedies that had been originally prescribed by physicians but could now be obtained almost anywhere. Add to this the great increase in the availability of patent medicines, many of which contained up to 50% morphine by volume. Of course, "Dr. Smith's oils, good for what ails you" would make almost anyone feel better, making the consumer believe that the medicine worked and thus buy more. Certainly up until the past 2–3 years, Gee's Linctus, a cough medicine containing tincture of opium, could be bought over the counter at any chemist shop in the United Kingdom and other former Commonwealth countries (personal experience) (Fig. 1.12). Widespread prescribing by physicians and easy availability of the opiate medications made addiction a frequent result of medical therapeutics.

The advent of anesthesia owes as much to self-experimentation as to scientific research. In 1798, Humphrey Davy, the superintendent of the Medical Pneumatic Institution founded by Dr. Thomas Beddoes in Bristol, England, performed considerable experiments on himself on the gas identified by Joseph Priestley as nitrous oxide [16] (Fig. 1.13). He described in detail his addiction to the inhalation of nitrous oxide and of the pleasurable sensations he obtained. He noted also "as nitrous oxide in its extensive operation seems capable of destroying pain, it may probably

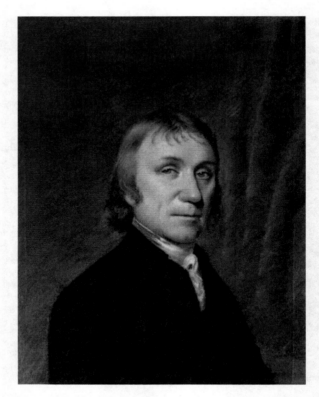

Fig. 1.13 Joseph Priestley, a dissenting English theologian, educator, and natural philosopher, is best known for his discovery of dephlogisticated air (oxygen). Living next to a brewery, he experimented widely in all "airs" that might be released from different substances and isolated eight gases, including nitrous oxide. From: http://en.wikipedia.org/wiki/File:Priestley.jpg

be used with advantage during surgical operations in which no great effusion of blood takes place." Nevertheless, he found more use for nitrous oxide as a means for amusement and ladies and gentlemen of England flocked to the Pneumatic Institute to inhale the wonderful gas (Fig. 1.14 and 1.15).

In the early 1800s, the European attitude of stern admiration for the arts and sciences differed somewhat from the freer, less didactic American way of learning. Pharmacology experiments were often designed to amuse students and nitrous oxide was considered an academic plaything. A medical student at the University of Pennsylvania wrote "A dissertation on the chemical properties and exhilarating effects of nitrous oxide gas" in 1808 (Edgar F. South collection, University of Pennsylvania). The captions on the illustrations read "What a concatenation of ideas" and "Nothing exists but thought" (both of these remarks are quoted in Davy's book) and "This world's a little dirty planet and I'll no longer help to man it," "I feel disposed to merriment" and "The effects of breathing nitrous oxide, the only genteel way of getting drunk" (Fig. 1.16). It was while at this same university that Dr Crawford Long (1815–1878) experimented with ether frolics, which gave him the idea to use

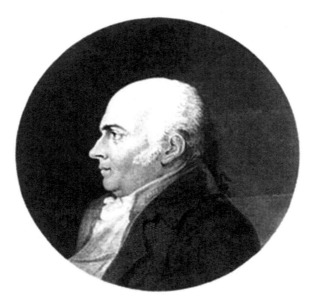

Fig. 1.14 Thomas Beddoes, an English physician and writer, established the Pneumatic Institute at Dowry Square, Hotwells, Bristol, to treat diseases by the inhalation of different gases. From: http://en.wikipedia.org/wiki/File:Thomas-beddoes.jpg

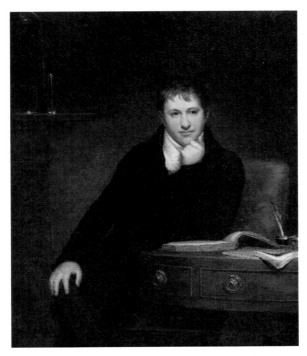

Fig. 1.15 Sir Humphrey Davy, a British chemist and inventor, was recruited by Dr. Beddoes to superintend the laboratory at the Pneumatic Institute in 1798. Davy is depicted in the background on the right behind the counter. From: http://en.wikipedia.org/wiki/File:Davy_Humphry_desk_color_Howard.jpg

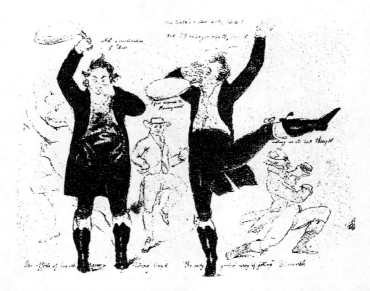

Fig. 1.16 In this cartoon by a medical student at the University of Pennsylvania, inhalation of nitrous oxide is shown to be most beneficial. Crawford Long may have been influenced by this extracurricular behavior

this drug in March 30th 1842 when he excised a tumor from the neck of James Venables (Fig. 1.17) [17].

Itinerant exhibitions of the effects of the inhalation of laughing gas and ether were common in the nineteenth century. It was at just that sort of meeting, run by Gardner Colton, a "so called" professor of chemistry, *a Grand exhibition of Laughing Gas*, on December 10th 1844 (Fig. 1.18) that Horace Wells (Fig. 1.19) observed an injury sustained but unnoticed by Samuel Cooley, one of the 12 young men recruited to inhale the gas [18]. Wells convinced that he had found a revolutionary new approach to pain relief in his dental practice, experimented on himself and others. Rather prematurely, he took his experiment to the Massachusetts General Hospital in Boston in 1845 where the patient did not experience adequate pain relief and he, Wells, was declared a humbug; Wells left the practice of dentistry, traveling to Europe and later returning to the United States. Addicted first to nitrous oxide, he then preferred ether and finally chloroform [19]. In 1848, after a week's binge on chloroform, he threw sulfuric acid on two prostitutes. He was committed to the Tombs in New York, but in accordance with the times was permitted to return home to gather his personal effects. He collected more chloroform and, under the pain-relieving effects of the vapor, he committed suicide by slitting his femoral artery. Wells had shared his findings with another dentist, William Morton (1819–1868) (Fig. 1.20), who on October 16, 1846 gave the first public demonstration of the effects of sulfuric ether anesthesia on Gilbert Abbott from whom, John Collins Warren (1778–1856), professor of surgery at Harvard Medical School, removed a vascular tumor of the neck, also at the Massachusetts General Hospital (Fig. 1.21).

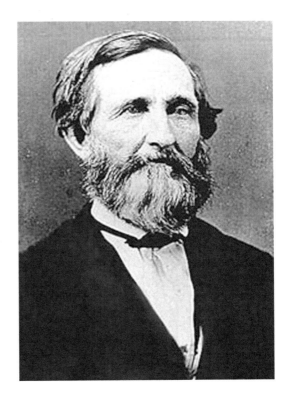

Fig. 1.17 Crawford Long, a country physician in Athens, Georgia, anesthetized a friend for the removal of a tumor in 1842. However, he did not publish his discovery. From: http://en.wikipedia.org/wiki/Crawford_Long

During the operation, the patient muttered and afterward stated the pain was considerable although mitigated, as though the skin had been scratched with a hoe [20]. On the following day, the vapor was administered to another patient for removal of a fatty tumor from the arm with more success. Greatly impressed with the new discovery, Warren uttered his famous words: "Gentlemen, this is no humbug." A new epoch in surgery had begun. Operations could be performed more efficaciously, and haste was no longer of primary concern. The inhalation and ingestion of the ethers had been recommended at least since the beginning of the nineteenth century for various maladies such as gastric problems, tuberculosis, and asthma but usually coupled with a caution against abuse [20]. Several cases of extreme lethargy, seizures, and even death were described and the inhalation of ether was largely abandoned by 1832. A few years later, Morton, after much experimentation on himself and animals, introduced his inhaler, a small two-necked glass globe with sponges to enlarge the evaporating vapor and a valve to divert the expired gas to the atmosphere (Fig. 1.22). In his review of the inhalation of ether, Bigelow (the junior surgeon who had arranged the ether demonstration with Morton and Warren) concluded that:

1. (Ether) is capable of abuse and can readily be applied to nefarious ends
2. Its action is not yet thoroughly understood and its use should be restricted to responsible persons and

Fig. 1.18 A poster, such
as this one, advertised the
exhibition of the effects
of nitrous oxide

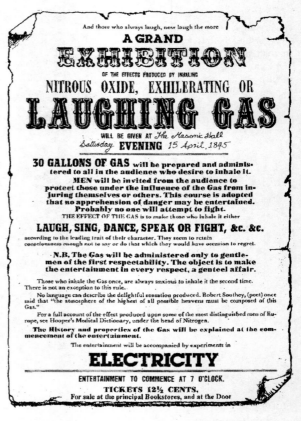

Early experiments in pharmacology were not always didactic.

3. One of the greatest fields is the mechanical art of dentistry many of whose
   processes are by convention, secret, or protected by patent rights [20].

Word of the discovery of the capability of ether to allow painless surgery spread
around the world in weeks. Sir James Simpson (1811–1870) in Edinburgh heard of
this and applied it in his practice (Fig. 1.23). He found the pungency less than
desirable. In a search for something better than ether, he enticed his colleagues
(Drs Keith and Duncan) to sniff several vapors, including chloroform, after dinner,
as was their custom. His guests fell asleep awakening many hours later. Simpson
used chloroform the next day in his obstetrical practice. (November 4th 1847). Six
days later, he reported to the Edinburgh Medico Chirurgical Society on more than
30 painless deliveries [21].

The Scottish Church opposed the use of chloroform, for God said, "Unto the
woman, I will greatly multiply thy sorrow and thy conception; in sorrow thou shalt

Fig. 1.19 Horace Wells, a Connecticut dentist, attended a display of the effects of nitrous oxide and realized the potential for pain relief in his practice. He tried the gas on himself and later became addicted to several agents. From: http://en.wikipedia.org/wiki/Horace_Wells

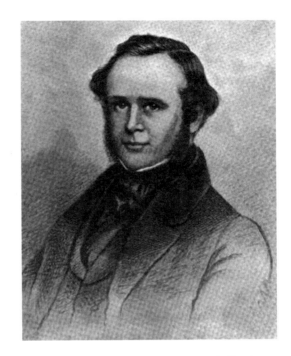

Fig. 1.20 William Morton, an American dentist alerted by Wells to the beneficial effects of inhaled agents for pain relief, first publicly demonstrated the effects of ether in 1846. From: http://en.wikipedia.org/wiki/File:WilliamMorton.jpg

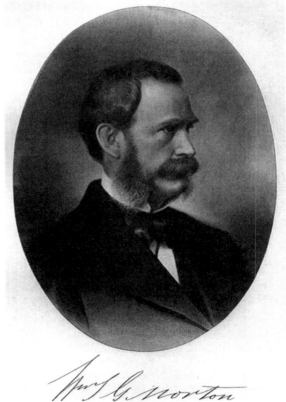

bring forth children and thy desire shall be to thy husband and he shall rule over thee." (Genesis 111:16) In Edinburgh in 1591, a young lady Euphemia Maclean, asked a midwife, Agnes Samson, known as the Wise Woman of Keith, for relief from labor pains. She was publicly burned by the order of King James as a warning to any woman who wished to be relieved of this primal curse. Simpson was denounced from Scottish pulpits and in pamphlets. One clergyman proclaimed "Chloroform is a decoy of Satan, apparently offering itself to bless women; but in the end it will harden society and rob God of the deep, earnest cries which arise in time of trouble for help." [22] Snow countered in "Answers to the religious objections against the employment of anesthetic agents in midwifery and surgery" in 1847. He argued that the Hebrew word "sorrow" could be translated as "toil" or labor." Because of their erect position, childbirth in humans is much more laborious than in animals and the Bible was only recognizing a physiologic fact [22]. Queen Victoria scuttled this thinking when she insisted, on the advice of her accoucher, James Clark, that the surgeon/anesthetist, John Snow, administer chloroform for the birth of Prince Leopold in 1853 (Fig. 1.24). The lady was obviously satisfied and invited Dr Snow back in 1857 to attend during the birth of Princess Beatrice [23]. Snow, who had studied at the Hunterian school, was admitted to the Royal College of Surgeons in 1838. He figured in the initial safe development of anesthesia and arguably was the greatest anesthetist who ever lived. His broad use of both ether and chloroform for his own enjoyment and that of his guests led to the publication of two books which incidentally might be said to also describe office-based anesthesia [24, 25].

But not all self-experimentation by physicians resulted in monumental discoveries for mankind. The father of psychoanalysis, Dr Sigmund Freud, was an early user and proponent of cocaine as a stimulant and as an analgesic (Fig. 1.25). He wrote several articles on the antidepressant qualities of the drug and was influenced also by his friend, Wilhelm Flies, who advocated cocaine for "nasal reflex neurosis." Fliess operated on the nose of Freud as well as on several of the latter's patients [26]; Freud believed that cocaine would work as a panacea. He prescribed it for his friend, Ernst von Fleischl-Marxow, for the treatment of morphine addiction and declared it curative, despite the fact that Fleischl-Marxow developed acute cocaine psychosis and subsequently died, apparently still addicted to both cocaine and morphine. Despite increasing reports of overdose and addiction to cocaine from around the world, Freud continued to use the drug. Some critics have suggested that most of Freud's psychoanalytic theory was merely a by-product of his cocaine use [27]. In addition to cocaine, Freud also abused tobacco, smoking some 20 cigars a day. He developed a squamous cell carcinoma of the mouth and underwent over 30 surgeries. His suffering was intense but he continued to smoke until he died in a morphine coma, induced to relieve the pain [28].

The *Strange Case of Dr. Jekyll and Mr. Hyde* relates the good and evil in everyone (Fig. 1.26). Taking a "potion," described as a white powder, led Dr. Jekyll into a wonderful state of disinhibition for a while until finally evil took over and he

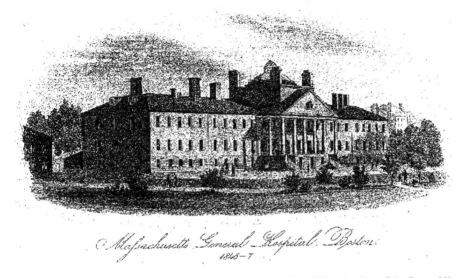

Fig. 1.21 The Massachusetts General Hospital as it appeared in 1846 at the time of the first public demonstration of anesthesia. From: Warren JC. The influence of anesthesia on the surgery of the 19th century. Boston: Privately printed; 1897:Opposite p24

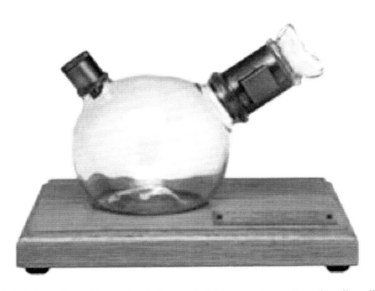

Fig. 1.22 Inhaler as devised by Morton for better administration of ether. From: http://en.wikipedia.org/wiki/File:Morton_inhaler.jpg

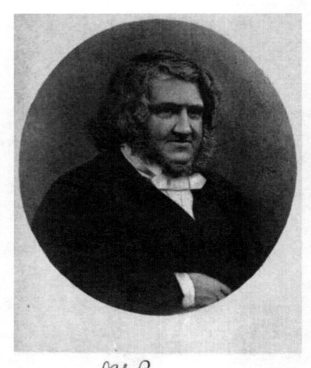

Fig. 1.23 Sir James Simpson, a Scottish obstetrician, used chloroform, first on his guests after dinner and on the following day for his laboring patients. From http://en.wikipedia.org/wiki/File:Simpson_James_Young_signature_picture.jpg

committed suicide [29]. Robert Louis Stevenson (1850–1894), who had a long history of drug use including opium and hashish, confronted his own cocaine-induced demons in this novella which he is said to have written in about 3 days while under the influence of the drug (Fig. 1.27) [30]. Another Scottish writer and also physician, Sir Arthur Conan Doyle (1859–1930), also wrote of the effects of cocaine in 1890 (Fig. 1.28). The first scene of *The Sign of the Four* relates:

> Sherlock Holmes took his bottle from the corner of the mantelpiece and his hypodermic syringe from its neat morocco case. With his long, white, nervous fingers he adjusted the delicate needle, and rolled back his left shirt-cuff. For some little time his eyes rested thoughtfully upon the sinewy forearm and wrist all dotted and scarred with innumerable puncture-marks. Finally he thrust the sharp point home, pressed down the tiny piston, and sank back into the velvet-lined armchair with a long sigh of satisfaction.

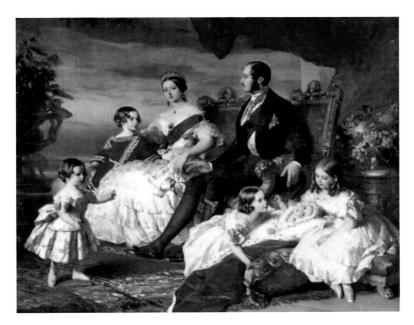

Fig. 1.24 Queen Victoria with her husband Prince Albert and some of their children. With her acceptance and endorsement of pain relief for childbirth, obstetrical anesthesia was born. From: http://commons.wikimedia.org/wiki/File:Queen_Victoria,_Prince_Albert,_and_children_by_ Franz_Xaver_Winterhalter.jpg

A little later in the story Holmes states:

It is cocaine," he said, "a seven-per-cent solution. Would you care to try it?

Professor William Halsted (1852–1922) was a very influential American surgeon. By 1884, he had read Dr. Carl Koller's report on the anesthetic properties of cocaine (Fig. 1.29). Halsted with his students began to experiment by injecting each other's nerves and demonstrated that safe and reversible local anesthesia could be produced. In the process, Halsted became addicted to cocaine and was later sent to the Butler Sanatorium in Rhode Island in 1886. There a cure was attempted by converting his addiction from cocaine to morphine, a not uncommon practice (Fig. 1.30) [31]. Halsted remained addicted to morphine (around 180 mg/day) until the end of his life. At this dosage level, he was able to function well and establish what is the core of American surgery today. He was appointed surgeon-in-chief at Johns Hopkins Hospital when it opened in 1889.

Other uses and abuses of cocaine were related to the desire of army leaders to both force their soldiers to avoid exhaustion and fear of fighting. Dr. Theodor Ashenbrandt, a German army physician, secured a supply of pure cocaine from the pharmaceutical firm of Merck and issued it to his Bavarian soldiers during

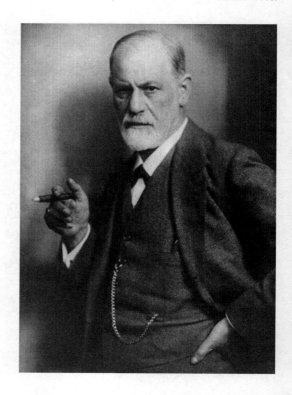

Fig. 1.25 Sigmund Freud was an Austrian neurologist who founded the school of psychoanalysis. He became addicted to several drugs throughout his life. From: http://en.wikipedia.org/wiki/Sigmund_Freud

maneuvers [32]. He reported the beneficial effects of the drug in increasing the ability of the men to endure fatigue. The use of morphine on the battlefield was so extensive that by 1880 so many Union veterans were addicted that the press regarded morphinism as the "soldiers' disease." [33] History relates that the Confederate army was so poor that the anesthetic of choice for amputations was whiskey [33]. Drug abuse has remained a problem in the military of all nations, although now it is self-administered rather than dictated by the leaders.

It is estimated that by 1900 nearly 2–5% of the adult population of the United Sates was addicted to drugs, mainly morphine and cocaine. The principal reason for morphine dependence related to hospital experience. Morphine was liberally prescribed for pain relief during and after surgery and hospital stays were often prolonged [33]. As recently as 1975, average hospital stay following hysterectomy was 14 days, breast mass excision 7 days, and tubal ligation 8 days [34]. Only with the advent of ambulatory surgery and developments in anesthesia with greater use of regional techniques and nonsteroidal agents have patients returned to their homes relatively pain and narcotic free.

Although it was believed that cocaine was a drug associated with privilege and the higher social classes, and a drug immune from serious problems, it is clear that

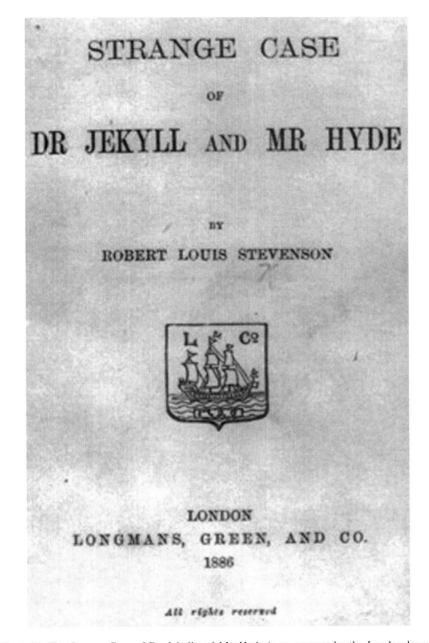

Fig. 1.26 The Strange Case of Dr. Jekyll and Mr. Hyde is an account by the London lawyer, Gabriel Utterson of the odd occurrences between his friend Dr. Henry Jekyll and the misanthropic Mr. Edward Hyde. From: http://en.wikipedia.org/wiki/File:Jekyll_and_Hyde_Title.jpg

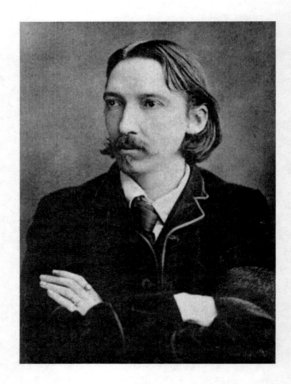

Fig. 1.27 Robert Louis Stevenson was a Scottish author who was addicted to drugs and liberally passed the addiction on to his characters, including physicians. From: http://en.wikipedia.org/wiki/File:Robert_Louis_Stevenson_Knox_Series.jpg

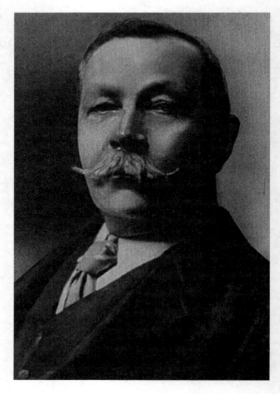

Fig. 1.28 Sir Arthur Conan Doyle, a British author and physician, dabbled in drugs and wrote their use into some of his books. From: http://en.wikipedia.org/wiki/File:Conan_doyle.jpg

Fig. 1.29 A prominent American surgeon, William Halsted, required ever-increasing amounts of morphine throughout his life to deal with his addictions. From: http://en.wikipedia.org/wiki/File:William_Stewart_Halsted_Yale_College_class_of_1874.jpg

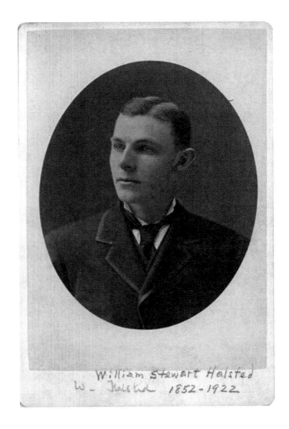

those were not the sole motivating factors for abuse. Imagination, scientific curiosity, ignorance of its addictive qualities, a search for better means to pain relief, and a desire to improve the efficiency of the war model all played a part [35].

A Changing Picture

Because narcotics and alcohol were prescribed freely, taken socially, sometimes mandated or part of a religious rite, overuse and dependence on these substances were not considered to be a disease and thus treatment and legislation as to use were not indicated. Thomas Trotter, an Edinburgh physician, published an essay in 1804 in which he stated that he considered drunkenness to be a disease [36]. However, in 1822 Thomas De Quincey in the famous "Confessions of an opium eater" proclaimed that the opium habit must be learned and "on Saturday you are an opium eater, on Sunday no longer such" (Fig. 1.31) [37].

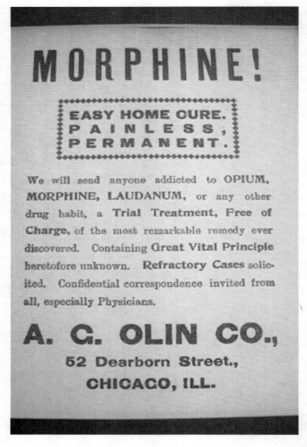

Fig. 1.30 Advertisements such as this promised that morphine addiction could be cured usually by substitution of another narcotic. Similarly, giving morphine could cure cocaine addiction

Perhaps because of the ubiquitous consumption of alcohol by people of all ages, the recognition of alcoholism as such came sooner. The American Society for the Promotion of Temperance was founded in Boston in 1826 and by 1833 there were some 6,000 local Temperance societies with over one million members. Benjamin Parsons, an English clergyman, listed 42 distinct diseases caused by alcohol, including nephritis, gout, encephalitis, and dropsy [36]. Although the American Medical Association (AMA) was founded in 1847, it appears to have had little early or substantial involvement in any form of addiction recognition or treatment. Rather with the growing movement of temperance (especially with women's movements, such as that driven by Susan B. Anthony, Fig. 1.32) and the passage of the 18th amendment to the US Constitution in 1919, it was in the interests of physicians to support prohibition and garner the ability to control alcohol and narcotics. It is estimated

Fig. 1.31 Thomas de Quincey (1785–1859) was an English author and intellectual who is best known for "Confessions of an English Opium Eater" written in 1821. From: http://en.wikipedia.org/wiki/File:Thomas_de_Quincey_-_Project_Gutenberg_eText_16026.jpg

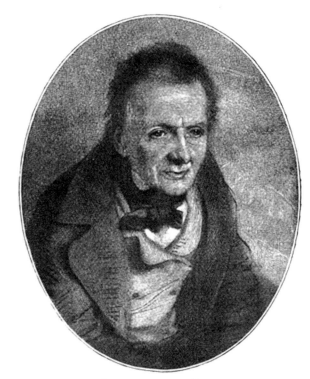

Fig. 1.32 Susan B. Anthony (1820–1906) was a prominent American civil rights leader and activist for women who strongly opposed drug and alcohol addiction. She lectured extensively throughout the United States, averaging 75–100 lectures a year. From: http://en.wikipedia.org/wiki/File:SusanBAnthony-sig.png

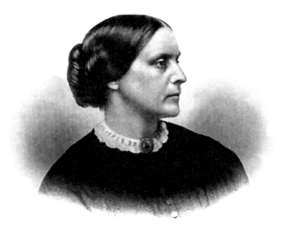

that by 1928, US physicians made $40 million annually writing prescriptions for whiskey and brandy [38]. With the founding of the American Pharmaceutical Association in 1856, a stated goal was "To as much as possible restrict the dispensing and sale of medicines to regularly educated druggists and apothecaries"… a rather vague statement as the education of said professionals was not subject to much scrutiny [39].

An inquiry, the report of the Indian hemp drug, a 3,000-page document, was commissioned by the British Government in 1894 and concluded that "there is no evidence of any weight regarding the mental and moral injuries from the moderate use of these drugs"…also "Moslem and Hindu custom forbid taxing anything that gives pleasure to the poor." [40]. (The first statement was still supported by the American Medical Association during the debate over the Marihuana Tax Act of 1937 [33]).

So with many fits and starts, the problems of addiction were slowly recognized and not necessarily by the medical profession. Legal measures against drug abuse were first established in 1875 when opium smoking was outlawed in the city limits in San Francisco and confined to neighboring Chinatowns and their opium dens (see Fig. 1.8). The second Opium War between Britain, France, and China had ended in 1860, leaving China open to enormous abuse of the drug. Many immigrants had fled to the United States and the Californian settlement was a haven for opium users. Enforcement of the law was very difficult.

In a somewhat backward step for the war on addiction, diacetylmorphine was synthesized in 1874 by C. R. Alder Wright, an English chemist working in London. He had been experimenting with combining morphine with various acids. The compound was acquired by the German company Bayer, who named its new over-the-counter drug "Heroin" in 1895. The name was derived from the German "*heroisch*" (heroic) due to its perceived "heroic" effects upon a user. It was chiefly developed as a morphine substitute for cough suppressants that did not have morphine's addictive side effects. Morphine at the time was a popular recreational drug, and Bayer wished to find a similar but nonaddictive substitute to market. However, contrary to Bayer's advertising it as a "nonaddictive morphine substitute," heroin would soon have one of the highest rates of dependence amongst its users.

The first national drug law, the Pure Food and Drug Act of 1906, no longer allowed medicines containing narcotics to be obtained over the counter or by mail order without proper labeling. The Act also established the Food and Drug Administration and required that all drugs that may be habit forming should be so labeled [33, 41].

The 16th Amendment created the legal authority for federal income tax. Between 1870 and 1915, the tax imposed on liquor provide an estimated one-half to two-thirds of the entire internal revenue of the United States, or about $200 million annually [42].

The Harrison Narcotics Tax Act followed in 1914 and was the first Federal law to criminalize the nonmedical use of drugs in the United States. The Act forbade the sale of substantial doses of cocaine or opiates, except by licensed doctors and pharmacies. Because Congress feared that the bill might not pass as it was doubtful if the government could actually regulate a profession and probably did not have the power to pass a general criminal law, the Act was presented as two taxes. For a small fee, doctors would purchase a stamp that would allow them to prescribe narcotics for patients. The second tax imposed a large sum on anyone exchanging any of the drugs listed for nonmedical reasons; in other words, persons caught in possession of the drug and who had not paid the tax were guilty of tax evasion [33]. Shortly thereafter, heroin was also banned and subsequent Supreme Court decisions made it illegal for doctors to prescribe narcotics to addicts; physicians who prescribed maintenance doses as part of addiction therapy were jailed and thus all attempts at cure were abandoned.

In 1917, the AMA had endorsed national prohibition and declared that one of the methods for controlling syphilis was by controlling alcohol. However, the Council of the AMA refused to confirm these earlier resolutions and thus, in the 6 months after the enactment of the Volstead Act (the statute passed in 1919 to define the terms and implementation of the 18th Amendment, which was not repealed until 1933), more than 15,000 physicians and 57,000 drug manufacturers applied for licenses to prescribe and sell liquor [43]. Bootlegging and crime increased. Dr Prentice of the Committee on Narcotic Drugs of the AMA spoke of the "propaganda in the press… and…. shallow pretense that drug addiction is 'disease' [44]." It was not until 1935 that the AMA passed a resolution that "alcoholics are valid patients [45]." Finally, in 1966 Congress enacted the "Narcotics Addict and Rehabilitation Act" that formally inaugurated a federal civil commitment program for addicts.

Conclusion

Spanning at least 7,000 years, the association between drugs of addiction and the healing professions is complex. While some physicians, often by chance, turned their use and abuse of drugs to the benefit of mankind, others profited by the control they maintained over society. Huge financial gains were possible and organized medicine in the United States was slow to turn this tide and recognize drug addiction for the disease that it is.

References

1. Lindesmith AR. Addiction and opiates. New York: Aldine; 1968. p. 207.
2. Hamarneh S. The physician and the health professions in medieval Islam. Bull N Y Acad Med. 1971;47:1088–110.
3. Sigerist HE. A history of medicine 1. Primitive and archaic medicine. New York: Oxford University Press; 1951. 203:341:485:489.
4. Hamarneh S. Pharmacy in medieval Islam and the history of drug addiction. In: Anees MA, editor. Health sciences in early Islam, Collected papers, vol. 2. Blanco, TX: Zahra Pub; 1983. p. 226–37. Accessed at Yale Library Call no Hist R 143 H 355.

5. Adams F. The seven books of Paulus Aegineta, trans, vol. 3. London: The Sydenham Society; 1847. p. 247–8.
6. Smith M. Studies in early mysteries in the near and middle east, vol. 47. London: Sheldon; 1931. p. 160–6.
7. Fort J. The pleasure seekers; the drug crisis, youth and society. Indianapolis, IN: Bobs Merrill; 1969. p. 14.
8. Crafts WF. Intoxicating drinks and drugs in all lands and times. Washington, DC: The International Reform Bureau; 1911. p. 5.
9. Adams F. The genuine works of Hippocrates, trans. London: The Sydenham Society; 1849. p. 298–9.
10. Brecher EM. Licit and illicit drugs. New York: Little Brown and Comany; 1974. p. 212.
11. Goodman L, Gilman A. The pharmacologic basis of therapeutics. 1st ed. New York: Macmillan; 1941. p. 186.
12. Boyes JH. Dover's powder and Robinson Crusoe. N Engl J Med. 1931;204:440–3.
13. Duke M. Thomas Dover – physician, pirate and powder, as seen through the looking glass of the 20th-centuryphysician. Conn Med. 1985;49:179–82.
14. Osler W. Thomas Dover, M. B. (of Dover's Powder), physician and buccaneer. Bull Johns Hopkins Hosp. 1896;7:1–6.
15. Musto D. The American disease; origins of narcotic control. Oxford: Oxford University Press; 1999. p. 71–2.
16. Davy H. Researches chemical and philosophical chiefly concerning nitrous oxide. London: Biggs and Cottle, Bristol; 1800. p. 453–96.
17. Long CW. An account of the first use of sulphuric ether by inhalation as an anaesthetic in surgical operations. Southern Med Surg J. 1849;5:705–13.
18. Raper HR. Man against pain. New York: Prentice-Hall; 1945. p. 68–78.
19. Ardher WH. Life and letters on Horace Wells. Discoverer of anesthesia. J Am Coll Dent. 1944;11:80–210.
20. Bigelow HJ. Insensibility during surgical operations produced by inhalation. Boston Med J. 1846;35:309–17.
21. Simpson JY. On a new anaesthetic agent, more efficient than sulphuric ether. Lancet. 1847;2: 549–50.
22. Haggard HA. Devils, drugs and doctors. New York: Blue Ribbon Books; 1929. p. 107–9.
23. Ball C. James Young Simpson 1811–1870. Anaesth Intensive Care. 1996;24(6):639.
24. Snow J. On chloroform and other anaesthetics: their action and administration. London: John Churchill, New Burlington Street; 1858. p. 1–443.
25. Snow J. On the inhalation of the vapour of ether in surgical operations: containing a description of the various stages of etherization, and a statement of the result of nearly eighty operations in which ether has been employed in St. George's and University College Hospitals. London: John Churchill; 1847. p. 1–88.
26. Masson JM. The assault on truth: Freud's suppression of the seduction theory. New York: Pocket books (Division of Simon and Schuster); 1998. p. 233–50.
27. Borch-Jacobsen M. How a fabrication differs from a lie. London Rev Books. 2000;22(8):3–7.
28. Hafner JW, Sturgis EM. The famous faces with oral cavity and pharyngeal cancer. Tex Dent J. 2008;125(5):410–29.
29. Stevenson RL. The strange case of Dr. Jekyll and Mr. Hyde. London: Longmans, Green and Co; 1886.
30. Schultz M. The strange case of Robert Louis Stevenson: a tale of toxicology. JAMA. 1971;216(1):90–4.
31. Penfield W. Halsted of Johns Hopkins. The man and his problem as described in the secret records of William Osler. JAMA. 1969;210:2214–8.
32. Brecher EM. Licit and illicit drugs. New York: Little Brown and Co; 1974. p. 272.
33. Whitebread C. The history of the non-medical use of drugs in the United States. Address to the California Judges association 1995. http://www.druglibrary.org/schaffer/History/whiteb1.htm. Accessed 7 Aug 2010.

34. Frost E. Outpatient evaluation. A new role for the anesthesiologist. Anesth Analg. 1976;55(3): 307–10.
35. Siegel RK. Cocaine and the privileged class: a review of historical and contemporary images. Adv Alcohol Subst Abuse. 1984;4(2):37–49.
36. Roueche B. Alcohol: the neutral spirit. New York: Berkeley Pub Corp (Penguin Group); 1971. p. 87–8.
37. DeQuincy T. Confessions of an English opium eater, 1822. London: Pomona Press; 2005. 143.
38. The Lectric Law Library. A history of drug use and prohibition, p 21. http://www.lectlaw.com/files/drg09.htm. Accessed 8 July 2010.
39. Musto D. The American disease; origins of narcotic control. Oxford: Oxford University Press; 1999. p. 258.
40. Taylor N. The pleasant assassin; the story of marijuana. In: Solomon D, editor. The Marijuana Papers. Milwaukee, WI: Panther Books; 1970. p. 31–47.
41. Pure Food and Drug Act of 1906. http://www.druglibrary.prg/schaffer/history/e1900/pfdn.htm. Accessed 8 July 2010.
42. The Lectric Law Library. A history of drug use and prohibition, p 20. http://www.lectlaw.com/files/drg09.htm. Accessed 8 July 2010.
43. Sinclair A. Era of excess: a social history of the prohibition movement. New York: Harper Colophon Books; 1964. p. 492.
44. Prentice AC. The problem of the narcotic drug addict. JAMA. 1921;76:1551–6.
45. Kessel N, Walton H. Alcoholism. New York: Penguin Book; 1966. p. 21.

Chapter 2
The Genetic Basis of Addiction

Chad Epps and Elizabeth Laura Wright

Introduction

Addiction is a complex disease influenced by genetic, environmental, developmental, and social factors. Once viewed as a moral weakness in character, substance use disorders are now defined as maladaptive patterns of substance use leading to inability to control use despite significant consequences in the American Psychiatric Association's Diagnostic and Statistical Manual of Mental Disorders (DSM-IV) [1]. Family, adoption, and twin studies support the importance of biologic factors and prompted the search for an inherited link. Because addiction is a heterogeneous and complex disorder without a clear Mendelian pattern, identification of specific genes has proved challenging.

This chapter reviews the role of genetic factors, molecular mechanisms, and related imaging of the addicted brain. Although drug dependency is commonly associated with illegal substances (e.g., opioids, cocaine, marijuana, and methamphetamine), legal substances such as alcohol and nicotine must also be considered. Because there is a preponderance of data on alcohol and tobacco use, these drugs are emphasized throughout the chapter though the concepts are, in many cases, applicable to other substances.

Genetic Factors in Substance Abuse

Two primary strategies exist for identifying genetic factors in substance abuse. The first is the candidate gene approach in which techniques are developed to target

C. Epps (✉)
Department of Anesthesiology, University of Alabama at Birmingham, Birmingham, AL, USA

Department of Clinical and Diagnostic Sciences, University of Alabama at Birmingham, Birmingham, AL, USA
e-mail: cepps@uab.edu

E.O. Bryson and E.A.M. Frost (eds.), *Perioperative Addiction:*
Clinical Management of the Addicted Patient, DOI 10.1007/978-1-4614-0170-4_2,
© Springer Science+Business Media, LLC 2012

specific genes that may determine susceptibility to addiction. The details of these techniques are beyond the scope of this chapter but involve dissection of deoxyribonucleic acid (DNA) into specific nucleotide patterns called markers [2]. These markers are then examined to determine if there is a linkage (when the marker is transmitted along with the disease in families) or an association (when a marker allele is seen more commonly among diseased individuals in a population). The second approach is the genome-wide linkage approach in which the whole genome is studied blindly to determine points of integration among addicted phenotypes.

Candidate Genes

Candidate genes thought to influence the pathogenesis of dependence and addiction have been postulated to include genes that act on neural mechanisms involved in reward and behavior (e.g., dopamine receptor and catechol-O-methyltransferase) and genes that encode enzymes involved in alcohol metabolism (alcohol dehydrogenase and aldehyde dehydrogenase).

The first report of an "alcoholism gene" occurred in 1990. Blum et al. [3]. identified a gene for the D_2 dopamine receptor (DRD2) that was thought to be associated with risk for developing alcoholism. Dopamine's role in the mesolimbic reward circuit had been clearly established at this point; so, Blum's idea was widely received. Since then, the role of DRD2 has been the subject of much debate and remains controversial [4, 5]. Gamma-aminobutyric acid (GABA) is the major central inhibitory neurotransmitter and the genes for its receptor are also implicated in alcoholism. Studies have determined that GABA receptors play an important role in the depressant effects of alcoholism [6]. It appears that two $GABA_A$ receptor genes are related to the risk of developing alcoholism [7]. In addition to the dopaminergic and GABAergic systems, the serotonergic system also appears to be a source of genetic variation favoring addiction. Various genes that encode serotonin receptors and transporters have also been implicated in the development of addiction [8, 9].

Catechol-O-methyltransferase (COMT) is one of several enzymes responsible for metabolizing and inactivating the catecholamine neurotransmitters, including dopamine and norepinephrine. The COMT protein is coded by gene *COMT* in which G to A polymorphisms are common at codon position 158 resulting in the amino acids valine (Val158) or methionine (Met158), respectively. The allelic variant, Val158, is well studied and is known to result in a fourfold increase in enzyme activity [10]. The prefrontal cortex, known to be closely linked to a person's personality and executive function, is highly dependent on COMT for regulation of dopamine activity as there are few dopamine transporters [11]. The Val158 allele results in lower dopamine concentrations in the prefrontal cortex and is associated with inefficient frontal lobe function and behavior disinhibition leading to impulsive behavior

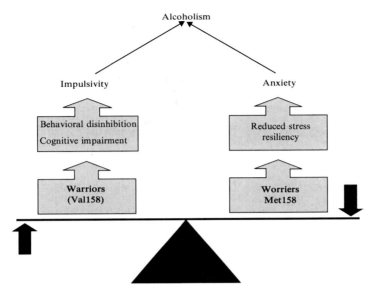

Fig. 2.1 Catechol-O-Methyltransferase (COMT): the warrior (Val158) versus worrier (Met158) model (From Ducci F. Genetic approaches to addiction: genes and alcohol. *Addiction.* 2008;103:1414–1428)

[12, 13]. The Met158 allele is associated with better cognitive performance but less stress resiliency, increased levels of anxiety [14], and increased reactivity of the amygdala to unpleasant stimuli [15]. For any given individual, a balance exists between "warriors" (Val158) and 'worriers' (Met158) (Fig. 2.1) and though Val158 is most commonly associated with addiction there are subpopulations in which risk appears to be associated with Met158 [16]. Numerous studies have examined the potential association of COMT with personality traits and psychiatric disorders, including obsessive–compulsive disorder, bipolar disorder, and drug dependence with somewhat inconsistent results [17].

Polymorphisms of alcohol metabolizing-enzyme genes have consistently demonstrated an association with alcohol susceptibility and include alcohol dehydrogenase IB (*ADH1B*) and aldehyde dehydrogenase (*ALDH2*). Ethanol is metabolized by the enzyme alcohol dehydrogenase to a toxic intermediate, acetaldehyde. Acetaldehyde is then metabolized by the enzyme aldehyde dehydrogenase to acetate. Acetaldehyde accumulation occurs with high activity of ADH1B or low activity of ALDH2 which results in flushing reaction with hypotension, palpitations, and tachycardia. These disulfiram [ANTIBUSE]-like reaction seems to confer protection against the development of alcoholism. Slower-metabolizing forms ADH1B and faster-metabolizing forms of ALDH2 appear to confer an increased risk of alcoholism and drug dependence [18].

Genome-Wide Scans

To detect genetic differentiation among populations, genome linkage and genome association studies are performed to identify chromosomal regions and genes implicated in addiction. Genome-wide linkage studies attempt to identify risk loci from a panel of polymorphisms in family-based samples. These studies identify chromosomal regions for risk-influencing loci that are shared within the family. To be complete, these studies employ markers that map throughout the entire genome. Genome-wide association studies are performed in very large data sets using panels of more than 500,000 polymorphisms. These association studies have increased power for detecting smaller chromosomal areas compared to the family-based linkage studies [16].

In response to the positive genetic correlations evidenced by twin, family, and adoption studies, the National Institute on Alcohol Abuse and Alcoholism funded the Collaborative Studies on Genetics of Alcoholism (COGA) [19]. Since 1989, the COGA investigators have been performing genetic linkage studies to identify genes that affect the risk for alcoholism in over 300 densely affected families. The COGA has successfully detected at least three genes within linked chromosomal regions (*GABRA2*, *CHRM2*, and *ADH4*) that contribute to predisposition to alcoholism and related disorders [20].

It is most likely that most of the genetic risk associated with drug dependency is not attributed to individual alleles. Genome-wide studies, once thought to hold all the answers, are also somewhat problematic. Association studies are complicated by other co-morbid traits such as bipolar affective disorder and schizophrenia, and appear to be falling short of the definitive results. In addition, a strong genetic association is sometimes difficult to identify in linkage studies [21]. This is most likely explained by the heterogeneity of addiction, population variation, and random variation.

Heritability

It is thought that genetics account for at least 50% of alcohol addiction, although the biologic effects of genetic factors are less well understood [22]. Early twin adoption studies reveal a 54% risk of an identical twin developing alcoholism if the other twin is alcoholic. [23] More recent research confirms the heritability of alcoholism, especially in men [24]. Although not as strong as alcoholism, similar twin studies indicate a genetic predisposition toward cocaine and opiate addictions [25]. Some work has been done on the genetics of opiate addiction, and although the genetic component plays a role, a single causative gene has not been isolated [26]. Other research finds genetic neuroelectric brain-wave differences in sons of alcoholics, who are not alcoholics, which are identical to that in the alcoholic fathers. These brain-wave alterations were not seen in the nonalcoholic control population [27].

Studies to date highlight at least three important points regarding the genetic influence on addiction [2]. First, a family history of addiction is a strong predictor of risk regardless of socioeconomic status. Second, factors that may trigger addictive behavior are diverse and differ from individual to individual. For example, social isolation may trigger addictive behavior in some, while large social gatherings serve as a trigger in others. Third, there is likely no one gene that confers the risk of addiction but rather an interaction of multiple genes along with other environmental factors.

Shared Etiology

Addiction frequently occurs with other disorders in the same patient. The comorbidities may include co-addiction (tobacco, alcohol, illicit drugs, eating, gambling, or even sex) or other mental disorders. There appear to be genetic factors in common between nicotine and alcohol abuse that may partially explain why the two substances are often used concurrently [28, 29]. Persons with mental illness are about twice as likely to smoke as compared to controls [30] and the prevalence of nicotine dependence is 5–6 times higher in persons with psychiatric disorders as compared to the general population [31]. Persons with mental illness are about twice as likely to smoke as compared to controls [30] and the prevalence of nicotine dependence is 5–6 times higher in persons with psychiatric disorders as compared to the general population [31]. Twin studies support a shared genetic vulnerability to and significant genetic correlation between alcohol and tobacco use [28].

Up to 60% of persons diagnosed with alcoholism have evidence of other preexisting psychiatric disorders [32]. Borderline personality disorder [33] and major depression [34] have been associated with a high rate of nicotine dependence. In addition, twin studies reveal a genetic link between alcoholism and externalizing disorders, such as attention-deficit and hyperactivity disorder and antisocial personality disorder [35]. Like addiction, these other psychiatric disorders share a high heritability, suggesting that the genes responsible are likely pleiotropic (i.e., a single gene determining multiple phenotypes) and stress the importance of integrating the study of addiction with other psychiatric illnesses.

Brain-Reward Mechanisms

The most popular theories of addiction involve activation of the brain reinforcement circuit (Fig. 2.2), which is naturally activated by behaviors involving food and sex. Although drugs of abuse produce effects through many receptor systems in the brain, their effect on the mesolimbic dopaminergic system (Fig. 2.3) is critical and most often implicated in producing the rewarding effects. Dysfunction of this system contributes to several pathologic conditions including schizophrenia, attention-deficit and hyperactivity disorder, and Parkinson's disease and is thought to be critical to the

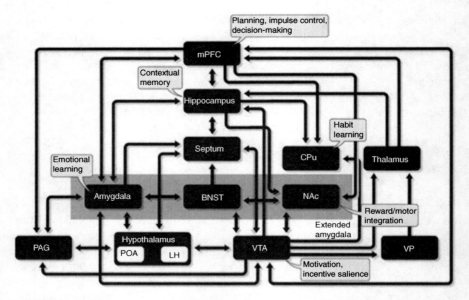

Fig. 2.2 Schematic representation of the brain reinforcement circuit. Brain sties of reinforcement are integrated in a circuit based on their connectivity and putative functional roles. *BNST* bed nucleus of the stria terminalis, *CPu* caudate putamen, *LH* lateral hypothalamus, *mPFC* medial prefrontal cortex, *NAc* nucleus accumbens, *PAG* periaqueductal gray, *POA* preoptic area, *VP* ventral pallidum, *VTA* ventral tegmental area (Reprinted from Le Merrer J, Becker JAJ, Befort K, Kieffer BL. Reward Processing by the opioid system in the brain. *Physiol Review.* 2009;89:1383)

addictive properties of abused substances [36]. Drugs of abuse increase extracellular dopamine concentration overriding the control of motivated and goal-directed behavior, contributing to compulsive drug seeking and taking [37]. Cocaine is known to alter dopamine release and reuptake which, with chronic use, alters the reward system in a way that leads to addiction and, possibly, relapse [38, 39].

The opioid system is also thought to play a key role in brain reinforcement circuits [40]. Brain opioid receptors are expressed primarily in the limbic system, cortex, and brain stem and are central in the mediation of nociception as well as other physiologic functions, including stress, endocrine function, and immune function. In recent years, the role of the brain opioid system in modulating mood and addictive behaviors has also become apparent [41, 42]. Pharmacologic activation or blockade of opioid receptors at several sites has demonstrated the role of these receptors in both the "pleasure" natural reward system and the reinforcing properties of abused drugs [40]. Brain sites where opioid agonists or antagonists modulate drug reinforcement include the ventral tegmental area (VTA) and nucleus accumbens (NAc). Mu and delta receptors found in the VTA and NAc modulate positive reinforcement for both opioid and nonopioid drugs of abuse, including ethanol [43], cocaine, and nicotine. In addition, mu and delta receptor blockade leads to a decreased response when drugs of abuse are administered [44].

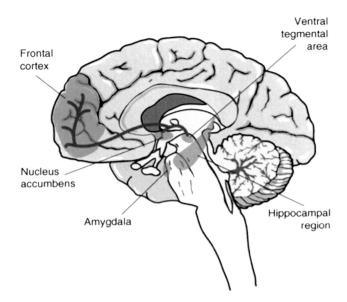

Fig. 2.3 The mesolimbic dopamine (reward) pathway in the brain. The dopamine pathway originates in the ventral tegmental area (VTA) and projects into the nucleus accumbens (NAC) and the prefrontal cortex (PFT). The VTA consists of dopaminergic neurons, which respond to glutamate, whereas the NAC consists primarily of medium spiny neurons, which are GABA-ergic neurons. The hippocampus is involved in learning and memory (From Kalsi G, Prescott CA, Kendler KS, Riley BP. Unraveling the molecular mechanisms of alcohol dependence. *Trends Genet.* 2008;25(1):50)

In addition to dopamine and opioids, other neurotransmitters, including glutamate, serotonin, and acetylcholine, are involved in the experience and progression of drug use [45, 46]. It is clear that these neurotransmitters share a neurobiologic interconnectiveness but further investigations are needed to investigate the full scope of relevance.

Imaging the Addicted Brain

The imaging of genetically different brains is fairly new, but may play a larger role in the future as genetic research expands. In the area of addiction, investigators have focused on genes that modulate dopamine in the reward system. This type of research may help determine whether addiction causes neuroplasticity or the genetic differences lead to the neuroplasticity associated with addiction.

Dopamine$_2$ (D$_2$) receptor polymorphism affects reward system processing. The presence of an A1 variant allele on post-synaptic D$_2$ receptor results in less expression of D$_2$ receptors in areas of the ventral striatum and putamen. These receptors are also

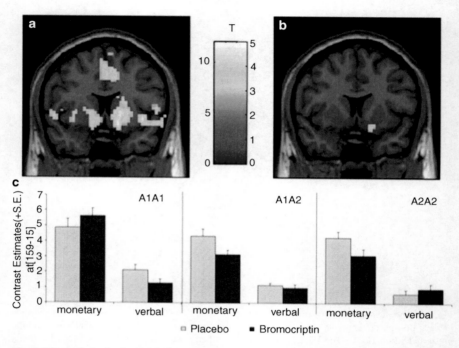

Fig. 2.4 Increased striatal activation during the anticipation of reward varies by genotype. (**a**) Main affect in all groups. (**b**) Stronger activation to bromocriptine in the NAc varied by genotype, with greatest activation by A1 genotype. (**c**) Response to anticipated monetary reward greatest with A1 allele after bromocriptine administration (Reprinted from Kirsch P, Reuter M, et al. Imaging gene-substance interactions: the effect of the DRD2 TaqIA polymorphism and the dopamine agonist bromocriptine on the brain activation during the anticipation of reward. *Neurosci Lett.* 2006;405:199, with permission)

associated with less dopamine binding. It is thought that decreased numbers of receptors and less dopamine binding lead to reduced dopamine release in the nucleus accumbens. In addicts, this reduced sensitivity to dopamine causes an urge to increase dopamine levels with their substance of choice; hence, craving results. In a sense, this allele rewards substances that increase dopamine levels. Kirsch et al. have demonstrated differences in blood oxygen level-dependent (BOLD) activation in functional magnetic resonance imaging (fMRI) of the nucleus accumbens between those with the A1 gene and those without [47]. This difference was in response to the anticipation of a monetary reward after the administration of a dopamine agonist. Initially, participants with the A1 allele performed worse on a monetary reward task than the non-A1 participants ($P < 0.05$), supporting genetically altered reward system processing. After administration of a dopamine agonist, the A1 participants significantly increased their ability to obtain monetary rewards as well as activation of the striatum in response to reward anticipation ($P < 0.05$) (Fig. 2.4) [48]. This genetic difference may help explain the overinflated anticipation associated with addiction.

On the other hand, the described work of van Eimeren et al. demonstrated that increased dopamine activity in the lateral orbitofrontal and ventral striatum altered

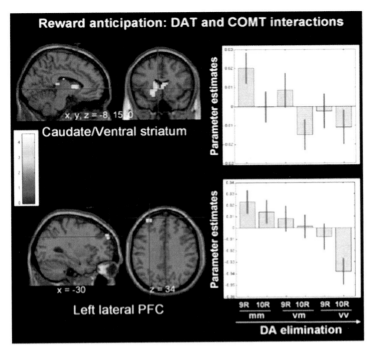

Fig. 2.5 Interaction between COMT and DAT1 genotypes with COMT and DAT variant showing those (*left*) augmented neural response in the caudate, ventral striatum, and prefrontal cortex and (*right*) reduced elimination of dopamine in anticipation of an uncertain reward in those with the variants (Reprinted from Dreher JC, Kohn P, Kolachana B, et al. Variation in dopamine genes influences responsivity of the human reward system. *Proc Natl Acad Sci USA.* 2009;106:619)

reward processing [49]. This phenomenon could have a genetic basis. Genetic influences on the reward system may also involve the modulation by the enzymes responsible for catabolism of synaptic dopamine and its re-uptake into the presynaptic membrane in the prefrontal cortex and ventral striatum [48]. Synaptic dopamine levels are maintained by (COMT), which catabolizes synaptic dopamine, and the dopamine transporter enzyme (DAT1), which transports synaptic dopamine back into the presynaptic vesicle. COMT is very active in the prefrontal cortex, where little DAT1 is found and vice versa, although COMT likely plays some role in modulating dopamine in the ventral striatum via downstream neural connections. Specific variants of either of these genes cause reduced expression and activity of these enzymes, ultimately resulting in increased synaptic dopamine and increased activity in the prefrontal cortex and ventral striatum [48]. A genetic difference was demonstrated in brain activity with BOLD activation on an fMRI in response to uncertain reward anticipation and reward outcome. Participants with the COMT variant had a significant increase in activity of the lateral prefrontal in anticipation of uncertain reward ($P < 0.001$, uncorrected) and orbitofrontal cortex in response to reward ($P < 0.005$) and reduced dopamine elimination in these areas (Fig. 2.5) [48]. Those with the DAT1 variant had increased activity in the caudate nucleus and the

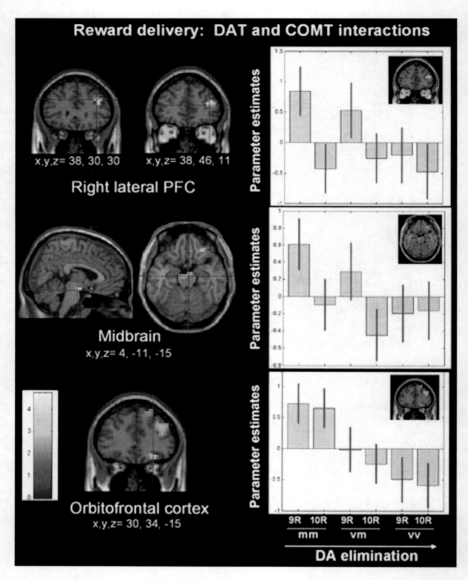

Fig. 2.6 Interaction between COMT and DAT1 genotypes with COMT and DAT variant showing (*left*) augmented neural response in the right lateral prefrontal cortex and midbrain and (*right*) reduced elimination of dopamine in response to reward in those with the variants (Reprinted from Dreher JC, Kohn P, Kolachana B, et al. Variation in dopamine genes influences responsivity of the human reward system. *Proc Natl Acad Sci USA*. 2009;106:621)

striatum. An interaction effect was also noted between the COMT and DAT1 genotypes in the ventral striatum, caudate nucleus, and lateral prefrontal cortex ($P<0.01$). This interaction resulted in a hyper-responsivity of reward system (Fig. 2.6) [48]. These results support van Emerein and colleague's work that revealed increased dopamine via administration of a dopamine agonist in the ventral striatum and lateral orbitofrontal cortex was associated with increased risk-taking behaviors. It should be noted that neither of studies looked specifically at the addicted brain; however, these results provide a foundation for understanding how genetics play a role in brain reinforcement circuits and risk-taking behavior associated with addiction.

Summary

Substance abuse and addiction are heritable disorders often found concurrently with psychiatric comorbidities. The causes are complex and multifactorial but recent studies suggest multiple genetic influences. Linkage studies have identified genes likely involved in the pathogenesis, but only a fraction of the entire genetic risk has been accounted for. Newer methodologies including genome-wide scans will assist in identifying more rare risk variants.

Activation of the brain reinforcement circuit is integral to the addictive process and drug-seeking behavior. Recent advances in imaging have greatly contributed to our understanding of addictive behavior, the genetic influence, and underlying mechanisms.

Spotlight on the Role of the Opiate System in Addiction

Michelle M. Jacobs, PhD

The μ-opioid receptor (OPRM1) is the primary receptor target for both endogenous opioid peptides and exogenous opioid analgesics. There is individual variability for response to opioid analgesics as well as a likelihood to become tolerant and/or dependent on these agents. As such, it is important to understand the genetic and biological basis for individual differences that may guide better pain management with reduced side effects.

The OPRM1 gene is a large, highly complex gene located on chromosome 6q24–25. Currently, there are over 800 single nucleotide polymorphisms (SNPs) associated with this gene. However, the most frequently studied SNP has been the A118G SNP located within exon 1 that results in a substitution of asparagine for aspartate at position 40 in the receptor's extracellular domain

(N40D). This SNP is relatively common in individuals of European (10–15%) and Asian ancestry (36–50%), but much less frequent in African American (0–4%) populations. In vitro studies have produced conflicting results as to the functional relevance of this substitution. Initial studies indicated that the human G118 variant had an increased binding affinity for β-endorphin and enhanced activation of G-protein coupled potassium channels [50], suggesting a gain of function as a result of A118G mutation. Other studies have failed to replicate the original findings [51]. Additional studies performed in postmortem brain tissue have supported a loss of function role for the mutation with G118 subjects demonstrating a 1.5-fold reduction in mRNA expression [52].

A118G in Substance Abuse
Various human genetic studies have highlighted the importance of the A118G SNP in substance abuse. It has been associated with opioid dependence in several different ethnic populations including Han Chinese [53], Indian [54, 55] and European Caucasian [56, 57]. Several studies have also found a role for A118G and alcohol abuse across many populations including Korean [58–60], Japanese [61] and Caucasian [62–64]. In addition to substance abuse, individual differences have also been reported for responses to pain. Individuals carrying the 118G allele report an elevated pain response as well as decreased pain threshold [65, 66]. Chronic pain patients and those who have undergone surgery who are 118G carriers consume more morphine or other opioids as compared to A118A homozygote subjects [67, 68]. Of interest, 118G individuals often have reduced side effects such as lower levels of nausea and respiratory depression [66, 69].

Treatment for Substance Abuse and Relevance of A118G
Two main classes of drugs are available to treat opioid addiction; opioid receptor antagonists including naloxone and naltrexone, and opioid receptor agonists or partial agonists such as methadone, levomethadyl acetate (LAAM) and buprenorphine. These drugs act on the μ-opioid receptor and can block the effects of an ingested opioid. However, each of these drugs varies in treatment efficacy as well as adherence rates. Risk of overdose on methadone and LAAM is also a concern as these drugs are full agonists of the μ-opioid receptor and considered highly addictive themselves.

Given the differences and difficulties in treatment efficacy and adherence and the known functional role of A118G in OPRM1, recent studies have questioned if individual genetic variability at A118G can predict therapeutic outcomes to opioid receptor agonists and antagonists. One of the best characterized examples of this theory is the response to naltrexone in alcohol dependent subjects. 118G subjects reported more sensitivity to alcohol while naltrexone blocked this alcohol-induced "high" [70, 72]. Numerous clinical trials have reported A118G's effects on responses to naltrexone [60, 70–73]. 118G subjects were more likely to respond to naltrexone than A118A subjects and most importantly, 118G subjects had longer rates of relapse [71]. In addition, cue-induced craving is also greater in 118G-carrying individuals. Clearly, these studies have highlighted the importance of including individual genetic analysis when determining optimal therapy for addiction and the need for additional studies for opioid antagonists/agonists.

References

1. American Psychiatric Association. Diagnostic criteria from DSM-IV-TR. Washington, DC: American Psychiatric Association; 2000.
2. Lowinson JH. Substance abuse: a comprehensive textbook. 4th ed. Philadelphia: Lippincott Williams & Wilkins; 2005. 37.
3. Blum K, Noble EP, Sheridan PJ, et al. Allelic association of human dopamine D2 receptor gene in alcoholism. JAMA. 1990;263(15):2055–60.
4. Le Foll B, Gallo A, Le Strat Y, Lu L, Gorwood P. Genetics of dopamine receptors and drug addiction: a comprehensive review. Behav Pharmacol. 2009;20(1):1–17.
5. Bowirrat A, Oscar-Berman M. Relationship between dopaminergic neurotransmission, alcoholism, and reward deficiency syndrome. Am J Med Genet B Neuropsychiatr Genet. 2005;132B(1):29–37.
6. Maccioni P, Colombo G. Role of the GABA(B) receptor in alcohol-seeking and drinking behavior. Alcohol. 2009;43(7):555–8.
7. Lobo IA, Harris RA. GABA(A) receptors and alcohol. Pharmacol Biochem Behav. 2008;90(1):90–4.
8. McHugh RK, Hofmann SG, Asnaani A, Sawyer AT, Otto MW. The serotonin transporter gene and risk for alcohol dependence: a meta-analytic review. Drug Alcohol Depend. 2010;108(1–2):1–6.
9. Enoch MA, Gorodetsky E, Hodgkinson C, Roy A, Goldman D. Functional genetic variants that increase synaptic serotonin and 5-HT3 receptor sensitivity predict alcohol and drug dependence. Mol Psychiatry. 2010. doi: 10.1038/mp.2010.94.http://www.nature.com/mp/journal/vaop/ncurrent/full/mp201094a.html.
10. Chen J, Lipska BK, Halim N, et al. Functional analysis of genetic variation in catechol-O-methyltransferase (COMT): effects on mRNA, protein, and enzyme activity in postmortem human brain. Am J Hum Genet. 2004;75(5):807–21.
11. Mazei MS, Pluto CP, Kirkbride B, Pehek EA. Effects of catecholamine uptake blockers in the caudate-putamen and subregions of the medial prefrontal cortex of the rat. Brain Res. 2002;936(1–2):58–67.
12. Egan MF, Goldberg TE, Kolachana BS, et al. Effect of COMT Val108/158 Met genotype on frontal lobe function and risk for schizophrenia. Proc Natl Acad Sci USA. 2001;98(12):6917–22.
13. Malhotra AK, Kestler LJ, Mazzanti C, Bates JA, Goldberg T, Goldman D. A functional polymorphism in the COMT gene and performance on a test of prefrontal cognition. Am J Psychiatry. 2002;159(4):652–4.
14. Enoch MA, Xu K, Ferro E, Harris CR, Goldman D. Genetic origins of anxiety in women: a role for a functional catechol-O-methyltransferase polymorphism. Psychiatr Genet. 2003;13(1):33–41.
15. Smolka MN, Schumann G, Wrase J, et al. Catechol-O-methyltransferase val158met genotype affects processing of emotional stimuli in the amygdala and prefrontal cortex. J Neurosci. 2005;25(4):836–42.

16. Ducci F, Goldman D. Genetic approaches to addiction: genes and alcohol. Addiction. 2008;103(9):1414–28.
17. Craddock N, Owen MJ, O'Donovan MC. The catechol-O-methyl transferase (COMT) gene as a candidate for psychiatric phenotypes: evidence and lessons. Mol Psychiatry. 2006;11(5):446–58.
18. Sher KJ, Grekin ER, Williams NA. The development of alcohol use disorders. Annu Rev Clin Psychol. 2005;1:493–523.
19. National Institute on Alcohol Abuse and Alcoholism. http://www.niaaa.nih.gov/ResearchInformation/ExtramuralResearch/SharedResources/projcoga.htm. Accessed 1 Oct 2010.
20. Edenberg HJ, Foroud T. The genetics of alcoholism: identifying specific genes through family studies. Addict Biol. 2006;11(3–4):386–96.
21. Gelernter J, Kranzler HR. Genetics of drug dependence. Dialogues Clin Neurosci. 2010;12(1):77–84.
22. Renner JA. Alcoholism and alcohol abuse. In: Stern A, Herman J, editors. Massachusetts General Hospital Psychiatry and Board Preparation. 2nd ed. New York: McGraw Hill; 2004. p. 73–84.
23. Cloninger CR, Bohman M, Sigvardsson S. Inheritance of alcohol abuse. Cross-fostering analysis of adopted men. Arch Gen Psychiatry. 1981;38(8):861–8.
24. Prescott CA, Caldwell CB, Carey G, Vogler GP, Trumbetta SL, Gottesman II. The Washington University Twin Study of alcoholism. Am J Med Genet B Neuropsychiatr Genet. 2005;134B(1):48–55.
25. Matthews J, Moylan A. Substance-related disorders; cocaine and narcotics. In: Stern A, Herman J, editors. Massachusetts General Hospital Psychiatry and Board Preparation. 2nd ed. New York: McGraw Hill; 2004. p. 85–96.
26. Mahajan SD, Aalinkeel R, Reynolds JL, et al. Therapeutic targeting of "DARPP-32": a key signaling molecule in the dopiminergic pathway for the treatment of opiate addiction. Int Rev Neurobiol. 2009;88:199–222.
27. Begleiter H, Porjesz B. What is inherited in the predisposition toward alcoholism? A proposed model. Alcohol Clin Exp Res. 1999;23(7):1125–35.
28. Hopfer CJ, Stallings MC, Hewitt JK. Common genetic and environmental vulnerability for alcohol and tobacco use in a volunteer sample of older female twins. J Stud Alcohol. 2001;62(6):717–23.
29. Schlaepfer IR, Hoft NR, Ehringer MA. The genetic components of alcohol and nicotine co-addiction: from genes to behavior. Curr Drug Abuse Rev. 2008;1(2):124–34.
30. Lasser K, Boyd JW, Woolhandler S, Himmelstein DU, McCormick D, Bor DH. Smoking and mental illness: a population-based prevalence study. JAMA. 2000;284(20):2606–10.
31. Grant BF, Hasin DS, Chou SP, Stinson FS, Dawson DA. Nicotine dependence and psychiatric disorders in the United States: results from the national epidemiologic survey on alcohol and related conditions. Arch Gen Psychiatry. 2004;61(11):1107–15.
32. Di Sclafani V, Finn P, Fein G. Treatment-naive active alcoholics have greater psychiatric comorbidity than normal controls but less than treated abstinent alcoholics. Drug Alcohol Depend. 2008;98(1–2):115–22.
33. Eaton NR, Krueger RF, Keyes KM, et al. Borderline personality disorder co-morbidity: relationship to the internalizing? Externalizing structure of common mental disorders. Psychol Med. 2011;41:1041–50.
34. Klungsoyr O, Nygard JF, Sorensen T, Sandanger I. Cigarette smoking and incidence of first depressive episode: an 11-year, population-based follow-up study. Am J Epidemiol. 2006;163(5):421–32.
35. Grant BF, Stinson FS, Dawson DA, Chou SP, Ruan WJ, Pickering RP. Co-occurrence of 12-month alcohol and drug use disorders and personality disorders in the United States: results from the national epidemiologic survey on alcohol and related conditions. Arch Gen Psychiatry. 2004;61(4):361–8.
36. Gonzales RA, Job MO, Doyon WM. The role of mesolimbic dopamine in the development and maintenance of ethanol reinforcement. Pharmacol Ther. 2004;103(2):121–46.
37. Di Chiara G, Bassareo V. Reward system and addiction: what dopamine does and doesn't do. Curr Opin Pharmacol. 2007;7(1):69–76.

38. Dackis CA, O'Brien CP. Cocaine dependence: a disease of the brain's reward centers. J Subst Abuse Treat. 2001;21(3):111–7.
39. Cohen BM, Carlezon Jr WA. Can't get enough of that dopamine. Am J Psychiatry. 2007; 164(4):543–6.
40. Le Merrer J, Becker JAJ, Befort K, Kieffer BL. Reward processing by the opioid system in the brain. Physiol Rev. 2009;89(4):1379–412.
41. Williams JT, Christie MJ, Manzoni O. Cellular and synaptic adaptations mediating opioid dependence. Physiol Rev. 2001;81(1):299–343.
42. Gerrits MA, Lesscher HB, van Ree JM. Drug dependence and the endogenous opioid system. Eur Neuropsychopharmacol. 2003;13(6):424–34.
43. Margolis EB, Fields HL, Hjelmstad GO, Mitchell JM. Delta-opioid receptor expression in the ventral tegmental area protects against elevated alcohol consumption. J Neurosci. 2008;28(48):12672–81.
44. Ward SJ, Roberts DC. Microinjection of the delta-opioid receptor selective antagonist naltrindole 5'-isothiocyanate site specifically affects cocaine self-administration in rats responding under a progressive ratio schedule of reinforcement. Behav Brain Res. 2007;182(1):140–4.
45. Bonson KR, Grant SJ, Contoreggi CS, et al. Neural systems and cue-induced cocaine craving. Neuropsychopharmacology. 2002;26(3):376–86.
46. Williams MJ, Adinoff B. The role of acetylcholine in cocaine addiction. Neuropsychopharmacology. 2008;33(8):1779–97.
47. Kirsch P, Reuter M, Mier D, et al. Imaging gene-substance interactions: the effect of the DRD2 TaqIA polymorphism and the dopamine agonist bromocriptine on the brain activation during the anticipation of reward. Neurosci Lett. 2006;405(3):196–201.
48. Dreher JC, Kohn P, Kolachana B, Weinberger DR, Berman KF. Variation in dopamine genes influences responsivity of the human reward system. Proc Natl Acad Sci USA. 2009; 106(2):617–22.
49. van Eimeren T, Ballanger B, Pellecchia G, Miyasaki JM, Lang AE, Strafella AP. Dopamine agonists diminish value sensitivity of the orbitofrontal cortex: a trigger for pathological gambling in Parkinson's disease? Neuropsychopharmacology. 2009;34(13):2758–66.
50. Bond C, LaForge KS, Tian M, Melia D, Zhang S, Borg L, et al. Single-nucleotide polymorphism in the human mu opioid receptor gene alters beta-endorphin binding and activity: possible implications for opiate addiction. Proc Natl Acad Sci USA. 1998;95(16):9608–13.
51. Beyer A, Koch T, Schroder H, Schulz S, Hollt V. Effect of the A118G polymorphism on binding affinity, potency and agonist-mediated endocytosis, desensitization, and resensitization of the human mu-opioid receptor. J Neurochem. 2004;89(3):553–60.
52. Zhang Y, Wang D, Johnson AD, Papp AC, Sadee W. Allelic expression imbalance of human mu opioid receptor (OPRM1) caused by variant A118G. J Biol Chem. 2005;280(38):32618–24.
53. Szeto CY, Tang NL, Lee DT, Stadlin A. Association between mu opioid receptor gene polymorphisms and Chinese heroin addicts. Neuroreport. 2001;12(6):1103–6.
54. Tan EC, Tan CH, Karupathivan U, Yap EP. Mu opioid receptor gene polymorphisms and heroin dependence in Asian populations. Neuroreport. 2003;14(4):569–72.
55. Kapur S, Sharad S, Singh RA, Gupta AK. A118g polymorphism in mu opioid receptor gene (oprm1): association with opiate addiction in subjects of Indian origin. J Integr Neurosci. 2007;6(4):511–22.
56. Bart G, Heilig M, LaForge KS, Pollak L, Leal SM, Ott J, et al. Substantial attributable risk related to a functional mu-opioid receptor gene polymorphism in association with heroin addiction in central Sweden. Mol Psychiatry. 2004;9(6):547–9.
57. Drakenberg K, Nikoshkov A, Horvath MC, Fagergren P, Gharibyan A, Saarelainen K, et al. Mu opioid receptor A118G polymorphism in association with striatal opioid neuropeptide gene expression in heroin abusers. Proc Natl Acad Sci USA. 2006;103(20):7883–8.
58. Kim SA, Kim JW, Song JY, Park S, Lee HJ, Chung JH. Association of polymorphisms in nicotinic acetylcholine receptor alpha 4 subunit gene (CHRNA4), mu-opioid receptor gene (OPRM1), and ethanol-metabolizing enzyme genes with alcoholism in Korean patients. Alcohol. 2004;34(2–3):115–20.

59. Kim SG. Gender differences in the genetic risk for alcohol dependence – the results of a pharmacogenetic study in Korean alcoholics. Nihon Arukoru Yakubutsu Igakkai Zasshi. 2009;44(6):680–5.
60. Kim SG, Kim CM, Choi SW, Jae YM, Lee HG, Son BK, et al. A micro opioid receptor gene polymorphism (A118G) and naltrexone treatment response in adherent Korean alcohol-dependent patients. Psychopharmacology (Berl). 2009;201(4):611–8.
61. Nishizawa D, Han W, Hasegawa J, Ishida T, Numata Y, Sato T, et al. Association of mu-opioid receptor gene polymorphism A118G with alcohol dependence in a Japanese population. Neuropsychobiology. 2006;53(3):137–41.
62. Bart G, Kreek MJ, Ott J, LaForge KS, Proudnikov D, Pollak L, et al. Increased attributable risk related to a functional mu-opioid receptor gene polymorphism in association with alcohol dependence in central Sweden. Neuropsychopharmacology. 2005;30(2):417–22.
63. van den Wildenberg E, Wiers RW, Dessers J, Janssen RG, Lambrichs EH, Smeets HJ, et al. A functional polymorphism of the mu-opioid receptor gene (OPRM1) influences cue-induced craving for alcohol in male heavy drinkers. Alcohol Clin Exp Res. 2007;31(1):1–10.
64. Miranda R, Ray L, Justus A, Meyerson LA, Knopik VS, McGeary J, et al. Initial evidence of an association between OPRM1 and adolescent alcohol misuse. Alcohol Clin Exp Res. 2010;34(1):112–22.
65. Sia AT, Lim Y, Lim EC, Goh RW, Law HY, Landau R, et al. A118G single nucleotide polymorphism of human mu-opioid receptor gene influences pain perception and patient-controlled intravenous morphine consumption after intrathecal morphine for postcesarean analgesia. Anesthesiology. 2008;109(3):520–6.
66. Tan EC, Lim EC, Teo YY, Lim Y, Law HY, Sia AT. Ethnicity and OPRM variant independently predict pain perception and patient-controlled analgesia usage for post-operative pain. Mol Pain. 2009;5:32.
67. Chou WY, Yang LC, Lu HF, Ko JY, Wang CH, Lin SH, et al. Association of mu-opioid receptor gene polymorphism (A118G) with variations in morphine consumption for analgesia after total knee arthroplasty. Acta Anaesthesiol Scand. 2006;50(7):787–92.
68. Campa D, Gioia A, Tomei A, Poli P, Barale R. Association of ABCB1/MDR1 and OPRM1 gene polymorphisms with morphine pain relief. Clin Pharmacol Ther. 2008;83(4):559–66.
69. Oertel BG, Schmidt R, Schneider A, Geisslinger G, Lotsch J. The mu-opioid receptor gene polymorphism 118A>G depletes alfentanil-induced analgesia and protects against respiratory depression in homozygous carriers. Pharmacogenet Genomics. 2006;16(9):625–36.
70. Ray LA, Hutchison KE. A polymorphism of the mu-opioid receptor gene (OPRM1) and sensitivity to the effects of alcohol in humans. Alcohol Clin Exp Res. 2004;28(12):1789–95.
71. Oslin DW, Berrettini WH, O'Brien CP. Targeting treatments for alcohol dependence: the pharmacogenetics of naltrexone. Addict Biol. 2006;11(3–4):397–403.
72. Ray LA, Hutchison KE. Effects of naltrexone on alcohol sensitivity and genetic moderators of medication response: a double-blind placebo-controlled study. Arch Gen Psychiatry. 2007;64(9):1069–77.
73. Anton RF, Oroszi G, O'Malley S, Couper D, Swift R, Pettinati H, et al. An evaluation of mu-opioid receptor (OPRM1) as a predictor of naltrexone response in the treatment of alcohol dependence: results from the Combined Pharmacotherapies and Behavioral Interventions for Alcohol Dependence (COMBINE) study. Arch Gen Psychiatry. 2008;65(2):135–44.

Chapter 3
Pharmacologic Treatments for Addiction

Clifford Gevirtz, Ethan O. Bryson, and Elizabeth A.M. Frost

Introduction

Prescription drug abuse, especially the illegal use of opiates such as Oxycontin®, has reached epidemic proportions in the United States. Patients who are opiate dependent can be very challenging to care for. Chronic opiate use significantly alters neurophysiology and limits the effectiveness of many anesthetic medications. Similarly, many of the agents now used to attempt to detoxify patients may also alter anesthetic responsiveness. A detailed knowledge of the pharmacology of the agents used to maintain and detoxify addicts is essential for successful perioperative management of these challenging patients.

Buprenorphine

It is estimated that only 12–15% of the opioid-dependent population in the United States are enrolled in a methadone-maintenance program [1]. A significant change occurred with passage of the Drug Addiction Treatment Act of 2000 (DATA 2000). Now for the first time in some 90 years, physicians can legally prescribe opioid medications for the treatment of opiate addiction. The opiate designated by the Drug Enforcement Agency was buprenorphine (Subutex®, Reckitt Benckiser, Bristol, UK). Subsequently, the US Food and Drug Administration (FDA) approved buprenorphine/naloxone (Suboxone, Reckitt Benckiser), a sublingual preparation

C. Gevirtz (✉)
Somnia Pain Management, New Rochelle, NY, USA
e-mail: cliffgevirtzmd@yahoo.com

E.O. Bryson and E.A.M. Frost (eds.), *Perioperative Addiction:*
Clinical Management of the Addicted Patient, DOI 10.1007/978-1-4614-0170-4_3,
© Springer Science+Business Media, LLC 2012

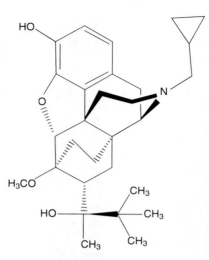

Fig. 3.1 Structural formula for buprenorphine. Buprenorphine hydrochloride is a white powder, weakly acidic with limited solubility in water (17 mg/mL). Chemically, buprenorphine is 17-(cyclopropylmethyl)-α-(1,1-dimethylethyl)-4,5-epoxy-18,19-dihydro-3-hydroxy-6-methoxy-α-methyl-6,14-ethenomorphinan-7-methanol, hydrochloride [5α,7α(S)]-. Buprenorphine hydrochloride has the molecular formula $C_{29}H_{41}NO_4$ HCl and the molecular weight is 504.10

of buprenorphine and naloxone, intended for the treatment of opioid-dependent individuals [2]. Unlike other opioid-abuse treatments, these formulations can be legally prescribed and managed by specially trained clinicians in an office-based setting, as opposed to the intense ongoing monitoring and observation required for methadone-maintenance programs. While methadone administration must be witnessed and dispensed one dose at a time initially, patients taking buprenorphine maintenance may obtain a month's supply at a time and self-administer the drug (Fig. 3.1).

In addressing the void of medications with documented effectiveness for detoxification, buprenorphine is nearly ideal, as it can be adjusted rapidly with minimal risk for inducing severe consequences. Buprenorphine also has a low abuse potential, especially when combined with naloxone. In this combination product, attempts to use the drug by snorting, injecting, or cooking the tablet releases the antagonist drug naloxone into the systemic circulation, which, in turn, results in the development of the withdrawal syndrome in opioid-dependent patients. Both the increased access to treatment and the improved safety profile make buprenorphine/naloxone an attractive and significant treatment option for addicts.

The expanded safety profile of buprenorphine has made it the first opioid treatment option that can be managed and prescribed by trained physicians in an office-based setting. This management allows patients to live a more regular life while getting treatment for their addiction. It also avoids the stigma involved in the use of methadone.

Characteristics of Buprenorphine/Naloxone

Buprenorphine is gaining widespread acceptance. While there are an estimated 1.2 million patients dependent on opioids in 2005 [3], approximately 100,000 have been placed on buprenorphine treatment [4]. According to the manufacturer, by 2008, the estimate for use worldwide had risen to 400,000 patients [5]. Currently, buprenorphine is sold under the trade name of Suboxone, which is a formulation of buprenorphine and naloxone, in a 4:1 ratio. Subutex is a formulation that contains only buprenorphine and is used as the first induction onto the partial agonist drug during the detoxification process from illicit or prescription pain medications.

In the combination form, naloxone is added to the buprenorphine formulation that serves to prevent diversion and subsequent misuse via the parenteral or intranasal routes. The naloxone is not absorbed in clinically relevant amounts by the patient if taken sublingually as directed, thus leaving the opioid agonist effects of buprenorphine to predominate. However, naloxone does not necessarily prevent diversion; in fact, the buprenorphine/naloxone product has some value on the street for mitigating the effects of withdrawal associated with opioid abuse when opioids of choice are not available. When taken parenterally by patients physically dependent on full agonist opioids, the opioid antagonist naloxone will cause the withdrawal syndrome.

Suboxone is deemed to be a Schedule III drug under the Controlled Substances Act. Just prior to approval by the FDA, Suboxone was rescheduled from Schedule V, the schedule with the lowest restriction and penalties for misuse, to Schedule III, to reflect its potential for diversion and abuse. Under this classification, any doctor who becomes certified to prescribe buprenorphine/naloxone may treat opioid addiction in the office. The certification process is simple and requires practitioners to participate in a defined 8-h continuing medical educational program and then send a formal notice to the Department of Health and Human Services that he/she intends to prescribe these medications for detoxification purposes. A separate registration is not required if the medication is prescribed for intra-operative or pain-management purposes only. Similarly, the intravenous form is specifically labeled "not for detoxification."

Buprenorphine, a semi-synthetic opioid, acts as a partial mu-opioid agonist and as an antagonist at the k-opioid receptors. While buprenorphine has a very high potency, 25-fold to 50-fold higher than morphine at low doses, its full opioid agonist effects are lower. As such, it has an improved safety profile when compared to methadone [6]. The affinity of buprenorphine for mu and kappa receptors is high, 1,000-fold higher then morphine, and dissociation from the receptors is extremely slow. This pharmacology explains the fact that naloxone cannot reliably reverse the respiratory depression effect of As compared to fentanyl, which has a dissociation half-time of 7 min, the dissociation half-time for buprenorphine from mu-receptor is 166 min. These traits of buprenorphine limit the opioid "high" associated with pure mu agonists such as methadone. At higher doses, the agonist effects of the drug plateau, providing a ceiling effect, allowing a larger therapeutic window.

Starting doses of 4–8 mg sublingually are appropriate to treat moderate to severe pain. The usual maximum recommended dose is 24 mg per day, and is required only for the rare patient previously on large doses of opiates, e.g., greater than 120 mg of methadone or 200 mg of morphine per day. The pharmacodynamics of buprenorphine require a slower titration for pain relief, i.e., adding 4 mg every 20 min, rather than resorting immediately straight to the maximum dose.

Use During Pregnancy

Because there is a lack of comprehensive data on the safety of buprenorphine during pregnancy, pregnant women who conceive while on buprenorphine treatment should be transferred to methadone maintenance. However, some pregnant women may decline this option. There may arise clinical situations where it appears "less unsafe" for a pregnant woman to continue buprenorphine during pregnancy than to relapse to dependent heroin use. This unsettling balance of risk for pregnant women who use intravenous heroin is the risk of seroconversion with HIV and hepatitis versus the potential unknown dangers of buprenorphine. The dangers of maintaining illicit heroin use, during pregnancy thus may well be significantly greater than the risks of buprenorphine maintenance for these women and their babies. The substantial body of knowledge of the safety of methadone treatment during pregnancy must also be added to the calculus of decision making.

Johnson et al. [7] discerned an advantage for the newborn by conducting a meta-analysis of the incidence of withdrawal symptoms when born to a mother dependent on buprenorphine. While an estimated 55–94% of infants born to opioid-dependent mothers in US show signs of opioid withdrawal, buprenorphine has been reported to produce little or no autonomic signs or symptoms of opioid withdrawal following abrupt termination in adults. The authors conducted a meta-analysis with 21 published reports representing approximately 15 evaluable cohorts of infants exposed to buprenorphine in utero. The neonatal abstinence syndrome (NAS) was reported in 62% infants of the 309 infants exposed, with 48% requiring treatment; apparently, greater than 40% of these cases are confounded by use of other illicit drugs. The NAS associated with buprenorphine generally appears within 12–48 h, peaks at approximately 72–96 h, and lasts for 120–168 h. These symptoms appear similar to or less severe than those observed following in utero exposure to methadone. Based on this review of the literature, buprenorphine appears to be safe and effective in both mother and infant, with an NAS that may differ from methadone both qualitatively and quantitatively.

Pediatric Use

Michel et al. [8] reviewed pediatric pharmacologic data on buprenorphine, especially with respect to the long-term application in children suffering chronic pain after repeated sublingual or long-term transdermal administration. Compared to adults, after single-dose buprenorphine, children exhibit a larger clearance to body weight ratio but a paradoxically longer duration of action.

If combined with other opioids or sedatives or if the metabolite norbuprenorphine (norBUP) cumulates, it is difficult to predict the risk of respiratory depression. It is emphasized that clear-cut evidence is missing in children that there is a ceiling of buprenorphine-induced respiratory depression. Due to its various application routes, long duration of action, and metabolism largely independent of renal function, buprenorphine is of special clinical interest in pediatrics, especially for postoperative pain and cancer pain control. Geib et al. [9] published a case series of five toddlers with respiratory and mental-status depression after unintentional buprenorphine exposure. Despite buprenorphine's partial agonist activity and ceiling effect on respiratory depression, all children required hospital admission and either opioid-antagonist therapy or mechanical ventilation. The results of routine urine toxicology screening for opioids were negative in all cases. Confirmatory testing for buprenorphine ingestion was only sent for one child and returned with a positive result. As the use of buprenorphine in home-based therapy for opioid addiction increases in the United States, a public health concern for the pediatric population arises and patients need to be warned to specifically take precautions to prevent the accidental ingestion by children.

Use in Renal Failure

Hand et al. [10] studied buprenorphine clearance in patients with normal and impaired renal function and found that it was similar (934 and 1,102 ml min^{-1}, respectively), as were dose-corrected plasma concentrations of buprenorphine. In patients with renal failure, plasma concentrations of norBUP were increased by a median of four times, and buprenorphine 3-gluconate concentrations by a median of 15 times. But since these metabolites are not clinically active, there is no need to modify the doses in patients with in renal failure.

Use in Liver Disease

Berson et al. [11] reported four cases of former heroin addicts infected with hepatitis C virus and who had been placed on substitution therapy with buprenorphine. These patients exhibited a marked increase in serum alanine amino transferase after injecting buprenorphine intravenously and three of them also became jaundiced. Stopping these buprenorphine injections was associated with prompt recovery, even though two of these patients continued ingesting buprenorphine by the sublingual route. A fifth patient infected with both hepatitis C and human immunodeficiency viruses, developed jaundice and asterixis with panlobular liver necrosis and microvesicular steatosis after using sublingual buprenorphine along with small doses of paracetamol and aspirin. They concluded that while buprenorphine hepatitis is uncommon even after intravenous misuse, addicts placed on buprenorphine should be repeatedly warned not to use it intravenously. In sum, higher drug concentrations can trigger hepatitis in intravenous users, possibly if mitochondrial function is already impaired by viral infections and other factors.

This issue was further examined by Petry et al. [12], who assessed changes in liver enzyme levels among opioid-dependent patients treated with buprenorphine. Liver enzyme levels were evaluated in 120 individuals before and following a minimum of 40 days of buprenorphine treatment (2, 4, or 8 mg/70 kg/day). In patients with a history of hepatitis, AST and ALT levels significantly increased ($p < 0.05$) with buprenorphine treatment. The odds of observing an increase in AST were directly correlated with increasing buprenorphine dose ($p < 0.05$; odds ratio = 1.23 per 1 mg increase in dose). These results suggest that liver enzyme levels should be monitored frequently when patients with hepatitis are treated with buprenorphine. Anesthesiologists would be well advised to use agents that are not extensively metabolized by the liver and to use techniques that maintain hepatic blood flow.

Special Considerations for Acute and Chronic Pain Control

Limited published data are available involving patients on buprenorphine who present for procedures or surgery requiring anesthesia; case reports lend guidance for the management of perioperative pain.

The successful management of post-cesarean section pain in two patients maintained on buprenorphine was achieved using intravenous morphine patient-controlled analgesia (PCA) with oral oxycodone for breakthrough pain at markedly elevated doses [13]. In both cases, the patients were able to continue buprenorphine therapy throughout their hospital stay. Each patient was able to achieve acceptable levels of pain control with a total dose of 180 mg per day of morphine. When switched to oral medications, one patient was able to achieve pain relief with 60 mg per day of oxycodone and 6 g of acetaminophen; however, the second patient required 600 mg of ibuprofen every 8 h in addition to this regimen.

Supplemental doses of sublingual buprenorphine have successfully been used to control postoperative pain in a patient maintained on buprenorphine [14]. This patient received general anesthesia for the removal of breast implants and was instructed to take supplemental buprenorphine, 2–4 mg every 4–6 h, in addition to her 24 mg-per-day maintenance dose, as needed for pain. She was able to achieve adequate pain relief with supplemental buprenorphine, requiring a total dose of 72 mg on post-op day 1, and tapering back to 24 mg per day by post-op day 11.

Recommendations have been proposed for the control of acute pain in the patient maintained on buprenorphine by using shorter-acting opioid analgesics in addition to the maintenance dose of buprenorphine and titrating to effective pain control [15]. By dividing the buprenorphine-maintenance dose over the course of 24 h and relying on the analgesic properties of buprenorphine, replacing the buprenorphine with methadone and then adding another opioid analgesic, or replacing the buprenorphine with another opioid analgesic altogether, adequate pain relief can be achieved in the acute setting. However, patients maintained on buprenorphine typically require much higher doses of opioid agonists to achieve adequate pain relief.

The use of epidural and intrathecal buprenorphine has been reported anecdotally only. The danger here is that accidental respiratory depression cannot be reliably reversed with either naloxone or nalmefene.

Options for Postoperative Pain Control in Buprenorphine-Maintenance Patients

Some patients on buprenorphine may wish to avoid opioids, if at all possible, because of the perceived risk of relapse into opiate addiction. If a patient is on buprenorphine-maintenance therapy, several options for intraoperative and post-operative pain control can be considered, including pre-emptive administration of celecoxib or pregabalin, preloading of the incision sites with local anesthetic prior to incision, placement of an epidural catheter for intraoperative as well as post-operative use, and postoperative ketorolac administration.

High-dose buprenorphine used for opioid substitution has a long half-life, which combines with its strong affinity for the mu-opioid receptor and slow receptor dissociation to account for the long duration of action of the drug [16]. Studies have demonstrated that the opioid-blocking action of buprenorphine can persist for several days following discontinuation of the medication, which would make conventional opiate pain therapy difficult or impossible. In one study of male subjects with a recent history of opioid addiction, sublingual buprenorphine, at a dose of 8 mg daily for 1 week, blocked the subjective and respiratory depressant effects of hydromorphone 4mg intramuscularly for up to 5 days following discontinuation of the buprenorphine [17].

Because buprenorphine is a partial agonist, patients maintained on this drug have a significantly increased tolerance for opioids and may require extremely high doses to achieve analgesia. This affinity of buprenorphine for mu-receptors is so high that it has been reportedly used to reverse heroin overdose [18]. No controlled trials have been conducted which demonstrate the extent to which doses of particular opioid agonists required to achieve analgesia are increased for patients maintained on buprenorphine. One option for treatment of acute pain is to increase the dose of buprenorphine itself, though there is a ceiling effect, and, if analgesia is not achieved, other options need to be considered. The use of nonopioid analgesics, local or regional techniques, or a combination of techniques or other partial agonists may prove effective.

Methadone

Patients who are participating in formal methadone-maintenance programs present special challenges perioperatively. These patients may be difficult to manage as they are often very opioid tolerant and can be hyperalgesic or pain intolerant. Indeed, it is not unusual to administer multiple doses of opiates in the post-operative period with little effect. When high doses of opioids are administered or when these drugs are administered for a long time, it seems that, among other phenomena, upregulation of pronociceptive systems occurs, and eventually leads to a change in sensitivity to pain or opioid-induced hyperalgesia. A better understanding of the pharmacology of methadone is necessary to achieve better patient care.

Methadone Pharmacology

Methadone's pharmacology is characterized by high variability between individuals, a strong potential for interaction with other medications, and a long elimination half-life (Fig. 3.2).

Totah et al. [19] demonstrated the primary role of CYP2B6 in the metabolism of methadone, while other authors [20] ascribe the metabolism to other CYP isozymes. Using a series of pharmacologic tools and a rigorous analytical strategy, Totah et al. were able to identify the CYP2B6 enzyme as being primarily responsible for the bulk of methadone metabolism in humans, particularly the S-methadone isomer which is the pharmacologically active isomer. Therefore, they concluded that CYP 2B6 controls both the overall plasma levels and also the ratio of plasma methadone isomers. Further, they elucidated that methadone has an exceedingly variable but generally slow hepatic clearance. This wide variation along with its very long half-life raises serious concern over the potential for overdose.

The chief hazard associated with methadone used for perioperative pain management is respiratory depression. What makes the drug particularly problematic is that the accumulation to a steady state can take a week or more when the drug is first started. This slow climb to steady-state levels brings with it the possibility that side effects of respiratory depression and sedation can also appear gradually. These side effects are detailed in Table 3.1.

The elderly or those prone to abuse of medications may be at particular risk for delayed respiratory depression by methadone. State mortality data strongly support the notion that methadone's slow accumulation can have lethal consequences. Sims et al. [21] found that the number of methadone deaths in Utah increased 1,770% from 5 in 1997 to 110 in 2003. Similar increases in methadone-related deaths across the United States have resulted in a generally recommended theme of a "start low, go slow" approach [22]. Also of import are the genetic factors impacting metabolism through the CYP enzyme system, particularly the CYP2B6 isoforms important for hepatic methadone metabolism. These genes are polymorphic in humans, and this polymorphic nature has been demonstrated to affect the rates of clearance, production of metabolites, and probability of reaching clinical endpoints for various drugs, including methadone. Zanger et al. [23] have demonstrated the CYP2B6 enzyme to be highly polymorphic, and more detailed studies will be required to determine which haplotypes of the more than 100 single-nucleotide polymorphisms are associated with altered enzymatic activity. In sum, the impact of this polymorphism

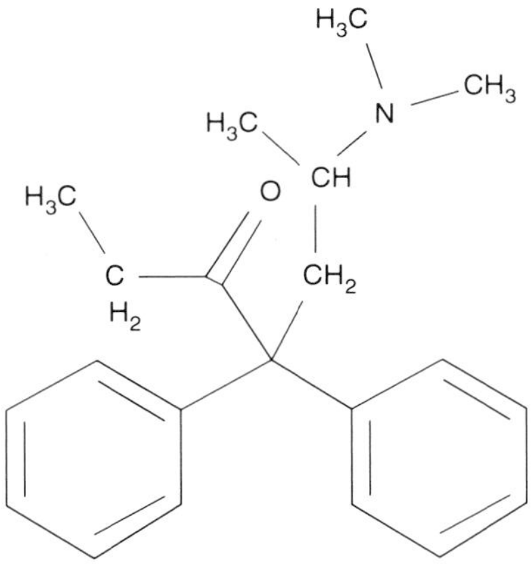

Fig. 3.2 Structural formula of Methadone. Methadone is a white powder, lipophilic, basic with limited solubility in water. Its chemical structure is 6-dimethylamino-4,4-diphenyl-3-heptanone. Methadone has the molecular formula $C_{21}H_{27}NO$ and the molecular weight is 309.44

Table 3.1 Adverse effects of methadone

- Somnolence
- Sedation
- Constipation
- Delirium
- Myoclonic jerking
- Hypertension
- Bradypnea
- Bradycardia

is to require a very cautious approach: low dose to start and then very gradual increases as the individual response to the drug is evaluated.

The management plan for patients taking methadone may differ depending on the type of surgery and the associated perioperative differences in fasting status and gastrointestinal function.

Methadone and Drug Interactions

Methadone causes QT interval prolongation in patients at high doses, usually only of concern in patients with concomitant cardioarrhythmic medications such as tricyclic antidepressants or in patients with congenital long QT syndrome. Cytochrome P450 (CYP) inducers, which may reduce methadone serum levels as well as analgesia, include phenobarbital, phenytoin, carbamazepine, and neveripine, a non-nucleoside reverse transcriptase inhibitor used in combination with other medications to treat human immunodeficiency virus (HIV) infection in patients with or without acquired immunodeficiency syndrome (AIDS). In contrast, CYP inhibitors, which may increase methadone serum levels, analgesia, and the risk of toxicity, include erythromycin, ketoconazole, and itraconazole. Caution is also needed when methadone

Table 3.2 Methadone conversion ratios

Current daily oral morphine equivalent dose	Conversion ratio (morphine to methadone)	Conversion factor (approximate percentage of morphine dose)
≤100 mg	3–1	33.3
101–300 mg	5–1	20.0
301–600 mg	10–1	10.0
601–800 mg	12–1	8.3
801–1,000 mg	15–1	6.7

Adapted from Ayonrinde OT, Bridge DT. The rediscovery of methadone for cancer pain management Med J Aust. 2000;173:536–40

is administered with other central nervous system-depressing medications and substances, such as benzodiazepines, alcohol, and concomitant opioids.

Conversion Ratio Issues

Many opiate conversion programs give a single numerical ratio when converting from one opiate to another in a single-dose acute care situation. When dealing with methadone, the issue is substantially more complex since the drug accumulates. With this risk in mind, the conversion ratio changes with increasing dosage. Table 3.2 is meant to serve as an initial conversion from opioids to methadone in healthy patients. The final dose must be carefully individualized. It must also be emphasized that this is a one-way conversion; the ratios do not necessarily hold in the opposite direction. Short-acting opioids should be available for the treatment of breakthrough pain during the titration period.

Postoperative Analgesia Requirements in Methadone Patients

In one study [24] of patients undergoing liver transplantation who were on methadone pre-operatively, anesthesia and pain control requirements were tallied from operating room records. Postoperative pain medication requirements were calculated by converting doses of opiate analgesia recorded in the charts to equivalent average daily doses of intravenously administered morphine. Methadone doses on each day of transplant for the patients receiving MMT were compared with the dose at the time of discharge from the hospital. Postoperative analgesia administered to patients in the surgical intensive care unit immediately after surgery was noted to be highly variable. Most patients received intravenous morphine sulfate on an as-needed basis in the surgical intensive care unit, but, after transfer to the recovery floor, most patients used patient-controlled analgesia (PCA) with good results. The mean daily postoperative analgesia doses were unequivocally higher in the MMT group (67.86 mg/d intravenous morphine, SD = 38.84) compared with the non-MMT group

(12.17 mg/d intravenous morphine, SD = 10.24). When preoperative and postoperative oral methadone dose at hospital discharge were compared, they found on the day before transplant patients receiving MMT averaged 65 mg/d of methadone (range: 30–120 mg) compared with 82 mg/d (range: 45–160 mg) on the day of discharge post-transplant. They concluded that 50% of patients receiving MMT required an average increase of 60% of their methadone dose by the day of discharge from the hospital.

Methadone-Maintenance Programs and Anesthesia

There is a potential for problems as a result of the intra-operative use of opioids or other substances in the continued enrollment of patients in MMP. Because patients are subjected to frequent toxicology screenings, and need to be able to document medications they have received, it is important to provide this documentation to the patient in the form of a readable list of medications (for example, electronic record). Failure to do so may result in a patient who fails out of a program for having medications in his/her system that were reasonably prescribed in the course of delivering an anesthetic.

Ibogaine

In the early 1960s, anecdotal reports appeared concerning the ability of ibogaine to interrupt addictions to methadone, heroin, alcohol, and cocaine [25]. In the past decade, several reports have appeared suggesting that ibogaine can alleviate the withdrawal syndrome associated with cessation of opioid use, decrease cravings, and assist formerly addicted individuals in maintaining abstinence. It was thought that ibogaine might have the potential to facilitate introspection, helping to elucidate the psychological issues and behavior patterns that drive addictions or other problems. However, ibogaine therapy for drug addiction is the subject of controversy, despite its recent citation on an episode of a popular crime series ("Users," the seventh episode of the eleventh season of Law and Order: Special Victims Unit. In the episode, Doctor George Huang administers ibogaine to an end-stage teenage heroin addict and within hours the boy is completely cured and sober and is able to testify against a therapist who raped a girl under his care). No other claims have been made for such miraculous results.

Ibogaine is not an opiate replacement or blocker. Unlike other detoxification agents, it appears to act on two important neurotransmitters in the brain (NMDA and serotonin), giving it an LSD-like action. It may also stimulate the production of brain-derived neurotrophic factor (BDNF). Ibogaine is an indole alkaloid found in the roots of a rain forest shrub native to West Africa (Fig. 3.3). Tabernanthe Iboga (Apocynaceae family) has been used by indigenous peoples in low doses to combat

Fig. 3.3 Structural formula
of Ibogaine. The complex
ring structure (**a**) along with
a 3D representation (**b**)
accounts for this molecules
actions at several different
receptor sites

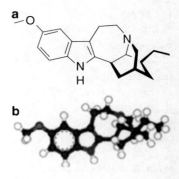

fatigue, hunger, and thirst, and in higher doses as a sacrament in religious rituals. Members of self-help groups such as narcotics anonymous in both Europe and America have claimed that ibogaine promotes long-term drug abstinence from addictive substances, with reports suggesting that all that is needed is a single dose of the agent to eliminate withdrawal symptoms and reduce drug craving. Addicts in recovery report that this ibogaine effect lasts for extended periods of time.

The purported efficacy of ibogaine for the treatment of drug dependence may be due in part to the active metabolite noribogaine. Ibogaine biotransformation proceeds primarily via CYP2D6 with the O-demethylation of ibogaine to 12-hydroxyibogamine (noribogaine). Blood concentration versus time profiles of ibogaine and noribogaine obtained for individual subjects after single oral dose administrations demonstrate a complex pharmacokinetic profile.

Ibogaine has shown preliminary efficacy for opiate detoxification and for short-term stabilization of drug-dependent persons as they prepare to enter substance abuse treatment. Mash et al. reported that ibogaine significantly decreased craving for cocaine and heroin during inpatient detoxification [26]. Self-reports of depressive symptoms were also significantly lower after ibogaine treatment and at 30 days after program discharge. Further, levels of self-reported depressive symptoms and craving were significantly decreased following ibogaine administration. A limitation of the study was that it is based on reports in only 27 subjects; thus, replication is needed in future studies to determine the stability of the findings. It is not known whether the symptoms experienced in the treatment setting are unique; however, subjects were evaluated at 1 month after program discharge, having returned to their normal environment or following entry to residential sober living in a community setting.

Despite significant positive outcomes, ibogaine use is not without risk. The drug has been placed in strict drug prohibition schedules in the United States and a handful of other countries due to its many side effects, including ataxia, prolonged nausea and vomiting (it has been given by enema to avoid this complication), and marked cardiac dysrhythmias including QT prolongation [27]. Cerebellar toxicity has been documented in rat models when ibogaine is administered at high doses. Because of this, the FDA has listed ibogaine as a Schedule 1 drug and waivers must be obtained for future clinical studies to be performed. Due to safety concerns, the National Institute on Drug Abuse (NIDA) has decided not to support further ibogaine studies. Unfortunately, in the absence of private funding and rigorous research methodology, ibogaine is likely to remain a bit of a mystery and something for future researchers to evaluate.

While this prohibition in the US has slowed scientific research into its anti-addictive properties, the use of ibogaine for drug treatment has grown in the form of a large worldwide medical subculture [28]. Canada and Mexico both allow ibogaine therapy facilities and openly contribute to further understanding of the detoxification and therapeutic process that may facilitate. It is now used by treatment clinics in 12 countries on six continents to facilitate detoxification and relief of chemical dependence to substances such as methadone, heroin, alcohol, powder cocaine, crack cocaine, and methamphetamine, as well as by other cultures and groups to facilitate psychological introspection and spiritual exploration. It was also marketed in France as Lamborene, a drug used for weight loss.

Ultra-Rapid Opiate Detoxification

The process of precipitating withdrawal while unconscious under general anesthesia has been used to shorten the withdrawal period experienced by opioid-dependent patients and reduce the subjective discomfort responsible for the low success rates when traditional detoxification methods are used. The constellation of withdrawal symptoms experienced by the patient during detoxification (restlessness, rhinorrhea, lacrimation, diaphoresis, myosis, piloerection, and increased cardiovascular activity) is at best objectionable and frequently cited as the reason why conventional attempts at detoxification have such a low success rate [29]. While conventional treatments for opioid abuse involve substitution of the opioid of abuse with another opioid agonist such as methadone or partial agonist such as buprenorphine, ultra-rapid opiate detoxification (UROD) involves the acute precipitation of withdrawal with a pure antagonist such as naloxone, naltrexone, or nalmefeme. UROD is designed to detoxify patients rapidly while maintaining hemodynamic stability, lack of awareness, and analgesia.

Candidates for Detoxification

Only patients who have documented dependence on opiates, as indicated by history coupled with positive blood, urine, or hair testing, are candidates for UROD. Patients who are polysubstance abusers, especially patients who are also abusing cocaine or amphetamines, are at risk for serious cardiovascular complications during this process and should not be detoxified using this method. Chronic pain patients who undergo UROD for dependence on pain medication should be cautioned that this process can result in pain which is responsive only to local or regional placement of local anesthesia or neurolysis as opioid receptors are rendered unresponsive for a period of time.

There are a number of medical conditions which contraindicate the use of UROD as a detoxification modality. In general, patients who are acutely ill should not undergo this process. Acute hepatitis, recent myocardial infarction (within 6 months), and recent cerebrovascular accident (within 2 months) are relative contraindications. There is no evidence that UROD is safe for pregnant patients. Psychotic patients or patients who are unable to give informed consent should not be detoxified using this procedure. Psychiatric clearance is essential, since psychiatric illness frequently coexists with substance abuse. The patient must express a desire to become detoxified and voice understanding of the risks and benefits associated with UROD.

Methodology

Once the patient has been deemed an acceptable candidate and preanesthetic testing has defined the extent of any end-organ damage related to substance abuse, high-dose clonidine blockade is begun to attenuate the hemodynamic effects of withdrawal. Incremental doses of the drug are administered as premedication with the goal of reducing the blood pressure to the lower limits of normal. Other premedications include vitamin C to acidify the urine and accelerate opioid elimination from the body, anti-diarrheal suppositories, antiemetic medications, and sedatives as necessary. UROD must be administered in a setting with facilities available for the administration of general anesthesia and use of standard American Society of Anesthesiologists (ASA) monitoring is essential. Ideally, the process is conducted in the intensive care unit or post-anesthesia care unit, but a variety of settings have been successfully used. Once general anesthesia is induced, the patient is intubated and will remain so throughout the withdrawal process. After hemodynamic stability is established, withdrawal is precipitated with the antagonist of choice and supportive care is provided for the duration of the process (usually 4–6 h). The patient remains spontaneously breathing throughout the procedure which is deemed completed when minute ventilation declines to 80% of the peak value and there are no signs of withdrawal in response to a 0.4-mg dose of intravenous naloxone. Specific medications used for UROD are detailed in Table 3.3. The patient should ideally be observed overnight.

Complications

When adequate sympathetic blockade is achieved during the detoxification process, there is no catecholamine surge and no accompanying hemodynamic instability [30]. Complications such as pulmonary edema and myocardial infarction are rare. Immediately after the detoxification process, patients may experience emesis and diarrhea, requiring resuscitation with intravenous fluids. The subjective withdrawal

Table 3.3 Medications used during ultra-rapid opiate detoxification

Premedications:
- Clonidine (transdermal or oral)
- Vitamin C (1–2 g orally)
- Ondansetron (Chemotherapeutic doses)
- Glycopyrrolate (0.2–0.4 mg intravenously)
- Fluid replacement (3–4 times maintenance intravenously)

Intraprocedure:
- Propofol (for induction and/or maintenance of general anesthesia)
- Succinylcholine or Rocuronium (doses appropriate for rapid sequence induction)
- Volatile anesthetic or propofol infusion as maintenance
- Naloxone (up to 20 mg) or
- Naltrexone (up to 50 mg) or
- Nalmefeme (up to 8 mg)

Postprocedure:
- Naltrexone (depo injection or seeds for enforced abstinence)
- Ondansetron (for nausea or vomiting)[a]
- Octreotide (for diarrhea)[b]
- Melatonin (for disrupted sleep-wake cycle)
- NSAIDs (for muscle cramps, bone pain, lower back pain)

[a]Metoclopramide should not be used as its effects are antagonized by narcotics and is associated with hypertension due to catecholamine release
[b]Loperamide and other narcotic based anti-diarrheal medications should be avoided as there is some uptake into the central circulation which can increase withdrawal symptoms

syndrome, though attenuated, is not eliminated entirely, and restlessness, insomnia, irritability, and hypertension (symptoms of the protracted abstinence syndrome) may require treatment for up to 10 weeks following detoxification. Mood changes may require treatment with an antidepressant, and patients under the care of a psychiatrist should anticipate the need for additional medications post-procedure.

Naltrexone

The opioid receptor antagonist naltrexone has been used successfully in the management of opioid dependence and recently also as a treatment for alcohol abuse. It is manufactured as the hydrochloride salt, naltrexone hydrochloride, and sold under the trade names Revia, Depade, and in an extended-release formulation under the trade name Vivitrol. Both naltrexone and naloxone are full antagonists and will treat opioid overdose, but naltrexone is longer acting.

Naltrexone can be described as a substituted oxymorphone where the tertiary amine methyl-substituent is replaced with methylcyclopropane (see Fig. 3.4), which is the N-cyclopropylmethyl derivative of oxymorphone. Naltrexone and its active metabolite 6-β-naltrexol are competitive antagonists at μ- and κ-opioid receptors, and to a lesser extent at δ-opioid receptors [31]. The plasma half-life of naltrexone is about 4 h, and 13 h for 6-β-naltrexol.

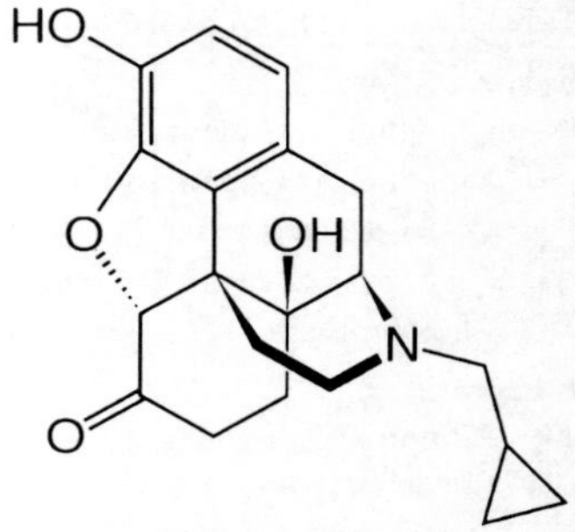

Fig. 3.4 Naltrexone

The blockade of opioid receptors by naltrexone prevents patients from experiencing the subjective "high" associated with opioid abuse and is the basis for its use in opioid-dependent patients in recovery. Interestingly, naltrexone has been shown to be effective in the treatment of alcoholics in recovery as well, though the mechanism of action is not fully understood [32]. It is possible that modulation of the dopaminergic mesolimbic pathway which ethanol is believed to activate is responsible for the effects of naltrexone on recovering alcoholics, specifically antagonism of endogenous opiates such as tetrahydropapaveroline, whose production is augmented in the presence of alcohol. Several studies dating back to 1992 have confirmed the efficacy of naltrexone in reducing the frequency and severity of relapse to drinking [33–35]. The multi-center COMBINE study has recently proven the usefulness of naltrexone in an ordinary, primary care setting, without adjunct psychotherapy [36].

For patients in recovery from alcohol abuse, the standard regimen is one 50 mg tablet per day. Initial problems of nausea usually disappear after a few days, and other side effects (e.g., liver enzyme induction) are rare. Drug interactions are not significant, although antagonism of opioid analgesics can present a problem if the patient develops pain and requires subsequent treatment with opioid analgesics. Naltrexone reduces cravings for alcohol in both the sober patient and the actively drinking patient who wishes to cut down but not stop entirely [37].

Depot injectable naltrexone (Vivitrol® Cephalon, Frazer, PA) was approved by the FDA on April 13, 2006 for the treatment of alcoholism. Although clinical trials focused mainly on alcohol, safety studies for the off-label use of the injection for opiate addicts were also performed [38]. The drug significantly reduced relapse rate and craving in single-drug abusers, though poly-drug abusers generally decreased their opiate use and increased their use of other drugs such as cocaine. Vivitrol is administered by intra-muscular injection resulting in clinically effective plasma levels of naltrexone for up to 30 days. While 70% of patients report a complete loss of cravings after six injections, patients with a genetic polymorphism of opioid receptor OPRM1 are far more likely to experience success at cutting back or discontinuing their alcohol intake altogether when naltrexone was included with the treatment regimen [39].

Conclusion

Suboxone in combination with naloxone has been prescribed to an increasing number of patients. Because buprenorphine is a partial opioid agonist with a high affinity for mu-receptors, patients maintained on this agent are prevented from experiencing the euphoria associated with opioid use, and require substantially higher doses of opioids to achieve the same level of pain control.

Methadone has a complex pharmacology. Much care must be taken to avoid complications when using this drug. While many pain specialists prescribe methadone as a cheap alternative to more expensive opioids for their patients, the costs of one hospitalization due to overdose almost certainly cancels out any pharmacoeconomic benefit.

When patients maintained on any of these agents present for procedures or surgery requiring anesthesia, standard opioid-based anesthetic techniques are not sufficient and alternate anesthetic agents must be employed. The anesthesiologist must be aware of this need and be prepared to adjust analgesic dosages accordingly.

Attempts to avoid the significantly distressing symptoms of opioid withdrawal, either through the use of alternative agents such as ibogaine or while under anesthesia as is done with ultra-rapid detoxification, present unique challenges. Perioperative care requires a team approach as well as an understanding of the process and possible complications.

References

1. Raisch DW, Fye CL, Boardman KD, Sather MR. Opioid dependence treatment, including buprenorphine/naloxone. Ann Pharmacother. 2002;36:312–21.
2. Ling W. Buprenorphine for opioid dependence. Expert Rev Neurother. 2009;9(5):609–16.
3. National Survey on Drug Use and Health, 2005. Rockville, MD, Substance Abuse and Mental Health Services Administration, Office of Applied Studies. 2006. Available at www.icpsr. umich.edu/cocoon/ICPSR/STUDY/04596.xml.
4. The Determinations Report: A Report on the Physician Waiver Program Established by the Drug Addiction Treatment Act of 2000 ("DATA"). Rockville, MD: Substance Abuse and Mental Health Services Administration, Center for Substance Abuse Treatment; 2006.
5. Patient Brochure. Suboxone Facts for Patients. Richmond, VA: Reckitt Benckiser Pharmaceuticals Inc; 2008. p. 23235.
6. Orman JS, Keating GM. Buprenorphine/Naloxone: a review of its use in the treatment of opioid dependence. Drugs. 2009;69(5):577–607.
7. Johnson RE, Jones HE, Fischer G. Use of buprenorphine in pregnancy: patient management and effects on the neonate. Drug Alcohol Depend. 2003;70 Suppl 1:S87–101.
8. Michel E, Zernikow B. Buprenorphine in children. A clinical and pharmacological review. Schmerz. 2006;20:40–50.
9. Geib AJ, Babu K, Burns M, et al. Adverse effects in children after unintentional buprenorphine exposure. Pediatrics. 2006;118:1746–51.
10. Hand CW, Sear JW, Uppington J. Buprenorphine disposition in patients with renal impairment: single and continuous dosing, with special reference to metabolites. Br J Anaesth. 1990;64:276–82.

11. Berson A, Gervais A, Cazals D, et al. Hepatitis after intravenous buprenorphine misuse in heroin addicts. J Hepatol. 2001;34:346–50.
12. Petry NM, Bickel WK, Piasecki D, et al. Elevated liver enzyme levels in opioid-dependent patients with hepatitis treated with buprenorphine. Am J Addict. 2000;9:265–9.
13. Jones HE, Johnson RE, Milio L. Post-cesarean pain management of patients maintained on methadone or buprenorphine. Am J Addict. 2006;15(3):258–9.
14. Book SW, Myrick H, Malcolm R, Strain EC. Buprenorphine for postoperative pain following general surgery in a buprenorphine-maintained patient. Am J Psychiatry. 2007;164:979.
15. Alford DP, Compton P, Samet JH. Acute pain management for patients receiving maintenance methadone or buprenorphine therapy. Ann Intern Med. 2006;144(2):127–34.
16. Robert DM, Meyer-Witting M. High-dose buprenorphine: perioperative precautions and management strategies. Anaesth Intensive Care. 2005;33:17–25.
17. Schuh KJ, Walsh SL, Stitzerr ML. Onset, magnitude and duration of opioid blockade produced by buprenorphine and naltrexone in humans. Psychopharmacology. 1999;145:162–74.
18. Welsh C, Sherman SG, Tobin KE. A case of heroin overdose reversed by sublingually administered buprenorphine/naloxone (Suboxone®). Addiction. 2008;103:1226–8.
19. Totah R, Sheffels P, Robert T, et al. Role of CYP2B6 in steroselective human methadone metabolism. Anesthesiology. 2008;108:363–74.
20. Mahajan G, Fishman SM. Opioids in Pain Management. In: Benzon HT, editor. Essentials of pain medicine and regional anesthesia. 2nd ed. Philadelphia, PA: Elsevier; 2005. Major Chapter 11.
21. Sims SA, Snow LA, Porucznik CA. Surveillance of Methadone related adverse drug events using multiple public health data sources. J Biomed Inform. 2007;40:382–9.
22. Glajchen M. Chronic pain: treatment barriers and strategies for clinical practice. J Am Board Fam Pract. 2001;14:211–8.
23. Zanger UM, Klein K, Saussele T. Polymorphic CYP2B6: molecular mechanisms and emerging clinical significance. Pharmacogenomics. 2007;8:743–59.
24. Peng PW, Tumber PS, Gourley D. Review article: perioperative pain management of patients on methadone therapy. Can J Anaesth. 2005;525:513–23.
25. Alper KR, Lotsof HS, Frenken GM, Luciano DJ, Bastiaans J. Treatment of acute opioid withdrawal with ibogaine. Am J Addict. 1999;8(3):234–42.
26. Mash DC, Kovera CA, Pablo J, et al. Ibogaine in the treatment of heroin withdrawal. Alkaloids. 2001;56:155–71.
27. Hoelen DW, Spiering W, Valk GD. Long-QT syndrome induced by the antiaddiction drug ibogaine. N Engl J Med. 2009;360(3):308–9.
28. Alper KR, Lotsof HS, Kaplan CD. The ibogaine medical subculture. J Ethnopharmacol. 2008;115(1):9–24.
29. Mattick RP, Breen C, Kinbler J, et al. Methadone maintenance therapy versus no opioid replacement therapy for opioid dependence. Cochrane Database Syst Rev. 2009;8(3):CD002209.
30. Kaye AD, Banister RE, Hoover JM, et al. Chronic pain and ultra rapid opioid detoxification. Pain Physician. 2005;5(1):33–42.
31. Shader RI. Antagonists, inverse agonists, and protagonists. J Clin Psychopharmacol. 2003;23(4):321–2.
32. Therapeutic Goods Administration. "Australian Register of Therapeutic Goods Medicines" (Online database of approved medicines). https://www.ebs.tga.gov.au/ebs/ANZTPAR/PublicWeb.nsf/cuMedicines?OpenView. Accessed 11 May 2010.
33. Latt NC, Jurd S, Houseman J, Wutzke SE. Naltrexone in alcohol dependence: a randomised controlled trial of effectiveness in a standard clinical setting. Med J Aust. 2002;176(11):530–4.
34. Heinälä P et al. Targeted use of naltrexone without prior detoxification in the treatment of alcohol dependence: a factorial double-blind placebo-controlled trial. J Clin Psychopharmacol. 2001;21:287–92.
35. O'Malley SS, Jaffe A, Chang G, Witte R, et al. Naltrexone in the treatment of alcohol dependence. In: Reid LD, editor. Opioids, bulimia, and alcohol abuse and alcoholism. New York, NY: Springer; 1990.

36. National Institutes of Health. Naltrexone or specialized alcohol counseling an effective treatment for alcohol dependence when delivered with medical management. Press release; May 2, 2006.
37. Sinclair JD. Evidence about the use of naltrexone and for different ways of using it in the treatment of alcoholism. Alcohol Alcohol. 2001;36(1):2–10.
38. Schmitz J, Stotts A, Rhoades H, Grabowski J. Naltrexone and relapse prevention treatment for cocaine-dependent patients. Addict Behav. 2001;26(2):167–80.
39. Anton R, Oroszi G, O'Malley S, et al. An evaluation of opioid receptor (OPRM1) as a predictor of naltrexone response in the treatment of alcohol dependence. Arch Gen Psychiatry. 2008;65(2):135–44.

Part II
Specific Drugs

Chapter 4
The Anesthetic Implications of Opioid Addiction

Michael Lewis and Fouad Souki

Introduction

Opioids have been used medicinally for thousands of years despite their known addictive nature. The increasing availability of these prescription pain relievers, and their psychological effects, makes such compounds prone to abuse, misuse, addiction, and diversion [1–3]. Today's opioid-addict no longer fits the classical image of a societal "drop-out" or "heroin user". Opioid abuse impacts all social strata and areas of medicinal care. Therefore, the opioid-using patient is frequently encountered by anesthesiologists in the perioperative and pain management settings. Adverse reactions during or following an anesthetic may be the result of opioid intoxication, tolerance, or withdrawal [4–6]. Clinicians must develop an appropriate anesthetic plan tailored to the non-opioid naïve patient, and immediately recognize and manage opioid abuse-related complications in the perioperative period.

Background

Opiates are extracted from the poppy plant (*Papaver somniferum*). They are naturally occurring compounds that belong to a larger class of drugs, the opioids, which also includes synthetic and semi-synthetic drugs. Opioids produce analgesia, euphoria, or both. These medications are highly addictive substances and may be abused orally, nasally, subcutaneously, or intravenously [7].

M. Lewis (✉)
Department of Anesthesiology, University of Miami Miller School of Medicine,
Miami, FL, USA
e-mail: mclewis@med.miami.edu

E.O. Bryson and E.A.M. Frost (eds.), *Perioperative Addiction:*
Clinical Management of the Addicted Patient, DOI 10.1007/978-1-4614-0170-4_4,
© Springer Science+Business Media, LLC 2012

Epidemiology

In the United States, opioids are among the most common class of prescribed drugs. The most frequently prescribed opioids include codeine, fentanyl, hydrocodone, hydromorphone, levorphanol, meperidine, methadone, morphine, and oxycodone [2]. Hydrocodone topped the list with 128 million prescriptions in 2009 [8].

Prescription opioid use has been steadily rising [1, 2] and is considered a public health issue. Misuse, addiction, and diversion for nonmedical uses are of concern with all prescription opioids. In 2008, an estimated 4.7 million Americans aged 12 or older were current nonmedical users of pain relievers, meaning they had used an illicit drug during the month prior to the survey interview. This number represents 2% of the population aged 12 or older [1]. Comparatively, only 200,000 are estimated to be current heroin users [1].

Most misused prescription medications come from a close acquaintance, friend, relative, or a lone prescribing physician [1, 2]. Only 4.3% obtained pain relievers from a drug dealer or stranger, and 0.4% were purchased over the Internet [1].

The pattern of opioid abuse differs among age groups. Rates of current (past month) use of prescription pain medication in 2008 were higher among young adults aged 18–25 (4.6%) than among youths aged 12–17 (2.3%) and adults aged 26 or older (~1%) [1]. Abuse of prescription drugs is also problematic among adolescents (see Chap. 13). According to the 2009 Monitoring the Future (MTF) survey, many 12th-grade students reported illicit use of Vicodin and OxyContin during the past year – 9.7% and 4.9%, respectively [9].

Abuse of prescription drugs can produce serious adverse health effects, including physical dependence and addiction. Daily administration of increasing doses results in physical dependence in as little as 2 weeks [6]. In 2008, an estimated 1.7 million persons aged 12 or older were classified with illicit opioid dependence in the past year based on criteria specified in the Diagnostic and Statistical Manual of Mental Disorders (DSM-IV) [10]. In terms of highest levels of past year dependence, pain relievers preceded cocaine and heroin but followed marijuana [1]. Between 2004 and 2008, the percentage and the number of persons dependent on pain relievers has increased (from 0.6 to 0.7%) [1].

A considerable proportion of emergency department visits related to medication (drug) abuse and suicide attempts is due to opioids. In 2007, Drug Abuse Warning Network (DAWN) estimated that 33.5% of emergency department (ED) visits related to pharmaceuticals and 16% of ED visits for suicide attempt involved the nonmedical use of opioids [11]. Methadone, oxycodone, and hydrocodone were most frequently implicated. ED visits related to nonmedical use of opioids and opioid-related suicide attempts increased 66% in the period from 2004 to 2007, respectively [11].

Elevated rates of high-risk behaviors, infectious diseases, and combination with other drugs and alcohol have been reported for those who abuse opioids. Serious mental illness seems to predispose to, rather than result from, drug abuse and dependence [1, 6].

Definitions

Prescription opioid abuse is defined as either the use of an opioid that is not specifically prescribed for an individual or taking the medication for reasons, or in dosages, other than prescribed. Physical dependence, tolerance, and addiction are discrete and different phenomena. Physical dependence may often be confused with addiction because the American Psychiatric Association and World Health Organization use the term "substance dependence" to connote "drug addiction" [10, 12]. Tolerance and physical dependence reflect physiological adaptation to the effects of a drug; they are neither necessary nor sufficient for a diagnosis of addiction.

The American Academy of Pain Medicine, the American Pain Society, and the American Society of Addiction Medicine have published a consensus document recognizing and recommending the following definitions [13]:

1. Tolerance is a state of adaptation in which exposure to a drug induces changes that result in a diminution of one or more of the drug's effects over time.
2. Physical dependence is a state of adaptation that is manifested by a drug classspecific withdrawal syndrome that can be produced by abrupt cessation, rapid dose reduction, decreasing blood level of the drug, and/or administration of an antagonist.
3. Addiction is a primary, chronic, neurobiologic disease, with genetic, psychosocial, and environmental factors influencing its development and manifestations. It is characterized by behaviors that include one or more of the following: impaired control over drug use, compulsive use, continued use despite harm, and craving.

Scientific Foundation and Mechanisms of Action

Opioid Abuse and Mechanism of Action

The mechanisms by which opioids produce euphoria, tranquility, and other alterations in mood (including rewarding properties) have been linked to specific dopaminergic pathways originating from the ventral tegmental area [12]. Similar to natural rewards (food, drink, and sex), opioids stimulate the release of dopamine from neurons of the presynaptic ventral tegmental area into the nucleus accumbens, causing euphoria, behavior reinforcement, craving, and emotional changes of withdrawal. The mesocortical dopamine circuit includes projections from the ventral tegmental area to the cortex and anterior cingulate. It is involved in the conscious experience of the effects of drugs, drug craving, and the compulsion to take drugs. Functional magnetic resonance imaging (fMRI) studies have demonstrated that a small intravenous dose (4 mg) of morphine induces positive signal changes in reward structures, including the nucleus accumbens, amygdala, cortex, and hippocampus, and decreases signal in cortical areas similar to the action of sedative-hypnotics [14].

All three opioid receptor types (μ, δ, and k) couple the $G_{i/o}$ protein and are present on the nucleus accumbens [15–17]. Selective μ- and δ-receptor agonists result in rewarding experience while selective κ-receptor agonists produce aversive effects. Receptor activation inhibits adenylate cyclase resulting in a reduction in cellular cyclic adenosine monophosphate (AMP) levels, decreases cAMP-dependent protein kinase A activity, and reduces phosphorylation of cytoplasmic and nuclear targets [12, 17, 18]. Electrophysiologically, activation of the opioid receptors reduces neuronal transmission by inhibiting the voltage-gated Ca^{2+} channel and activating the inwardly rectifying K^+ channels [17, 18].

The locus ceruleus contains both noradrenergic neurons and high concentrations of opioid receptors; it is postulated to play a critical role in feelings of alarm, panic, fear, and anxiety. Neural and adrenergic activity in the locus ceruleus is inhibited by both exogenous opioids' and endogenous opioid peptides' agonist action at the Mu receptor [12].

Risk of drug addiction has been associated with certain personality traits, mental disorders, and genetic factors. Risk-taking traits and psychiatric disorders favor the use of addictive drugs with an increased risk of abuse. Characteristics such as rapid onset and intensity of effect increase the potential for abuse of opioids [19]. Genetic factors influence the metabolism of drugs and consequently addiction potential. Cytochrome P polymorphisms cause variations in clinical effect of opioids. CYP2D6 partial activity occurs in approximately 5–10% of whites, 1% of Asians, 20% of African-Americans, and 3% of Mexican-Americans. A deficiency in CYP2D6 gene blocks the enzymatic conversion of codeine to morphine preventing codeine abuse [11, 20]. Equally, hydrocodone is metabolized to hydromorphone by CYP2D6.

Opioid Tolerance and Withdrawal

Repeated, regular exposure of the opioid receptors to agonists induces cellular adaptation mechanisms opposite to those of acute activation. Chronic activation of opioid receptors increases the phosphorylation of factors regulating gene transcription [21, 23]. It upregulates cAMP signaling pathways in nucleus accumbens and locus ceruleus [22] by increasing the activity of adenylyl cyclases, cAMP-dependent protein kinase A, and tyrosine hydroxylase. Also, decreases in the number of opioid receptors [23] have been related to the development of opioid tolerance. A substantial decrease in dopamine levels in the nucleus accumbens occurs during withdrawal [21]. These changes contribute to the negative emotions (dysphoria and anhedonia) present during the early phases of abstinence [18, 21].

Tolerance to the inhibitory effects of opioids occurs in the locus ceruleus during long-term administration. The presence of opioids brings these neurons toward their normal firing rates [23]. When opioid levels fall, the firing rates of neurons in the locus ceruleus are unopposed and lead to adrenergic overactivation. A direct relation between overactivity of the locus ceruleus neurons and the somatic expression of opioid withdrawal has been demonstrated, along with other mechanisms independent of the locus ceruleus [12].

Elevation of peripheral glucocorticoid levels and central corticotropin-releasing factor levels has been related to the rewarding properties of drug use. Drug administration and withdrawal activate central and peripheral stress systems [12]. Changes in corticotropin-releasing factor in the amygdala have been related to stress and negative effects of abstinence [24]. Activation of central glucocorticoid receptors (GRs) has also been implicated in modulating tolerance to morphine in rats [25].

Clinical Presentation of the Abuser by Organ System

Opioid-abusing patients may present with symptoms of opioid overdose or withdrawal (Table 4.1). The clinical manifestations of opioid intoxication involve several organ systems and are known as the "opioid toxidrome."

Neurologic Effects

Opioid intoxication causes altered mental status ranging from near normal to euphoria, hallucinations, lethargy, or coma. Seizures may present due to hypoxia or overdose of meperidine, tramadol, and propoxyphene. Serotonin toxicity reactions involving altered mentation, neuroexcitation, neuromuscular, and autonomic hyperactivity occur when opioids with weak serotonin re-uptake inhibition (meperidine, tramadol, methadone, dextromethorphan, and propoxyphene) interact with monoamine oxidase inhibitors (MAOs). During opioid withdrawal, patients may have normal mental status, restlessness, agitation, irritability, tremors, myoclonus, delirium, or dysphoria. Yawning, piloerection, rhinorrhea, myalgia, and arthralgia may also be seen during opioid withdrawal [7, 15, 26].

Ophthalmologic Effects

The pupils are characteristically miotic during opioid intoxication. Morphine and most μ- and κ-agonists cause constriction by an excitatory action on the parasympathetic nerve innervating the pupil. Opioids also abolish cortical inhibition of the Edinger-Westphal nucleus, resulting in pupillary constriction [15, 27]. At times, the changes in pupil size associated with opioid action may be too slight to be of clinical utility in assessing the degree of opioid effect. Normal pupil examination does not exclude opioid intoxication. Users of meperidine [15] and propoxyphene may present with normal or enlarged pupils. Mydriasis can also result from coingestants or may signal severe cerebral hypoxia. During opioid withdrawal, lacrimation and mydriasis may be seen [15, 26].

Table 4.1 Clinical features of opioid intoxication and withdrawal

	Opioids intoxication	Opioids withdrawal
Vital signs	Blood pressure decreased or unchanged	Blood pressure increased or unchanged; decreased if hypovolemic
	Heart rate decreased or unchanged	Heart rate increased or unchanged
	Respiratory rate decreased	Respiratory rate increased or unchanged
	Temperature decreased or unchanged	Temperature unchanged
Eye, nose	Miosis	Lacrimation, rhinorrhea, mydriasis
Central nervous system	Sedation or coma	Normal, Irritable, restlessness,
	Seizure (meperidine, propoxyphene, tramadol, or as a result of hypoxia)	seizures, tremor, yawning, muscle cramps
Gastrointestinal	Decreased bowel sounds, constipation	Nausea, vomiting, diarrhea
Skin		Piloerection, perspiration

Respiratory Effects

The respiratory depressant actions of opioids are their most notable and serious adverse effects. Opioids activating the μ-receptor cause dose-dependent depression of respiration, primarily through a direct action on brainstem respiratory centers. Patients may have hypopnea, bradypnea, or respiratory arrest. Clinical manifestations of opioid overdose also include increased tidal volume (VT); however, the increase in VT may not always be present. The best predictor of opioid poisoning is a respiratory rate (RR) less than 12. Noncardiogenic pulmonary edema occurs with methadone or acute withdrawal with opioid antagonists. Withdrawal manifests as normal to increased respiratory rate or hyperventilation [7, 15, 26].

Cardiac Effects

The predominant and usual effect of opioids is to produce bradycardia, from stimulation of the central vagal nucleus, and mild hypotension, due to histamine release or hypovolemia. AV block may occur. Patients may present with normal pulse and blood pressure. Electrocardiographic (ECG) changes, QRS and QTc prolongation, leading to torsades de pointes, can be seen with propoxyphene and meperidine. During withdrawal, normotension or hypertension and supraventricular tachycardia occur [7, 15, 26].

Metabolic Effects

Opioid abuse and withdrawal could cause rhabdomyolysis due to extreme agitation, hyperthermia, and shock. Rhabdomyolysis will result in a high anion gap metabolic acidosis from increased serum lactic acid concentrations. The excessive intake of prescription opioids formulated with acetaminophen may result in hepatotoxicity leading to liver failure and associated symptoms. Nausea and vomiting could result in electrolyte abnormalities and acid/base disturbances. Hypothermia, which results from a combination of environmental exposure and impaired thermogenesis, may be present [7, 15, 26].

Infectious Effects

Fever may be a sign of developing infection. Numerous infectious complications such as cellulitis, superficial skin abscesses, septic thrombophlebitis, hepatitis, auto-immune deficiency syndrome (AIDS), endocarditis, pneumonia, and malnutrition have been encountered with opioid abusers [7, 15, 26].

Gastrointestinal Effects

Gastrointestinal effects include decreased bowel sounds and constipation. Nausea, vomiting, diarrhea, or increased bowel sounds occur with withdrawal [7, 15, 26].

Management of the Patient Acutely Intoxicated with Opioids

Generally, opioid exposures will fall into one of several categories: therapeutic use, recreational use, intended self-harm, and accidental exposure through illegal activities (body stuffing/body packing) [28]. The anesthesiologist's likely encounter with a patient acutely intoxicated with opioids is limited to emergency situations. In the emergency room, the anesthesiologist is called to help stabilize the patient, secure the airway, and assess for possible surgery. Therefore, knowledge of the opioid toxidrome should help anticipate and manage perioperative problems that may arise.

Preoperative Evaluation

The history, physical examination, laboratory evaluations, and ancillary studies are used to establish and confirm the diagnosis of opioid poisoning, determine the extent of intoxication, and identify other conditions requiring treatment.

History

Careful pre-anesthetic evaluation of possible illicit substance intake is necessary. Many patients who abuse drugs may be unconscious, reluctant, or medically unable to give a reliable history to their physicians. During assessment, care should be exercised to maintain privacy and confidentiality. The patient needs to be clearly reassured that their drug history will not impact proper treatment. The clinician should attempt to identify the specific drug, dose, and formulation to which the patient was exposed, and the presence of nonopioid coexposures. History-taking should also determine the reason for poisoning and prior history of opioid use, which may help predict the expected duration of poisoning and influence post-overdose management.

Physical Examination

The mental status, vital signs, and pupillary examination are the most useful elements and allow classification of the patient into either a state of physiologic excitation or depression. Discrepancies between the physical examination and the history may reflect an inaccurate ingestion history, polydrug overdoses, or a brief or prolonged time interval between exposure and physical examination. The differential diagnosis of opioid overdose includes the effects of other agents such as sedatives, hypnotic agents, alcohol, clonidine, carbon monoxide, phenothiazines, or cholinergic and sympatholytic drug [29].

Complete exposure and examination of the patient and measurement of core temperature are essential. As noted, hypothermia, which results from a combination of environmental exposure and impaired thermogenesis, may be present in any patient more than mildly intoxicated. In a severely obtunded patient, room temperature may produce significant hypothermia. Elevated temperature may suggest early aspiration pneumonia or complications of injection drug use such as endocarditis. Examination of the skin may identify medication patches that must be removed, track marks suggesting history of chronic injection drug use, or coexisting soft tissue infections. Trauma, particularly to the head, should be ruled out. Not only do opioids predispose the patient to trauma but obtundation from traumatic brain injury can be misidentified as drug intoxication.

Respiratory failure can arise through alveolar hypoventilation, aspiration pneumonitis, or noncardiogenic pulmonary edema [30]. Chest auscultation for abnormal lung sounds and pulse oximetry should be performed in every patient. The clinician should be wary that hypercapnia can be present in the setting of normal oxygen saturation, particularly when the patient receives supplemental oxygen. Acute lung injury (ALI) may present as noncardiogenic pulmonary edema and typically includes rales, hypoxia, and occasionally frothy sputum [30]. Often, noncardiogenic pulmonary edema occurs as a patient is recovering from opioid-induced respiratory depression or iatrogenic reversal of opioid toxicity. Status asthmaticus may be triggered by inhaled heroin [31].

Laboratory and Ancillary Studies

Most patients with mild or moderate unintentional or recreational poisoning can be managed successfully without any further laboratory investigation. Symptomatic patients and those with an unreliable or unknown history should, at a minimum, undergo urinalysis and measurement of serum electrolytes, BUN, and creatinine. Measurements of serum osmolality, ketones, liver function tests, amylase, calcium, and magnesium should also be performed in significantly ill patients. Arterial blood gas and serum lactate measurements may be necessary in patients with acid–base, cardiovascular, neurologic, or respiratory disturbances. Further laboratory studies depend upon the results of initial results. Serum creatine phosphokinase concentration should be obtained to exclude rhabdomyolysis in the patient presenting after prolonged immobilization. After any overdose in which the opioid is formulated with acetaminophen or intended for self-harm, serum acetaminophen concentration should be obtained. A salicylate concentration should be sought when clinical suspicion or signs of overdose exist (e.g., tachypnea or increased anion gap). Hypoglycemia can be potentially confused with, and coexist alongside, opioid poisoning. A rapid serum glucose concentration should be obtained in all suspected cases of opioid overdose. Routine urine pregnancy testing is strongly recommended in all women of childbearing age.

Urine toxicology screens should not be routinely obtained. Acute opioid poisoning is a clinical diagnosis; the management is unchanged by the result of a urine opioid screen. Immunoassay screens can generally be used to detect opioids and other substances within 1 h. All normal or abnormal results should be regarded as presumptive and require confirmatory testing. The confirmatory tests (liquid and gas chromatography or mass spectrometry) are expensive, time consuming, often do not predict or define the severity of poisoning, detect unsuspected drugs in only a minority of patients, and are unlikely to affect patient outcome [32, 33]. A false positive test for opiates can be seen in patients taking rifampin, fluoroquinolones, poppy seeds, and quinine in tonic water.

Imaging studies are not required in every patient but may be useful in some situations [28, 34, 35]. Chest radiography is reserved for those patients with adventitious lung sounds or hypoxia that does not correct when ventilation is addressed [29].

ECG should be reserved for those exposed to potentially cardiotoxic opioids (propoxyphene and methadone), particularly after first exposure to methadone or a large increase in dosage [36]. ECG should also be performed on all patients with complaints suggesting dysrhythmia, such as palpitations or syncope.

Intraoperative Management

There is no ideal anesthetic approach for the chronic addict or a patient with an acute opiate overdose [15]. Substance abuse, whether acute or chronic, alters normal physiological responses. Supportive care is the most important aspect of treatment and frequently is sufficient to affect complete patient recovery. Initial management should focus on support of the patient's airway and breathing. Rapid sequence induction with in-line cervical immobilization should be performed early in the poisoned patient with depressed mental status because of the high risk for aspiration and possibility of occult trauma. Acute intake of opioids decreases anesthetic requirements (decreased MAC) [15]. If the patient cannot give consent because of poisoning, consent is inferred based on medical necessity.

Support of the circulatory system with fluids and monitoring of arterial blood gases and pulmonary function are important. Hypertension in agitated patients is best treated initially with nonspecific sedatives such as a benzodiazepine [16]. Vasopressors are required when hypotension does not resolve with volume expansion. Large bore intravenous access should be obtained. Advanced cardiac life-support measures must be provided as required. Bradyarrhythmias associated with hypotension should be treated in the standard fashion with atropine or temporary cardiac pacing. Ventricular tachycardias are generally treated with standard doses of lidocaine. Overdrive pacing with isoproterenol or a temporary pacemaker may be effective in patients with methadone-induced torsades de pointes and prolonged QTc on ECG [37, 38]. If the QTc remains prolonged, the patient should be observed by cardiac monitoring for a 24-h period and hypocalcemia, hypokalemia, and hypomagnesemia should be corrected. Class IA and III antiarrhythmic agents should be avoided because of a potential to prolong QTc [37–39]. Many of the anesthetic agents prolong QTc (inhaled anesthetics, droperidol, ondansetron, and succinylcholine) and should be administered with care [40–43]. Prolongation of the QT interval, intraventricular conduction disturbances, heart block, and ventricular bigeminy can occur with propoxyphene. These ECG changes may respond to sodium bicarbonate, but not naloxone, by overcoming the sodium channel blockade [44].

Opioid intoxication requires the intravenous administration 0.05–2.0 mg of naloxone. Opioid antagonism typically occurs within minutes of naloxone administration and lasts for 45–90 min [45, 46]. Repeat naloxone boluses may be needed for continuous infusion to sustain the opioid antagonistic effects [45, 46]. The goal of naloxone administration is not a normal level of consciousness, rather adequate ventilation. When spontaneous ventilations are present, an initial dose of 0.05 mg is titrated upward every few minutes until the respiratory rate is 12 [45]. Apneic patients should receive higher initial doses of naloxone (0.2–1 mg). Patients in cardiorespiratory arrest following possible opioid overdose should be given a minimum of naloxone 2 mg [45]. In general, a lack of response to 10 mg of naloxone is required to exclude opioid toxicity, although larger doses may be required to antagonize the effects of propoxyphene, diphenoxylate, methadone, levo-alpha-acetylmethadol (LAAM), pentazocine, oxycodone, and ingested leaking drug packets [29, 46–48].

One should be wary of the potentially severe side effects of naloxone which include pulmonary edema, seizures, or opioid withdrawal [46, 47]. Patients should be ventilated prior to and during naloxone administration to reduce the chance of noncardiogenic pulmonary edema [49, 50]. Management of opioid and naloxone-related acute lung injury (ALI) is supportive and the prognosis is generally good [49, 50]. Supplemental oxygen and mechanical ventilation with positive end-expiratory pressure may be required to achieve adequate arterial oxygen saturation. Since central venous pressure is low, treatment of pulmonary edema with diuresis may aggravate hypotension.

Seizures are most common with propoxyphene and meperidine [29, 47] and are best treated with intravenous benzodiazepines followed by barbiturates if necessary. Ongoing seizures suggest either body packing or body stuffing of heroin or a secondary process [47]. Drug-associated agitated behavior is generally best treated with benzodiazepine administration, supplemented with neuroleptics (e.g., haloperidol) as needed [47].

Clinical hypoglycemia may be present. Empiric administration of dextrose is recommended for the patient with altered consciousness [51].

In cases of oral ingestion, gastric lavage should be attempted after ensuring adequate airway protection [47]. Activated charcoal should follow gastric lavage. Gastrointestinal decontamination should be reserved for patients presenting with potentially life-threatening coingestants or ruptured ingested drug packets [29]. The large volume of distribution of the opioids precludes removal of a significant quantity of drug by hemodialysis.

Postoperative Care

Disposition of the patient postoperatively is based upon clinical criteria that relate to the stability of the airway, respiratory system, cardiovascular system, and the patient's level of consciousness. Patients who only develop mild toxicity can be observed for 4–6 h until they are asymptomatic [29]. Patients with significant toxicity, or after ingestion of a sustained release preparation, should be admitted to an intensive care unit [48–50, 52]. Patients should also be monitored for withdrawal symptoms postoperatively and managed accordingly.

Postoperative pain management may be complicated in the drug abuser. Tolerance should not be synonymous with addiction. In the setting of pain accompanied with withdrawal symptoms, supplemental opioids are indicated. Failure of a physician to appropriately treat a patient's pain may be considered medical malpractice [53–55]. Pain patients abusing opioids have longer hospital stays and may have psychiatric disease (major depression, dysthymia, generalized anxiety disorder, and panic disorder) [56]. All patients with intentional overdose require psychiatric assessment prior to discharge.

Management of Opioid Tolerance and Withdrawal

Many patients who present for surgery and anesthesia may be opioid dependent or at least moderately tolerant to the therapeutic effects of opioid analgesics [57, 58]. These patients may be dependent as a result of recreational abuse, long-term pain therapy, or opioid addiction programs. Perioperative management of opioid addicted patients poses a challenge [57, 58] due, in part, to the occurrence of drug-specific adaptations such as tolerance and physical dependence. These variables, alone, or in combination, may diminish opioid analgesic effectiveness in the perioperative setting and cause unwarranted physiologic changes.

Preoperative Period

In many cases, detection of opioid abuse and dependence occurs by the anesthesiologist, either in preadmission testing or in the moments just preceding the scheduled procedure. The goal of preoperative assessment is to identify the cause of opioid dependence and to anticipate, avoid, and treat the physiologic changes that may arise. A thorough substance abuse history should be obtained from the patient or, when warranted, the family. A urine toxicology screen might be necessary when a patient is unable or unwilling to cooperate.

Opioid withdrawal occurs when opioids are abruptly discontinued or when opioid use has diminished. Likewise, if the clinician "overshoots" the appropriate dose of naloxone in an opioid-dependent individual, withdrawal will ensue. Opioid withdrawal occurs not only in patients dependent on heroin or prescription opioid medications but also in chronic pain patients maintained on opioid medications.

The severity of opioid withdrawal varies with the dose and duration of prior drug use. The time course of withdrawal varies, depending on the opioid used [6] (Table 4.2). Withdrawal symptoms usually occur 4–6 h following the last opioid intake, and peak in 48–72 h. Opioid withdrawal reactions are very uncomfortable but are not of themselves life threatening [7]. Symptoms are initially mild but typically increase in severity over the course of a few hours. In the initial phase of opioid withdrawal, the patient experiences a range of symptoms including anxiety, insomnia, diaphoresis, drug craving, thermoregulation disturbances, and diffuse myalgia. Many patients report localized, aching pain in the back, abdomen, and legs. Hot and cold flashes are also common, and patients may request blankets. Craving for the drug is associated with lacrimation, rhinorrhea, yawning, and piloerection ("going cold turkey" or "gooseflesh"). Early findings of opioid withdrawal may include tachycardia and hypertension [6, 7, 15]. Pupillary dilation can be marked. Gastrointestinal symptoms, which initially may be mild (anorexia), can progress in moderate to severe withdrawal to include nausea, vomiting, and diarrhea leading to dehydration and electrolyte disturbances [59]. Bothersome central nervous system (CNS) symptoms may also occur and include dysphoria, shaking, leg jerking ("kicking the habit") [59], and unconsciousness. Long-term opioid administration causes adrenal hypertrophy and impairs corticosteroid secretion [7]. Complications in opioid-dependent patients may involve the cardiovascular and renal systems. Hepatitis, acquired immunodeficiency syndrome, osteomyelitis, anemia, muscle weakness, and psychological and neurologic complications may be found in addicted patients.

Table 4.2 Time course of opioid withdrawal syndrome

Drug	Onset	Peak intensity	Duration
Meperidine	2–6 h	8–12 h	4–5 days
Dihydromorphine			
Codeine	6–18 h	36–72 h	7–10 days
Morphine			
Heroin			
Methadone	24–48 h	3–21 days	6–7 weeks

Adapted with permission from: Stoelting RK, Dierdorf SF: Psychiatric illness and substance abuse. In: Stoelting RK, Dierdorf SF, editors, Anesthesia and co-existing disease, 4th edition. New York, NY: Churchill Livingstone; 2002. p. 629–54.

Polydrug use is frequent among those with drug addiction and many fulfill the criteria for dependence on, or abuse of, more than one substance [59, 60]. Should the anesthesiologist not account for the presence of coingestants such as benzodiazepines, cocaine, scopolamine, or alcohol, severe withdrawal reactions, including anxiety, agitation, and confusion, may occur [29].

Perioperative management of opioid-dependent patients begins with preoperative administration of their daily maintenance or baseline opioid dose before induction of general, spinal, or regional anesthesia [61]. Ideally, patients should be instructed to take their usual dose of oral opioid on the morning of surgery and maintain any transdermal fentanyl patch into the operating room. Because most sustained-release opioids provide 12 h or more of analgesic effect, baseline requirements will generally be maintained during preoperative and intraoperative periods. Patients who miss their dose of baseline opioids may be treated with an equivalent loading dose of morphine or hydromorphone, administered before anesthetic induction or during the operative procedure [61]. Some anesthesiologists prefer to slowly "front load" relatively large amounts of morphine or methadone to cover baseline and estimated intraoperative opioid requirements after applying full monitoring and mask oxygen. Others prefer administering one-half of the estimated dose during pre-induction and induction periods and titrating the remainder as the case progresses [61].

Intraoperative

The first step in caring for any opioid-dependent patient is to ensure adequate airway management, intravenous access, and application of general resuscitative measures [62]. The ability to protect the airway may be compromised and the risk of aspiration greatly increases. Delayed gastric emptying is common in opioid-dependent patients [15]. Peripheral IV access may be difficult and central venous access may be required.

Management of Opioid Tolerance

Chronic opioid use leads to cross-tolerance to other central nervous system (CNS) depressants, including anesthetic drugs. Reduced intravascular fluid volume, malnutrition, or liver disease may require appropriate dose adjustments of anesthetic drugs. Tolerance to any one opioid preparation, be it oxycodone or heroin, results in clinically measurable insensitivity to most others and a diminished response to intraoperative doses of fentanyl and postoperative doses of morphine.

Precise dosing guidelines have not been developed; however, opioid doses required to meet intraoperative and postsurgical analgesic requirements may need to be increased 30–100% in comparison to requirements in opioid-naive patients [63]. There is a significant interpatient variability in opioid dose requirements. The optimal intraoperative dose avoids undermedication and overmedication, both associated with negative perioperative outcomes [62]. At end stages of the general anesthetic, patients with respiratory rates greater than 20 breaths per minute who exhibit slight to markedly dilated pupils generally require additional opioid dosing. Intravenous boluses of morphine, fentanyl, or hydromorphone are titrated to maintain a respiratory rate of 12–14 breaths per minute [60]. Local anesthetic infiltration of the surgical site helps to reduce pain in the perioperative period. The patient may also be maintained in a mildly sedated state to avoid agitation and pain upon emergence from anesthesia [60], which may be accomplished by administering additional opioid as needed prior to transport to the postanesthetic care unit. Alternatively, a dexmedetomidine infusion may be started [64]. Nonopioid analgesic adjuvants [NSAIDS, cyclooxygenase-2 inhibitors, ketamine, clonidine (0.1 mg/h)] may be used to reduce opioid dose requirements and provide analgesia during and following surgery [65–69].

Regional anesthesia may be safely administered to the opioid-addicted. However, increased tendency for hypotension should be anticipated following the induction of spinal or epidural anesthesia. Increased incidence of spinal, epidural, and disk space infection has been reported in this patient population, irrespective of the technique used [4].

Management of Opioid Withdrawal

General principles regarding the management of substance withdrawal syndromes include use of a symptom-triggered approach, substitution of a long-acting replacement for the abused drug in gradual tapering doses, and establishing a plan for long-term abstinence [59].

General supportive measures are necessary for managing withdrawal. Substitution with a long-acting opioid in tapering doses is the treatment of choice for managing opioid withdrawal [59]. For short-acting opioids, the natural course of withdrawal is generally relatively brief, though more intense and associated with a higher degree of discomfort than with equivalent doses of long-acting opioids. It is important to note, however, that there is considerable individual variation. The usual starting methadone dose is 20 mg orally, or 10 mg subcutaneously/ intramuscularly, or 1.25 mg intravenously (every 5–10 min) titrated upward to diminish or to avoid withdrawal symptoms [59, 60, 62, 70]. Larger methadone doses are required to treat patients who have larger opioid habits; for such patients, a routine starting dose might be 30 mg [62]. Once a stabilizing dose has been reached, methadone is tapered by 20% a day for inpatients, leading to a 1- to 2-week procedure. Close monitoring for treatment effectiveness and toxicity is required. No methadone should be administered to the habitual user until the appearance of withdrawal symptoms [29]. Symptoms of withdrawal due to naloxone administration should only be managed expectantly, and not with opioids. Hypertension associated with end-organ dysfunction can be treated with calcium-channel blockers, phentolamine, labetalol, or nitroprusside.

Patients with mild to moderate withdrawal may be successfully treated with clonidine, which has been demonstrated to decrease symptoms of opioid withdrawal [70–72], especially those relating to autonomic dysfunction. Typical clonidine doses used to treat opioid withdrawal range between 0.1 and 0.2 mg orally every 6 h [72]. A decrease in blood pressure and heart rate are useful markers of the drug effect on that particular patient. If no decrease in pain is reported and cardiovascular parameters remain unchanged, a further dose of clonidine is indicated. Heavy users of opioids may require 2–4 mcg/kg intravenously to produce a noticeable effect in 5–10 min [73]. Side effects include sedation, dry mouth, orthostatic hypotension, and constipation. Other alpha2-receptor agonists, such as dexmedetomidine, have been used for treating withdrawal symptoms [74–76]. Other medications that can help with withdrawal symptoms include nonopioid analgesics, anxiolytics (Librium), sleeping pills (temazepam, diphenhydramine), antiemetics (promethazine, hydroxyzine), and antidiarrheal agents [71].

Postoperative

The opioid-abusing patient seems to experience an exaggerated degree of post-operative pain and decreased pain tolerance [63, 77, 78]. Pain is often underestimated and under-treated; under-treatment may result in inadequate pain relief, withdrawal phenomena, and a prolonged hospital stay for pain management. It is noteworthy to understand that opioid seeking, when it arises during opioid treatment of pain, is not necessarily caused by addiction and could equally be caused by tolerance, withdrawal, or inadequate analgesia [12].

In opioid-dependent patients, it is important to have identified goals for acute pain management. Preexisting opioid usage should be continued as a baseline and additional multimodal analgesia ought to be provided as needed (local anesthesia, regional anesthesia, anti-inflammatory drugs, and short acting opioids) [60, 61]. Baseline requirements for oral opioids following surgery must generally be supplemented with additional doses (generally 20–50% increases above baseline) to accommodate pain associated with surgical injury [60, 61]. Opioid dosing may be increased, as needed, if patients do not experience adequate pain control. Opioid rotation may be a useful option. Evidence suggests that patient-controlled anesthesia (PCA) opioid doses can be expected to be significantly higher than in opioid-naive patients, requiring higher bolus doses and possibly a shortening of the lock-out interval [63].

To avoid withdrawal, baseline opioid dosing should be gradually tapered over 3–7 days as the intensity of acute pain diminishes following surgery [79]. In this setting, baseline doses may be reduced by 50% the day after surgery and tapered 25% every 24–48 h, depending on the opioid administered. When the dose has been decreased to 10–15 mg morphine equivalent per 24 h, it may be discontinued.

Several agents have been shown to enhance postoperative analgesia, or chronic pain control, and may serve as useful analgesic adjuncts in opioid-dependent patients. These include the alpha 2-adrenergic receptor agonist clonidine, dexmedetomidine [80], the NMDA receptor antagonist dextromethorphan [81–83], the anticonvulsant gabapentin [84], and the parenteral cyclooxygenase inhibitors [85] and ketamine [86].

Clonidine provides analgesia after surgery or trauma and is particularly useful when opioid withdrawal may be complicating the situation; clonidine acts synergistically with any background opioid, and, conveniently, does not promote nausea, vomiting, or respiratory depression. Application of a 0.1–0.2 mg/h clonidine transdermal patch may help to minimize some of the autonomic aspects of opioid withdrawal if symptoms should become distressing [73]. Prolonged use of alpha-2 agonists beyond 2–3 days in the perioperative period should be managed by pain management specialists [73].

It is worth emphasizing that the immediate perioperative period is not the optimal time to attempt detoxification or rehabilitation management of patients who are chronically using opioids [84]. After hospital discharge, opioid-dependent patients should be scheduled for a follow-up visit with a pain specialist who can optimize pain management during rehabilitation and facilitate opioid dose tapering.

Treatment Options

New treatment options for opioid tolerance and withdrawal involve use of buprenorphine, a strong affinity partial agonist at the mu opioid receptor (see Chap. 3). Buprenorphine and buprenorphine-naloxone are approved for the treatment of pain and opioid detoxification. A recent Cochrane systematic review of buprenorphine for opioid withdrawal [87] found that buprenorphine is more effective than clonidine for the management of opioid withdrawal. There appears to be no significant difference between buprenorphine and methadone in terms of completion of treatment, but withdrawal symptoms may resolve more quickly with buprenorphine. Therapy with buprenorphine-naloxone should start with a dose of 8 mg and should not begin until withdrawal symptoms occur because buprenorphine can precipitate opioid withdrawal if administered while opioids are still bound to the opiate receptor.

Limitations to the use of buprenorphine in the treatment of opioid dependence are its sublingual administration and issues with regard to pain control and sedation because opioids have little effect in patients receiving buprenorphine [62].

Another treatment modality for opioid dependence is ultrarapid inpatient detoxification using sedatives and anesthetics in combination with opiate antagonists [62] (see Chap. 3). However, a recent Cochrane systematic review [88] concluded that heavy sedation compared to light sedation does not confer additional benefits in terms of less severe withdrawal or increased rates of commencement on naltrexone maintenance treatment. Given that the adverse events are potentially life-threatening, the value of antagonist-induced withdrawal under heavy sedation or anesthesia is not supported. The high cost of anesthesia-based approaches, both in monetary terms and use of scarce intensive care resources, suggests that this form of treatment should not be pursued.

Conclusion

With the increasing availability and utilization of opioids, its abuse and dependence remain salient concerns for the anesthesiologist during the perioperative period. Anesthesiologists, more than ever, need to identify and treat underlying substance use disorders, and withdrawal symptoms, in patients presenting for surgery. A full preoperative assessment must be conducted followed by an individualized perioperative anesthetic plan tailored to the patient's unique level of dependence and/or syndrome. General principles regarding the treatment of substance intoxication and withdrawal include application of resuscitative measures (i.e., airway, breathing, and circulatory management). Metabolic and infectious changes can also impact care. Acute opioid intoxication can be reversed with judicious doses of naloxone; however, overdosing naloxone should be avoided. It is important to consider polysubstance use and harmful drug combinations in any patient presenting with a substance abuse issue.

In the opioid-dependent patient, baseline maintenance of opioid intake remains a rigid aspect of an anesthetic plan. Under-medicating these patients must be avoided. Patients should be advised to maintain their regular opioid intake the day of surgery. During opioid withdrawal, substitution of a long-acting agent, methadone, in tapering doses, is the general standard of care. Additionally, management of substance withdrawal syndromes includes use of a symptom-triggered approach. Clonidine has been shown to decrease symptoms of opioid withdrawal and aid in pain management. Successful perioperative pain in this pain-sensitive population requires maintaining baseline opioid levels, administering supplemental intraoperative and postoperative opioids, and providing nonopioid analgesics and neural blockade. As the postoperative course and stay of the opioid-dependent inpatient is usually extensive, the importance of consulting qualified pain management specialists, for long-term pain management, rehabilitation, and tapering cannot be stressed enough.

References

1. Substance Abuse and Mental Health Services Administration. Results from the 2008 National Survey on Drug Use and Health: National Findings (Office of Applied Studies, NSDUH Series H-36, HHS Publication No. SMA 09-4434). Rockville, MD; 2009. http://www.oas.samhsa. gov/nsduh/2k8nsduh/2k8Results.pdf. Accessed 30 Sep 2010.
2. Manchikanti L, Singh A. Therapeutic opioids. A ten-year perspective on the complexities and complications of the escalating use, abuse, and nonmedical use of opioids. Pain Physician. 2008;11(2 Suppl):S63–88.
3. Becker WC, Sullivan LE, Tetrault JM, Desai RA, Fiellin DA. Non-medical use, abuse and dependence on prescription opioids among U.S. adults: psychiatric, medical and substance use correlates. Drug Alcohol Depend. 2008;94(1–3):38–47.
4. Kuczkowski K. Anesthetic implications of drug abuse in pregnancy. J Clin Anesth. 2003;15:357–8.
5. Birnbach DJ, Browne IM, Kim A, Stein DJ, Thys DM. Identification of polysubstance abuse in the parturient. Br J Anaesth. 2001;87:488–90.
6. Stoelting RK, Dierdorf SF. Psychiatric illness and substance abuse. In: Stoelting RK, Dierdorf SF, editors. Anesthesia and co-existing disease. 4th ed. New York: Churchill Livingstone; 2002. p. 629–54.
7. Gutstein Howard B, Akil Huda. "Chapter 21. Opioid Analgesics". In: Brunton LL, Lazo JS, Parker KL, editors. Goodman & Gilman's the pharmacological basis of therapeutics, 11e: http://www.accessmedicine.com/content.aspx?aID=940653. Accessed 30 Sep 2010.
8. A narcotic painkiller tops Forbes' list of the most prescribed medicines. http://www.forbes. com/2010/05/11/narcotic-painkiller-vicodin-business-healthcare-popular-drugs.html. Accessed 30 Sep 2010.
9. Johnston LD, O'Malley PM, Bachman JG, et al. Monitoring the future national results on adolescent drug use: overview of key findings (NIH Publication No. 10-7583). Bethesda, MD: National Institute on Drug Abuse; 2009.
10. American Psychiatric Association. Diagnostic and statistical manual of mental disorders. 4th ed. Washington, DC: American Psychiatric Association; 2000. Text revision: DSM-IV-TR.
11. Substance Abuse and Mental Health Services Administration, Office of Applied Studies. Drug Abuse Warning Network, 2007. National Estimates of Drug-Related Emergency Department Visits. Rockville, MD; 2010.
12. Camí J, Farré M. Drug addiction. N Engl J Med. 2003;349:975–86.
13. Savage S, Covington EC, Heit HA, Hunt J, Joranson D, Schnoll SH. American Academy of Pain Medicine, American Pain Society and American Society of Addiction Medicine. Definitions Related to the Use of Opioids for the Treatment of Pain:Consensus document; 2001. http://www. painmed.org/Workarea/DownloadAsset.aspx?id=3204. Accessed 30 Sep 2010.
14. Becerra L, Harter K, Gonzalez RG, Borsook D. Functional magnetic resonance imaging measures of the effects of morphine on central nervous system circuitry in opioid-naive healthy volunteers. Anesth Analg. 2006;103:208–16.
15. Fukuda K. Intravenous opioid anesthetics. In: Miller RD, editor. Miller's anesthesia. 6th ed. Philadelphia, PA: Elsevier; 2005.
16. Stoelting RK. Opioids agonists and antagonists. In: Stoelting RK, Hillier S, editors. Pharmacology & physiology in anesthetic practice. 4th ed. Baltimore, MD: Lippincott Williams & Wilkins; 2006. p. 87–126.
17. Trescot A, Datta S, Lee M, Hansen H. Opioid pharmacology. Pain Physician. 2008;11:S133–53.
18. Nestler EJ. Molecular neurobiology of addiction. Am J Addict. 2001;10:201–17.
19. Roset P, Farre M, de la Torre R, et al. Modulation of rate of onset and intensity of drug effects reduces abuse potential in healthy males. Drug Alcohol Depend. 2001;64:285–98.
20. Kathiramalainathan K, Kaplan HL, Romach MK, et al. Inhibition of cytochrome P450 2D6 modifies codeine abuse liability. J Clin Psychopharmacol. 2000;20:435–44.

21. Nestler EJ. Molecular basis of long-term plasticity underlying addiction. Nat Rev Neurosci. 2001;2:119–28 [Erratum, Nat Rev Neurosci 2001;2:215].
22. Nestler EJ, Aghajanian GK. Molecular and cellular basis of addiction. Science. 1997;278:58–63.
23. Christie MJ. Cellular neuroadaptations to chronic opioids: tolerance, withdrawal and addiction. Br J Pharmacol. 2008;154:384–96.
24. Sarnyai Z, Shaham Y, Heinrichs SC. The role of corticotropin-releasing factor in drug addiction. Pharmacol Rev. 2001;53:209–43.
25. Lim G, Wang S, Zeng Q, et al. Spinal glucocorticoid receptors contribute to the development of morphine tolerance in rats. Anesthesiology. 2005;102:832–7.
26. O'Brien C. Chapter 23. Drug addiction and drug abuse (Chapter). In: Brunton LL, Lazo JS, Parker KL, editors. Goodman & Gilman's the pharmacological basis of therapeutics, 11e: http://www.accessmedicine.com/content.aspx?aID=941547. Accessed 30 Sep 2010.
27. Knaggs RD, Crighton IM, Cobby TF, et al. The pupillary effects of intravenous morphine, codeine, and tramadol in volunteers. Anesth Analg. 2004;99:108–12.
28. Traub SJ, Hoffman RS, Nelson LS. Body packing. The internal concealment of illicit drugs. N Engl J Med. 2003;349:2519.
29. Doyon S. Chapter 167. Opioids. In: Tintinalli JE, Kelen GD, Stapczynski JS, Ma OJ, Cline DM, editors. Tintinalli's emergency medicine: a comprehensive study guide, 6e: http://www.access-medicine.com.medlib.med.miami.edu:2048/content.aspx?aID=602227. Accessed 30 Sep 2010.
30. Sporer K, Dorn EA. Case series. Heroin-related noncardiogenic pulmonary. Chest. 2001;120:1628–32.
31. Cygan J, Trunsk M, Corbridge T. Inhaled heroin-induced status asthmaticus: five cases and a review of the literature. Chest. 2000;117:272–5.
32. Nafziger AN, Bertino Jr JS. Utility and application of urine drug testing in chronic pain management with opioids. Clin J Pain. 2009;25(1):73–9.
33. Moeller KE, Lee KC, Kissack JC. Urine drug screening: practical guide for clinicians. Mayo Clin Proc. 2008;83(1):66–76.
34. Amitai Y, Silver B, Leikin JG, et al. Detection of tablets in the gastrointestinal tract by ultrasound. Am J Emerg Med. 1992;10:18.
35. Florez MV, Evans JM, Daly TR. The radiodensity of medications seen on x-ray films. Mayo Clin Proc. 1998;73:516.
36. Krantz MJ, Kutinsky IB, Robertson AD, Mehler PS. Dose-related effects of methadone on QT prolongation in a series of patients with torsade de pointes. Pharmacotherapy. 2003;23:802.
37. Altmann D, Eggmann U, Ammann PW. Drug induced QT prolongation. Klin Wochenschr. 2008;120(5–6):128–35.
38. Gupta A, Lawrence AT, Krishnan K, et al. Current concepts in the mechanisms and management of drug-induced QT prolongation and torsade de pointes. Am Heart J. 2007;153(6):891–9.
39. Letsas KP, Efremidis M, Kounas SP, et al. Clinical characteristics of patients with drug-induced QT interval prolongation and torsade de pointes: identification of risk factors. Clin Res Cardiol. 2009;98(4):208–12.
40. Kies SJ, Pabelick CM, Hurley HA, et al. Anesthesia for patients with congenital long QT syndrome. Anesthesiology. 2005;102(1):204–10.
41. Charbit B, Alvarez JC, Dasque E, et al. Droperidol and ondansetron-induced QT interval prolongation: a clinical drug interaction study. Anesthesiology. 2008;109(2):206–12.
42. Yildirim H, Adanir T, Atay A, et al. The effects of sevoflurane, isoflurane and desflurane on QT interval of the ECG. Eur J Anaesthesiol. 2004;21(7):566–70.
43. Nakao S. Sevoflurane causes greater QTc interval prolongation in elderly patients than in younger patients. Anesth Analg. 2010;110(3):775–9.
44. Stork CM, Redd JT, Fine K, Hoffman RS. Propoxyphene-induced wide QRS complex dysrhythmia responsive to sodium bicarbonate. A case report. J Toxicol Clin Toxicol. 1995;33:179.
45. Saybolta M, Altera S, Santosb F, et al. Naloxone in cardiac arrest with suspected opioid over-doses. Resuscitation. 2010;81:42–6.
46. Dahan A, Aarts L, Smith TW. Incidence, reversal, and prevention of opioid-induced respiratory depression. Anesthesiology. 2010;112(1):226–38.

47. Mokhlesi B, Leiken J, Murray P, et al. Adult toxicology in critical care: part II: specific poisonings. Chest. 2003;123:897–922.
48. Schneir AB, Vadeboncoeur TF, Offerman SR, et al. Massive OxyContin ingestion refractory to naloxone therapy. Ann Emerg Med. 2002;40(4):425–8.
49. Larpin R, Vincent A, Perret C. Hospital morbidity and mortality of acute opiate intoxication. Presse Med. 1990;19(30):1403–6.
50. Grigorakos L, Sakagianni K, Tsigou E, et al. Outcome of acute heroin overdose requiring intensive care unit admission. J Opioid Manag. 2010;6(3):227–31.
51. Hoffman RS, Goldfrank LR. The poisoned patient with altered consciousness: controversies in the use of a 'coma cocktail'. JAMA. 1995;274:562.
52. Hamad A, Al-Ghadban A, Carvounis C, et al. Predicting the need for medical intensive care. J Intensive Care Med. 2000;15(6):321–8.
53. Shapiro R. Liability issues in the management of pain. J Pain Symptom Manage. 1994;9(3): 146–52.
54. Lawrence L. Legal issues in pain management: striking the balance. Emerg Med Clin North Am. 2005;23(2):573–84.
55. Fitzgibbon D, Rathmell J, Michna E, et al. Malpractice claims associated with medication management for chronic pain. Anesthesiology. 2010;112:948–56.
56. Sullivan M, Edlund M, Zhang L, et al. Association between mental health disorders, problem drug use, and regular prescription opioid use. Arch Intern Med. 2006;166:2087–93.
57. May JA, White HC, Leonard-White A, et al. The patient recovering from alcohol or drug addiction: special issues for the anesthesiologist. Anesth Analg. 2001;92:160–1.
58. Jage J, Bey T. Postoperative analgesia in patients with substance use disorders. Acute Pain. 2000;3:140–55.
59. Kosten TR, O'Connor PG. Management of drug and alcohol withdrawal [see comment]. N Engl J Med. 2003;348(18):1786–95.
60. Mitra S, Sinatra RS. Perioperative management of acute pain in the opioid-dependent patient. Anesthesiology. 2004;101:212–27.
61. Mehta V, Langford RM. Pain management for opioid dependent patients. Anaesthesia. 2006;61:269–76.
62. Tetrault JM, O'Connor PJ. Substance abuse and withdrawal in the critical care setting. Crit Care Clin. 2008;24:767–88.
63. Rapp SE, Ready LB, Nessly ML. Acute pain management in patients with prior opioid consumption: a case controlled retrospective review. Pain. 1995;61:195–201.
64. Chrysostomou C, Schmitt CG. Dexmedetomidine: sedation, analgesia and beyond. Expert Opin Drug Metab Toxicol. 2008;4(5):619–27.
65. Buvanendran A, Kroin JS. Multimodal analgesia for controlling acute postoperative pain. Curr Opin Anaesthesiol. 2009;22(5):588–93.
66. Katz WA. Cyclooxygenase-2-selective inhibitors in the management of acute and perioperative pain. Cleve Clin J Med. 2002;69 Suppl 1:SI65–75.
67. Chen JY, Ko TL, Wen YR, et al. Opioid-sparing effects of ketorolac and its correlation with the recovery of postoperative bowel function in colorectal surgery patients: a prospective randomized double-blinded study. Clin J Pain. 2009;25(6):485–9.
68. Bell RF, Dahl JB, Moore RA, Kalso E. Peri-operative ketamine for acute post-operative pain: a quantitative and qualitative systematic review (Cochrane review). Acta Anaesthesiol Scand. 2005;49(10):1405–28.
69. Haller G, Waeber JL, Infante NK, Clergue F. Ketamine combined with morphine for the management of pain in an opioid addict. Anesthesiology. 2002;96:1265–6.
70. Nicholls L, Bragaw L, Ruetsch C. Opioid dependence treatment and guidelines. J Manag Care Pharm. 2010;16(1 Suppl B):S14–21.
71. Kleber HS. Opioids: detoxification. In: Galanter M, Kleber HD, editors. Textbook of substance abuse treatment. 2nd ed. Washington, DC: The American Psychiatric Press; 1999. p. 251–69.
72. O'Connor PG, Samet JH, Stein MD. Management of hospitalized intravenous drug users: role of the internist. Am J Med. 1994;96:551–8.

73. Mackenzie JW. Acute pain management for opioid dependent patients. Anaesthesia. 2006;61:907–8.
74. Honey BL, Benefield RJ, Miller JL, Johnson PN. Alpha2-receptor agonists for treatment and prevention of iatrogenic opioid abstinence syndrome in critically ill patients. Ann Pharmacother. 2009;43(9):1506–11.
75. Tobias JD. Dexmedetomidine to treat opioid withdrawal in infants following prolonged sedation in the pediatric ICU. J Opioid Manag. 2006;2:201–5.
76. Baddigam K, Russo P, Russo J, Tobias JD. Dexmedetomidine in the treatment of withdrawal syndromes in cardiothoracic surgery patients. J Intensive Care Med. 2005;20:118–23.
77. Compton P, Charuvastra VC, Kintaudi K, Ling W. Pain responses in methadone-maintained opioid abusers. J Pain Symptom Manage. 2000;20:237–45.
78. Laulin JP, Celerier E, Larcher A, et al. Opiate tolerance to daily heroin administration. An apparent phenomenon associated with enhanced pain sensitivity. Neuroscience. 1999;89:631–6.
79. Inturrisi CE. Clinical pharmacology of opioids for pain. Clin J Pain. 2002;18(Suppl):S3–13.
80. Coursin DB, Coursin DB, Maccioli GA. Dexmedetomidine. Curr Opin Crit Care. 2001;7:221–6.
81. Weinbroum AA, Gorodetzky A, Nirkin A, et al. Dextromethorphan for the reduction of immediate and late postoperative pain and morphine consumption in orthopedic oncology patients: a randomized, placebo-controlled, double-blind study. Cancer. 2002;95:1164–70.
82. Weinbroum AA. Dextromethorphan reduces immediate and late postoperative analgesic requirements and improves patients' subjective scorings after epidural lidocaine and general anesthesia. Anesth Analg. 2002;94:1547–52.
83. Helmy SA, Bali A. The effect of the preemptive use of the NMDA receptor antagonist dextromethorphan on postoperative analgesic requirements. Anesth Analg. 2001;92:739–44.
84. Dirks J, Fredensborg BB, Christensen D, et al. A randomized study of the effects of single-dose gabapentin versus placebo on postoperative pain and morphine consumption after mastectomy. Anesthesiology. 2002;97:560–4.
85. Barton SF, Langeland FF, Snabes MC, et al. Efficacy and safety of intravenous parecoxib sodium in relieving acute postoperative pain following gynecologic laparotomy surgery. Anesthesiology. 2002;97:306–14.
86. Angst MS, Clark JD. Ketamine for managing perioperative pain in opioid-dependent patients with chronic pain: a unique indication? Anesthesiology. 2010;113(3):514–5.
87. Gowing L, Ali R, White JM. Buprenorphine for the management of opioid withdrawal. Cochrane Database Syst Rev. 2009;(3):CD002025.
88. Gowing L, Ali R, White JM. Opioid antagonists under heavy sedation or anaesthesia for opioid withdrawal. Cochrane Database Syst Rev. 2010;(1):CD002022.

Chapter 5
The Cocaine-Addicted Patient

Alan D. Kaye and Julia L. Weinkauf

Introduction

Cocaine (benzoylmethylecgonine, $C_{17}H_{21}NO_4$), a natural alkaloid, is derived from Erythroxylon coca, a plant indigenous to parts of South America, Mexico, the West Indies, and Indonesia. It is a pharmacologically diverse drug with local anesthetic, central nervous system stimulant, and sympathomimetic properties. As a readily available herb, it has been used and abused for over 5,000 years. Initially ingested by the Andean people to treat high-altitude fatigue in South America, it had application also as a topical local anesthetic, for spinal anesthesia, and as a dilator of the pupil for cataract surgery [1]. In 1914, the Harrison Narcotic Act limited its medical use in the United States. Over the past 20 years, the abuse of cocaine has grown enormously because of ubiquitous availability and reduction in cost (When adjusted for inflation, cocaine is now approximately 20% of the 1980s street price) [2]. Today, some 0.7% adults use cocaine regularly in the US, with 1.7% of adults, ages 18–25, using cocaine more than once per month [3]. Also, trauma patients requiring surgery are particularly likely to be recent users of cocaine, with one study finding that 38% of casualty victims had serum or urine test positive for cocaine [4]. In addition, there has been an increasing usage in parturients, causing complications in pregnancy and newborns [5]. This makes cocaine abuse of particular importance to the anesthesiologist, as many anesthetics are likely administered unknowingly to users. While cocaine intoxication is the number one cause of drug-related death, usually cardiopulmonary related [5], there are numerous cocaine-mediated effects, beyond the heart and the lungs, impacting especially the central nervous system and the kidneys.

A.D. Kaye (✉)
Department of Anesthesiology, LSU School of Medicine,
Louisiana State University, New Orleans, LA, USA
e-mail: alankaye44@hotmail.com

E.O. Bryson and E.A.M. Frost (eds.), *Perioperative Addiction:*
Clinical Management of the Addicted Patient, DOI 10.1007/978-1-4614-0170-4_5,
© Springer Science+Business Media, LLC 2012

Historical Notes

Albert Niemann (1880–1921) separated the alkaloid cocaine from the dried leaves of the coca plant in 1860. He studied the white powder and named it cocaine, also noting the temporary numbing effect the compound had on his tongue. During the 1880s in Vienna, Austria, Sigmund Freud (1856–1939) studied cocaine as a treatment for morphine addiction. (He himself was addicted to cocaine). He also suggested the possible use of cocaine as a local anesthetic to Viennese colleagues Leopold Königstein, a professor of ophthalmology, and Carl Koller (1857–1944), another ophthalmologist. Koller experimented on animals and presented his findings to the Congress of Ophthalmology in Heidelberg, Germany, in 1884. He demonstrated the successful use of cocaine as a local anesthetic during eye surgery. Cocaine became used widely for ophthalmological procedures until it was discovered that it damaged the cornea.

William Halsted, the first professor of surgery at Johns Hopkins, together with nearly 20–30 trainees, experimented with the injection of cocaine to produce local anesthesia for surgery. By the end of 1885, Halsted had performed over 1,000 operations using cocaine as an anesthetic. Unfortunately, Halsted also discovered another of cocaine's properties. He became addicted to the substance and spent many years overcoming his dependence. Harvey Cushing (1869–1939), a student of Halsted's, coined the term "regional anesthesia" for this use of cocaine, in contrast to the "general anesthesia" produced by ether. In 1885, Leonard Corning (1855–1939), a New York neurologist, injected a 2% cocaine solution as a spinal anesthetic.

There was no general medical condemnation throughout the nineteenth century of cocaine, and the addictive properties went unrecognized despite deaths reported as early as 1891. As a pain reliever and stimulant, the drug was a common ingredient in the very popular patent medicines of the late 1800s and early 1900s. Doctors freely prescribed cocaine for any number of ailments. Even a retired Surgeon General of the US Army extolled its fatigue-reduction and mood-elevating properties, while others vigorously promoted cocaine as an anesthetic, and a cure for alcoholism and opium abuse. Freud's endorsement of cocaine at the time was extreme, suggesting that its therapeutic use might even do away with inebriate asylums. Once the addictive dangers became known, scientists concentrated on developing synthetic substitutes for the recognized valuable anesthetic properties of cocaine. One of the first of these was Novocain.

Cocaine has a dubious role in American history as a supposed ingredient of the original Coca-Cola recipe. John Pemberton touted his new drink as an "intellectual beverage...contain[ing] the...stimulant properties of the Coca plant...makes not only an...invigorating beverage...but a cure for all nervous affections." Whole coca leaves remained an ingredient until 1901, when cocaine was increasingly recognized as dangerous and addictive. Then-owner Asa Candler arranged to begin using a decocainized leaf and, shortly thereafter, launched a revision of Coca-Cola history, claiming that cocaine had never been an ingredient [6].

The prevalence of cocaine as a drug of abuse began to escalate during the 1960s, and reached its peak some 25 years later. In 1983, if the cocaine trade had been included in the Fortune 500 list of industries, it would have ranked seventh in domestic sales, between the Ford Motor Company and the Gulf Oil Corporation [1].

Pharmacology and Pathophysiology

Cocaine blocks the uptake of sympathomimetic neurotransmitters such as dopamine (DA), norepinephrine (NE), and serotonin through respective transporters; thus, it prolongs adrenergic stimulation, primarily in the synaptic terminal/ventral basal nuclei of DA neurons. It inhibits the dopamine transporter (DAT), decreasing DA uptake from the synaptic cleft, inducing an amplifying concentration of DA in synapses, which is responsible for its euphoric influence (Fig. 5.1) [1]. A euphoric "high" is felt, followed by a dysphoric "crash". To decrease the dysphoria, users often mix cocaine with other drugs such as heroin, phencyclidine, marijuana, amphetamines, and alcohol. Psychologic and physiologic tolerance develops after the first dose, resulting in tachyphylaxis of subjective effects, and the need for increasingly larger doses to achieve the same euphoria.

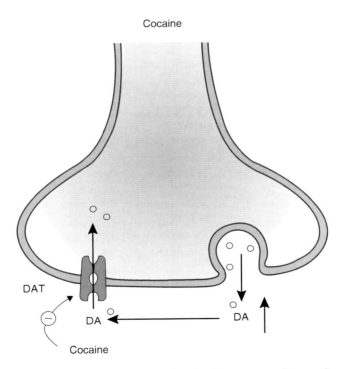

Fig. 5.1 Cocaine blocks the uptake of sympathomimetic neurotransmitters such as dopamine (DA), norepinephrine (NE), and serotonin through respective transporters. Reproduced with permission from: Katzung BG, Masters SB, Trevor AJ. 11th ed. New York, NY: McGraw-Hill companies; 2009

Another pharmacologic mechanism blocks catecholamine-binding sites, allowing free catecholamines, such as NE, to continue to stimulate the cardiovascular system [7]. This effect is considered secondary to the inhibition of the active reuptake of endogenously released NE from the adrenergic nerve fibers [8]. Thus, the increase in systolic, diastolic, and mean arterial blood pressure (BP), heart rate (HR), body temperature, and the risk of coronary artery vasospasm resulting in ischemia-induced cardiac arrhythmias are considered mainly to be caused by a sympathetic stimulation secondary to increased plasma levels of NE [8].

The effectiveness of cocaine as a local anesthetic is due to the ability to block sodium channels in neuronal cell membranes and halt propagation of nerve impulses [1]. Cocaine is lipophilic, and thus it diffuses across the blood–brain barrier to serve as a central stimulant by inhibiting the action of monoamine transport proteins on presynaptic nerve terminals. Furthermore, cocaine enhances calcium flux across cell membranes, produces hyper-responsive effector cells, inhibits monoamine oxidase, and functions as a potent vasoconstrictor [1].

Metabolism and Diagnosis

Cocaine is obtained by processing coca leaves with an organic solvent, yielding an alkaline coca paste of nearly 80% pure cocaine. Passing the alkaloid through an acidic aqueous solution creates the water-soluble crystalline form, cocaine hydrochloride, able to be ingested through multiple routes. The freebase form is created by dissolving the cocaine hydrochloride in an alkaline solution or in water and adding baking soda. The precipitate forms a soft mass that dries into "rocks" or "crack," which can be smoked. The term "crack cocaine" refers to the cracking sounds the crystalline form makes when heated. Various substances then are used to "cut" the pure form, including amphetamines, mannitol, lactose, dextrose, quinine, procaine, lidocaine, salicylamide, caffeine, talc, borax, Epsom salts, heroin, and plaster of Paris.

The onset of action, bioavailability, and duration of action are directly connected with the route of cocaine administration. Studies of the various routes indicate that the lower the bioavailability, the lower the peak effect [9]. Cocaine is prepared in many different forms, and may be consumed orally, rectally, nasally, and vaginally. Most deaths related to cocaine-induced myocardial infarction occur within three hours of ingestion and are directly linked to pharmacological uptake and the degree of bioavailability [10, 11].

Oral administration may take up to 30 min before the effects are experienced due to 30% bioavailability. Duration is up to 90 min. A common route of administration, intranasal, can create symptoms within 3 min that last 30–45 min, but it still only possesses a 30% bioavailability due to nasal vasoconstriction [12]. Intravascular injection takes 30 s to yield euphoria with almost 100% bioavailability. The peak effect can last 120 min [12].

Ingested cocaine is rapidly hydrolyzed primarily by plasma pseudocholinesterase and liver esterases to ecgonine methyl ester (EME) and benzoylecgonine [8, 13].

These metabolites are detected in urine by gas or liquid chromatography, mass spectrometry, and radioimmunoassay [14]. Because of the cholinesterase activity, the half-lives of EME and benzoylecgonine are much longer than that of cocaine (6 and 8 h, respectively, compared to 30–90 min for cocaine). These metabolites can be detected in urine for 60 h and up to 10 days following cocaine ingestion [8, 15]. The remaining cocaine is converted into the active metabolite, norcocaine, which is metabolized to N-hydroxynorcocaine, a hepatotoxin [16].

Urine tests, positive for cocaine metabolites, may be obtained even with normal physiologic variables and apparent emotional stability. An instant result for metabolites can be performed through OnTrak Abuscreen® assay, also known as a rapid latex agglutination test [14]. This test has comparable accuracy of 100% sensitivity and 100% specificity. Newborn meconium and maternal follicle hair can also be tested for cocaine to make the diagnosis of prior exposure [14].

Adverse Effects of Cocaine Abuse

The effects of acute and chronic cocaine use are many and involve every organ system. Acute deleterious clinical symptoms are primarily related to vasoconstriction and hypertension, effects that occur immediately due to inhibition of catecholamine reuptake and decreased production of the vasodilator nitric oxide. There is also a delayed vasoconstrictive effect probably due to production of active metabolites. Over time, the cocaine abuser develops pathology due to compensatory mechanisms of the various organ systems. Of note also is that cocaine abusers, including parturients, are prone to ingest other recreational drugs, such as tobacco and alcohol. These drug interactions may further increase hemodynamic instability in the cardiovascular system and cause even sudden death. Some of these effects are well understood, such as the case of coca-ethylene, an ethyl ester of benzoylecgonine, and a by-product of liver transesterification and ethanol. Coca-ethylene has a longer duration of action than cocaine alone and produces longer lasting euphoria but is significantly more neurotoxic and cardiotoxic [17].

Some of the actions of cocaine that are of particular concern to the anesthesiologist are described in the following section.

Cardiovascular System

Cocaine has profound cardiovascular effects due primarily to intense sympathetic overdrive. Acute actions include arrhythmias, systemic and pulmonary hypertension, coronary vasoconstriction, tachycardia, ischemia, and all of the consequences thereof, such as pulmonary edema, myocardial infarction, dissection of any artery including the coronaries and aorta, and death. Chronic changes include myocardial hypertrophy, hypertrophic cardiomyopathy, and accelerated atherosclerosis.

Like all local anesthetics, cocaine is a slow sodium channel blocker, and also a fast potassium blocker, which leads to biphasic electrocardiographic changes. At low concentrations, cocaine delays ventricular recovery and, at high concentrations, it speeds recovery, resulting in a wide spectrum of possible dysrhythmias and electrocardiographic findings, including QT prolongation, slow or fast ventricular tachycardias (including torsades de pointes), bundle-branch blocks, supraventricular tachycardias, Brugada syndrome, accelerated idioventricular rhythm, asystole, and ventricular fibrillation. Cocaine-induced ion channel blockade lengthens the QTc interval by prolongation of the action potential duration and is similar in action to the Vaughn-Williams antiarrhythmic Class 1c drug, flecainide [18]. Sodium and potassium channel blockade which results in QRS and QTc prolongation may be the primary underlying mechanism for the induction of arrhythmias, especially the polymorphic ventricular tachycardia type of torsades de pointes [19]. To support this concept, the administration of a concentrated solution of sodium ions (e.g., sodium bicarbonate) will effectively antagonize the intracardiac conduction slowing, thereby effectively treating ventricular arrhythmias [19].

Other potential mechanisms might explain cocaine-induced myocardial ischemia and infarct. Coronary artery vasospasm is a likely contributor, with frequent transient ST segment elevation noted in Holter monitoring of asymptomatic patients. Cocaine also accelerates atherosclerosis and microvascular disease. Development of a pro-thrombotic state is a potential contributor. Ultimately, oxygen delivery is inadequate to supply increased myocardial demand (due to hypertension, tachycardia, and increased contractility), and ischemia ensues.

Chronic cocaine use leads to left ventricular hypertrophy which can progress to hypertrophy cardimyopathy, pulmonary hypertension, and cor pulmonale. The exact mechanism is unclear; however, similar morphologic and histologic changes are seen in the hearts of patients with left ventricular hypertrophy from chronic hyper-tension and pheochromocytoma, suggesting that cocaine-induced hypertrophy is due to hypertension, increased afterload, and increased wall tension [20].

Cocaine users are at increased risk of sudden death. One recent prospective study found that 3% of sudden deaths are cocaine related [21]. The mechanism of this increased risk is not clearly understood. Most deaths in this study were attributed to myocardial infarction, but it is difficult to prove whether the infarction or an arrhythmia was the primary cause. Cocaine abuse leads to myocardial hypertrophy, an independent risk factor for sudden cardiac death. Hypertrophy is reflected in the electrocardiogram by QT prolongation, also a risk factor for ventricular arrhyth-mias, classically, torsades de pointes.

The theoretical mechanism to improve cocaine-induced intracardiac conduction slowing by sodium ion administration is pharmacologically similar in concept to the reversal of calcium channel blocker toxicity with ionized calcium [22]. Clinical studies that fail to observe any arrhythmic occurrence in cocaine users may be explained by the precise determination of an automated QTc interval duration before general anesthesia. Experimental studies with varying QTc prolongations seen electrocardiographically have been performed. Findings suggest prolonged QTc interval with greater than 450 ms in women and 440 ms in men significantly increases the risk of a fatal ventricular arrhythmia, implying the risk of any general anesthesia may be increased if the QTc interval exceeds 500 ms [23, 24]. The use of a 500 ms cutoff was defined by reports that ventricular arrhythmias occurring during electrolyte disturbances (e.g., hypokalemia) and noncardiac drug ingestion (including psychotherapeutic drugs such as amitriptyline, lithium, and chlorpromazine) were increased when there was a QTc interval exceeding 500 ms [25, 26]. Therefore, a QTc interval of less than 500 ms is suggested before proceeding with any surgery requiring general anesthesia.

Pulmonary System

Direct adverse effects of cocaine use on the pulmonary system include hypersensitivity pneumonitis ("crack lung"), pulmonary hemorrhage, cavitations, and pneumothorax [12, 27]. The etiology of pneumothorax seems to be deep inhalation followed by the valsalva maneuver to increase the effect of smoked cocaine. Alveoli rupture then allows air to dissect into the mediastinum, pericardium, pleural space, or subcutaneous tissues. If a tension Pneumothorax does not develop, resolution will occur spontaneously within 48–72 h with supportive management including monitoring and administration of high flow oxygen.

Cocaine can cause severe bronchospasm and exacerbation of asthma by its irritant properties. Secondary pulmonary complications include predisposition to infection (tuberculosis, staphylococcus), pulmonary edema, pulmonary infarction, and pulmonary hypertension [28–30].

The most common respiratory complaint of cocaine abusers is a productive cough of black colored sputum. Freebase users typically produce sputum, consisting of carbonaceous flecks and blood, and have burns throughout the upper and lower airways, occasionally leading to tracheal stenosis. Many chronic pulmonary changes develop. The diffusing capacity of the lung for carbon monoxide (DLCO) is reduced by 20–30% in chronic users, much like patients with restrictive lung diseases. Reasons for a decreased DLCO include direct damage to the pulmonary vascular bed, alveolar–capillary membrane, or secondary to interstitial disease as a result of intravenous drug use. Pulmonary complications are often combined and termed "crack lung syndrome." Features include pulmonary hemorrhage, pulmonary edema, chest pain, and interstitial infiltrates, probably due to cocaine-induced vasoconstriction of the pulmonary bed leading to hypoxia of epithelial and endothelial cells. Or pulmonary edema may be the result of left ventricular dysfunction caused by either myocardial ischemia from coronary vasospasm or intense peripheral vasoconstriction from sympathetic stimulation.

Chronic cocaine use by inhalation leads to progressive ischemic necrosis of the midfacial structures. Pathology ranging from simple, nasal, septal perforation to hard palate destruction and maxilla and orbital wall may result, making ventilation difficult and increasing the risk of aspiration.

Gastrointestinal System

Potential gastrointestinal complications of cocaine use are again primarily related to the intense vasoconstriction–ischemia phenomenon, and include ischemia and necrosis of any part of the bowel or stomach, perforation, ulcer formation, and hemorrhage [31–33]. It has also been suggested that the sympathomimetic effects of cocaine may act on medullary centers regulating gastric motility, delaying gastric emptying, and increasing the risk of aspiration [34].

Central Nervous System

Numerous studies have documented extensive central nervous system effects in the developing brain as well as the fully developed central nervous system. Some of the cocaine-related processes include behavioral effects, cerebral blood flow reduction, the potential for cocaine mediated cerebral vasculitis, and links to suicide. Complications include stroke from vasospastic ischemia, thrombosis, or cerebrovascular hemorrhage [35–38]. Cocaine can also precipitate seizures in previously unaffected patients, and lowers the seizure threshold in patients with epilepsy [39]. Preexisting movement disorders can be exacerbated by cocaine use, and new-onset movement disorders can develop [40].

Hematologic System

Cocaine increases plasminogen activator inhibitor (PA-I) activity and decreases protein C activity, both favoring a prothrombotic hematologic state [41]. Some studies indicate that cocaine increases platelet activation and aggregation; however, this finding is debatable, as there are studies that refute the claim [42].

The Cocaine-Abusing Parturient

In 2000, almost half of the obstetrical wards in New York City reported cocaine-related premature or ectopic pregnancies [43]. Complications of cocaine ingestion during pregnancy include all of the previously discussed pathology in the mother, in addition to premature onset of labor, placental abruption, uterine rupture, and fetal demise (Table 5.1). Because of the increasing sensitivity of progesterone and α adrenergic receptors from the heart, cocaine induces hypoxemia of epicardial coronary arteries and significantly causes myocardial infarction and tachycardia. In addition, because cocaine is highly lipophilic, transplacental simple diffusion causes direct vasoconstriction and ischemic effects to the fetus as well as indirect effects through decreased uterine blood flow, placing the fetus at risk of heart failure [44]. Prolonged cocaine toxicity can distress serotonin and catecholamine

Table 5.1 Cocaine abuse and the parturient

In the feto-maternal stage:
  Preterm labor
  Premature rupture of membranes
  Placental abruption
  Decreased utero-placental perfusion
  Fetal distress
  Fetal tachycardia
  Fetal hypertension
  Intra-uterine fetal demise
In the neonatal stage:
  Irritability
  Cocaine-withdrawal syndrome
  Myocardial ischemia
  Myocardial infarction
  Death

Modified from Skerman JH. The Cocaine-using Patient: perioperative concerns. MEJA 2005;18(1)

mechanisms which are involved in the development of fetal brain and central nervous system [43]. Alterations in urinary output and renal vascular resistance can be seen in the fetus [45]. Symptoms can be mistaken for pre-eclampsia, with hypertension, proteinuria, and possibly convulsions being characteristic of either situation. There is no clear recommendation for either general or regional anesthesia. Regional anesthesia in cocaine-abusing parturients can yield ephedrine-resistant hypotension, altered pain perception, and cocaine-induced thrombocytopenia [14]. Diluted phenylephrine usually restores blood pressure to normal if ephedrine does not successfully treat hypotension. Abnormalities in regional endorphin levels and changes in both mu (μ)- and kappa (κ)-opioid receptor densities, which are derived from cocaine-induced dopaminergic terminals, may result in sensation of pain despite normal spinal or epidural anesthesia sensory levels [46]. It has been reported that with the same concentration of intrathecal sufentanil, there is similar intrapartum analgesia with shorter duration of labor compared to noncocaine users [14].

As noted, the causes of cocaine-induced thrombocytopenia are controversial. Most experts believe that the elevated levels of plasma catecholamines (Epi and NE) cause an arterial vasoconstriction; α-adrenergic agonists bind to specific receptors and induce platelet activation. Thus, the complication of arterial vascular spasm and platelet activation increases thrombocytopenia in the cocaine-abusing parturients [46].

During general anesthesia of cocaine-abusing parturients, hypertension, arrhythmia, and myocardial ischemia are common. Propranolol, which is a β-adrenergic-blocking agent, is contraindicated because it transfers transplacentally into the fetal heart and can cause fetal bradycardia. On the other hand, esmolol yields effective control of tachycardia and hypertension, but enhances cocaine-induced coronary vasoconstriction [45]. The effects of hydralazine in gravid ewes with cocaine-induced hypertension have been studied and suggest that in the human patient cocaine elevates maternal mean arterial pressure (MAP) and diminishes uterine blood flow (UBF) through a

Table 5.2 ACOG recommendations for the potential cocaine abusing parturient

A drug history should be taken on all patients during the first prenatal meeting and should be
warned about the dangers of drug use during pregnancy

A woman acknowledging cocaine abuse should be counseled and offered support mechanisms to
aid in her abstinence

Periodic urine testing should be considered to encourage ongoing abstinence

Testing the mother and neonate may be useful in some clinical situations, such as unexplained
fetal growth restriction, prematurity, and placental abruption

Some state legislations consider the exposure of drug abuse in utero to be a form of child abuse
or neglect under the law and all positive drug tests need to be reported

When a maternal test is positive for cocaine, either pediatricians or neonatologists need to
monitor the infant at all time

Modified from Kuckowski KM. The cocaine-abusing parturient: a review of anesthetic consider-
ations. Obstetrical and Pediatric Anesthesia. Can J Anesth. 2004;51(2):145–154 and Chestnut DH.
"Substance Abuse". In: Obstetric anesthesia: principle and practice, 3rd ed. New York, NY:
Elsevier Mosby; 2004

decrease in systemic vascular resistance (SVR). Although hydralazine can help recover MAP, it can cause maternal tachycardia (120% increase after hydralazine) and fail to restore UBF [14]. In contrast to hydralazine, labetalol, which is a combined nonselective β and α-adrenergic blocker, can normalize maternal heart rate and UBF. However, it has been suggested that labetalol should not be used to manage cocaine-induced hypertension because the β-adrenergic receptors antagonism of labetalol is greater than its effect on α-adrenergic receptors [47].

The American College of Obstetricians and Gynecologists (ACOG) previously provided recommendations for the assessment of possible cocaine-abusing parturients (Table 5.2).

Under current law in Louisiana, parturients with positive urine test at the time of delivery in any hospital cannot claim the custody of their newborns and are immediately required to be counseled and treated.

In the past two decades, researchers have shown that over 80% of female smokers tend to continue to smoke when pregnant. It was also documented that more than one-third of parturients in the United States smoked cigarettes [44]. Nicotine aggravates vasoconstriction of the coronary arteries through α-adrenergic mechanisms similar to that of cocaine; thus, the combination of both substantially worsens the myocardial oxygen demand and supply in the heart. It follows that poly-substance interactions can additionally complicate anesthetic management, especially in pregnant patients.

General Anesthetic Considerations in Acute and Chronic Cocaine Abusers

Procedures on patients presenting for elective surgery who were found to be recent users of cocaine (by history or presence of urine cocaine metabolites) were traditionally cancelled and deferred until the patient had no evidence of recent use. Some argue, however, that asymptomatic, clinically "nontoxic" patients (normal blood pressure, heart rate, ECG, and temperature) may have elective surgeries performed without increased risk of complications [48]. Furthermore, most cocaine-related deaths are not due to overdose, but to pathophysiology developed from long-term use; thus, the risk would not decline by waiting for a negative test. It is reasonable to view chronic cocaine abuse as a risk factor for the physiologic consequences of long-term use, and patients should have a pre-operative work-up of specific organ–system complaints before elective cases. However, elective surgeries in a patient with normal vital signs, ECG, and a negative pertinent review of systems need not be delayed solely on the grounds of recent cocaine use. It is prudent to proceed at the discretion of the anesthesiologist, surgeon, and patient.

In the acutely intoxicated patient, management goals are focused around minimizing hemodynamic extremes and avoiding ischemic consequences of vasospasm. The overall treatment of the acutely cocaine-intoxicated patient is outlined in Table 5.3.

Regional anesthesia has been used successfully; however, considerations include a potentially intoxicated, uncooperative patient, and lack of airway control. With general anesthesia, the minimum alveolar concentration (MAC) may be decreased because of the depletion of catecholamines in chronic cocaine users. In acute usage, MAC is increased secondary to acute elevation of catecholamine concentration [14]. Cocaine-induced bronchospasm is common during periods of light anesthesia. The predicament of hypovolemia from cocaine-induced vasoconstriction and the increased MAC from chronic cocaine users is particularly difficult to manage [44]. Pulmonary edema is another obstacle to intubation in chronic abusers. Chronic cardiopulmonary consequences such as cardiomyopathy and pulmonary hypertension should be considered.

Cocaine smokers increase the lung permeability of cocaine with continuous exposure, an antigenic response leading to cough or asthma symptoms. Eosinophilia maybe observed in alveolar interstitial infiltrates and is associated with hemoptysis [49]. There is a greater probability to observe acute noncardiogenic pulmonary edema and acute alveolar hemorrhage [50]. In addition, cocaine use is associated with an increased incidence of renal failure and can therefore affect certain anesthetic elimination [51].

Administration of ketamine, atropine, or the older inhalational agents, halothane and enflurane, which can sensitize the myocardium to the effects of catecholamines, should be avoided [43]. Ketamine and atropine are phencyclidine analogs which elevate blood pressure, heart rate, and cardiac output (CO). Because of stimulation to the sympathetic central nervous system, they may exacerbate the cardiac effects of cocaine by further increasing catecholamines [45]. Symptoms of cocaine intoxication can include myoclonus, seizures, and hyperreflexia, which may be aggravated by disinhibiting effects of etomidate. In contrast, administration of propofol and thiopental for induction of anesthesia in cocaine-abusing patients, including parturients, appears safer and effective [45].

Cocaine induces vasoconstriction of coronary arteries, which is commonly seen with a complaint of chest pain from myocardial ischemia. It can be treated with the administration of phentolamine, an α-adrenergic blocking agent, or nitroglycerin with or without a calcium channel-blocking agent [10, 46]. Aspirin can prevent platelet aggregation and benzodiazepines can further reduce heart rate and systemic

Table 5.3 Treatment of acute cocaine effects

Ventricular arrhythmias:
  Sodium bicarbonate
  Lidocaine
  Cardioversion

Supraventricular tachyarrhythmias:
  Adenosine (stable SVT)
  DC cardioversion (avoid β-blockers)

Convulsions/seizures/tremors:
  Benzodiazepines
  Airway control

Hypertension/tachycardia:
  Nitroglycerin
  Benzodiazepines
  Phentolamine
  Verapamil
  +/− Hydralazine (avoid beta blockers)

Myocardial ischemia/infarction:
  Nitroglycerin
  Benzodiazepines
  Aspirin
  Phentolamine

blood pressure [10, 46]. Thrombolytic therapy may be indicated but should only be considered when coronary angiography and angioplasty are not available and should be secondary to treatment with oxygen, nitrates, aspirin, and benzodiazepines according to ACLS guidelines [51]. After much debate, it now seems clear that β-blockers should not be used in the setting of cocaine-induced hypertension or ischemia, due to the possibility of unopposed α-receptor activity [52]. Even mixed β-1 and β-2 receptor antagonists have been shown not to improve coronary blood flow. Dexmedetomidine and other newer drugs are currently being evaluated for treatment of hypertension.

The American Heart Association suggests the first-line agents of cocaine-induced myocardial ischemia or infarction to be nitroglycerin and benzodiazepines. Phentolamine is indicated as a second-line agent, followed by verapamil [53]. The use of lidocaine is controversial for the treatment of cocaine-induced arrhythmias because of CNS effects [54]. Sodium bicarbonate has demonstrated effectiveness in the treatment of ventricular arrhythmias.

Ongoing Research

The treatment of cocaine addiction with cocaine-specific vaccines has been studied in recent years. In theory, using vaccination to induce the production of anti-cocaine antibodies could prevent ingested cocaine from reaching the brain and may attenuate the negative inotropic and chronotropic effects on heart muscles. Despite promising early results, further investigations on the efficacy of cocaine vaccines are necessary [45, 46].

One of the challenges of the vaccine is that the cocaine molecule offers several sites for attachment of a "linker" structure; however, the drug-linker construct must be optimized with regard to both the placement of the linker molecule and the nature of the linker itself. The antibodies elicited by the vaccine should bind preferentially to the free drug rather than to the drug-linker molecule or to the linker itself [55].

Another area of research underway focuses on the pathways of cocaine-mediated arrhythmia, and to identify optimal therapeutic interventions.

Conclusions

The pharmacological actions and pathophysiological consequences of cocaine use are complicated and multifactorial. Many clinical interventions may have unpredictable outcomes in both the patient acutely intoxicated with cocaine and in the chronic cocaine abuser. Diagnosis is often difficult as, more often than not, patients will either attempt to downplay their actual use of cocaine or lie outright about recent use. In the obstetric patient, the pathophysiological consequences of cocaine use combined with the coexisting physiology of pregnancy may lead to lethal complications and significantly impact the management of obstetrical anesthesia. Even with ACOG anesthetic guidelines for cocaine-using parturients, the decision regarding the administration of peripartum analgesia or anesthesia should be conducted on a case-by-case basis.

The anesthesiologist called upon to anesthetize the acutely toxic cocaine-abusing patient emergently must be prepared to deal with the extreme hemodynamic and ischemic implications of acute cocaine use as well as other sequelae of chronic cocaine abuse. Many patients do well under general anesthesia, even with positive tests for cocaine, but practitioners should remain attentive to potential complications, as cocaine remains a dangerous drug of abuse with profound physiologic consequences.

References

1. Katzung BG. Drugs of abuse, Basic and clinical pharmacology. 10th ed. New York, NY: McGraw-Hill companies; 2007. p. 518–23.
2. Borden D. Editorial "Yes, the drug war really is still failing, DEA and ONDCP". http://stop-thedrugwar.org/chronicle/504/yes_the_drug_war_really_is_failing. Accessed 11 Apr 2010.
3. US Department of Health and Human Services. National survey on drug use and health. Washington DC: US Department of Health and Human Services; 2008. Figures 2.1, 2.6.
4. Brookoff D, Campbell EA, Shaw LM. The underreporting of cocaine-related trauma: drug abuse warning network reports vs hospital toxicology tests. Am J Public Health. 1993;83(3):369–71.

5. Feinstein L, Schmidt K. Cocaine users present unique anesthetic challenges: part 1. Anesthesiol News. 2010;36-2:8–9.
6. Pendergrast M. For god, country, and coca-cola. New York, NY: Charles Scribner's Sons; 1993. p. 32–3. 90–91, 355–56.
7. Hertting G, Axelrod J, Whitby LG. Effect of drugs on the uptake and metabolism of H^3-norepinephrine. J Pharmacol Exp Ther. 1961;134:146–53.
8. Jatlow PI. Drug of abuse profile: cocaine. Clin Chem. 1987;33:66B–71.
9. Bernards CM, Artru A, Visco E, et al. Chronic cocaine exposure alters carbon dioxide reactivity but does not affect cerebral blood flow autoregulation in anesthetized dogs. J Trauma. 2002;52:912–21.
10. Lange RA, Hillis LD. Cardiovascular complications in cocaine use. N Engl J Med. 2001;345(5):351–8.
11. Hollander JE, Hoffman RS. Cocaine-induced myocardial infarction: an analysis and review of the literature. J Emerg Med. 1992;10:169–77.
12. Meisels IS, Loke J. The pulmonary effects of free-base cocaine: a review. Cleve Clin J Med. 1993;60:325–9.
13. Jatlow P, Barash PG, Van Dyke C, et al. Cocaine and succinylcholine sensitivity: a new caution. Anesth Analg. 1979;58:235–8.
14. Chestnut DH. Substance abuse. In: Obstetric anesthesia: principle and practice, 3rd ed. New York, NY: Elsevier Mosby; 2004.
15. O'Brien CP. Drug addiction and drug abuse. In: Hardman JG, Limbird LE, editors. The pharmacological basis of therapeutics. New York, NY: McGraw-Hill; 2002. p. 621–42.
16. Ndikum-Moffor FM, Schoeb TR, Roberts SM. Liver toxicity from norcocaine nitroxide, an N-oxidative metabolite of cocaine. J Pharmacol Exp Ther. 1998;248:413–9.
17. Harris DS, Everhart ET, Mendelson J, Jones RT. The pharmacology of cocaethylene in humans following cocaine and ethanol administration. Drug Alcohol Depend. 2003;72:169–82.
18. Wang Z, Fermini B, Nattel S. Mechanism of flecainide's rate-dependent actions on action potential duration in canine atrial tissue. J Pharmacol Exp Ther. 1993;267:575–81.
19. Bauman JL, Grawe JJ, Winecoff AP, Hariman RJ. Cocaine-related sudden cardiac death: a hypothesis correlating basic science and clinical observations. J Clin Pharmacol. 1994;34:902–11.
20. Afonso L, Mohammad T, Thatai D. Crack whips the heart: a review of the cardiovascular toxicity of cocaine. Am J Cardiol. 2007;100(6):1040–3.
21. Lucena J, Blanco M, Jurado C, Rico A, Salguero M, Vazquez R, et al. Cocaine-related sudden death: a prospective investigation in south-west Spain. Eur Heart J. 2010;31(3):318–29. Epub 2010 Jan 12.
22. Kimura S, Bassett AL, Xi H, Myerburg RJ. Early after-depolarizations and triggered activity induced by cocaine. Circulation. 1992;85:2227–35.
23. DeWitt CR, Waksman JC. Pharmacology, pathophysiology and management of calcium channel blocker and beta-blocker toxicity. Toxicol Rev. 2004;23:223–38.
24. Charbit B, Samain E, Merckx P, Funck-Brentano C. QT interval measurement. Anesthesiology. 2006;104:255–60.
25. Khan IA, Long QT. Syndrome: diagnosis and management. Am Heart J. 2002;143:7–14.
26. Chvilicek JP, Hurlbert BJ, Hill GE. Diuretic-induced hypokalaemia inducing torsades de pointes. Can J Anaesth. 1995;42:1137–9.
27. Solaini L, Gourgiotis S, Salemis NS, Koukis I. Bilateral pneumothorax, lung cavitations, and pleural empyema in a cocaine addict. Gen Thorac Cardiovasc Surg. 2008;56(12):610–2.
28. Averbach M, Casey KK, Frank E. Near-fatal status asthmaticus induced by nasal insufflation of cocaine. South Med J. 1996;89(3):340–1.
29. Gotway MB, Marder SR, Hanks DK, Leung JW, Dawn SK, Gean AD, et al. Thoracic complications of illicit drug use: an organ system approach. Radiographics. 2002;22:S119–35.
30. Restrepo CS, Carrillo JA, Martínez S, Ojeda P, Rivera AL, Hatta A. Pulmonary complications from cocaine and cocaine-based substances: imaging manifestations. Radiographics. 2007;27(4):941–56.

31. Herrine SK, Park PK, Wechsler RJ. Acute mesenteric ischemia following intranasal cocaine use. Dig Dis Sci. 1998;43(3):586–9.
32. Lingamfelter DC, Knight LD. Sudden death from massive gastrointestinal hemorrhage associated with crack cocaine use: case report and review of the literature. Am J Forensic Med Pathol. 2010;31(1):98–9.
33. Nalbandian H, Sheth N, Dietrich R, Georgiou J. Intestinal ischemia caused by cocaine ingestion: report of two cases. Surgery. 1985;97(3):374–6.
34. Abramson DL, Gertler JP, Lewis T, Kral JG. Crack-related perforated gastropyloric ulcer. J Clin Gastroenterol. 1991;13(1):17–9.
35. Johnson BA, Dawes MA, Roache JD, Wells LT, Ait-Daoud N, Mauldin JB, et al. Acute intravenous low- and high-dose cocaine reduces quantitative global and regional cerebral blood flow in recently abstinent subjects with cocaine use disorder. J Cereb Blood Flow Metab. 2005;25(7):928–36.
36. Levine SR, Brust JC, Futrell N, Ho KL, Blake D, Millikan CH, et al. Cerebrovascular complications of the use of the "crack" form of alkaloidal cocaine. N Engl J Med. 1990;323(11):699–704.
37. Petty GW, Brust JC, Tatemichi TK, Barr ML. Embolic stroke after smoking "crack" cocaine. Stroke. 1990;21(11):1632–5.
38. MacEwen C, Ward M, Buchan A. A case of cocaine-induced basilar artery thrombosis. Nat Clin Pract Neurol. 2008;4(11):622–6.
39. Dhuna A, Pascual-Leone A, Langendorf F, Anderson DC. Epileptogenic properties of cocaine in humans. Neurotoxicology. 1991;12(3):621–6.
40. Daras M, Koppel BS, Atos-Radzion E. Cocaine-induced choreoathetoid movements ('crack dancing'). Neurology. 1994;44(4):751–2.
41. Heesch CM, Negus BH, Steiner M, et al. Effects of in vivo cocaine administration on human platelet aggregation. Am J Cardiol. 1996;78:237–9.
42. Kugelmass AD, Oda A, Monahan K, Cabral C, Ware JA. Activation of human platelets by cocaine. Circulation. 1993;88(3):876–83.
43. Kuckowski KM, Birnbach DJ, Van Zunder A. Drug abuse in the parturient. Semin Anesth Perioperat Med Pain. 2000;19:216–24.
44. Birnbach DJ, Stein DJ. The substance-abusing parturient: implications for analgesia and anesthesia management. Baillieres Clin Obstet Gynaecol. 1998;12:443–60.
45. Kuckowski KM. Anesthetic implications of drug abuse in pregnancy. J Clin Anesth. 2003;15:382–94.
46. Kuckowski KM. The cocaine abusing parturient: a review of anesthetic considerations. Can J Anaesth. 2004;51(2):145–54.
47. Hollander JE. The management of cocaine-associated myocardial ischemia. N Engl J Med. 1995;333:1267–72.
48. Hill GE, Ogunnaike BO, Johnson ER. General anaesthesia for the cocaine abusing patient: is it safe? Br J Anaesth. 2006;97:654–7.
49. Susskind H, Weber DA, Volkow ND, Hitzemann R. Increased lung permeability following long-term use of free-base cocaine (crack). Chest. 1991;100:903–9.
50. Baldwin GC, Choi R, Roth MD, et al. Evidence of chronic damage to the pulmonary microcirculation in habitual users of alkaloidal ("crack") cocaine. Chest. 2002;121:1231–8.
51. Norris KC, Thornhill-Joynes M, Robinson C, et al. Cocaine use, hypertension, and end-stage renal disease. Am J Kidney Dis. 2001;38:523–8.
52. Hoffman RS. Cocaine and beta-blockers: should the controversy continue? Ann Emerg Med. 2008;51(2):127–9. Epub 2007 Sep 24.
53. McCord J, Jneid H, Hollander JE, et al. Management of cocaine-associated chest pain and myocardial infarction: a scientific statement from the American Heart Association Acute Cardiac Care Committee of the Council on Clinical Cardiology. Circulation. 2008;117:1897–907.
54. Battaglia G, Napier TC. The effects of cocaine and the amphetamines on brain and behavior: a conference report. Drug Alcohol Depend. 1998;52:41–8.
55. Moreno AY, Janda KD. Immunopharmacotherapy: vaccination strategies as a treatment for drug abuse and dependence. Pharmacol Biochem Behav. 2009;92(2):199–205.

Chapter 6
Club Drugs

Samuel DeMaria

Introduction

The use of illicit substances in large dance parties ("raves") and nightclubs has become commonplace globally since the 1990s. Having now dispersed from rave sub-cultures, these drugs are available in college bars, house parties, and at concerts. Given this widespread availability, the "typical" club drug user is harder to classify than it had been in the 1990s. One large survey of New York City nightclub attendees attempted to characterize typical users: [1] 1,914 club-going adults aged 18–29 were sampled, of which 70% reported using club drugs at least once and 22% reported recent use. Men were more likely to abuse ketamine and GHB, while female gender was predictive of cocaine use. Gay/bisexual orientation and White race were predictive of use of several club drugs.

While most of the club drugs are not truly new substances, their increased prevalence (lifetime rates of use among US college students irrespective of nightclub attendance ranges from 10 to 15% in one survey) [2] makes them important. Also, the high likelihood of polysubstance intoxication, whether through choice or through impurities in the drugs, makes toxidromes often difficult to diagnose and treat.

The most commonly used club drugs include methylenedioxymethamphetamine or "Ecstasy", gamma-hydroxybutyrate, ketamine, and flunitrazepam (Table 6.1). As use of these substances has increased, acute and chronic effects have been more widely observed in the perioperative setting. Their effects and potential pitfalls for providers of anesthetic care are presented. Since GHB and flunitrazepam may be associated with physical dependence and withdrawal, these issues are introduced in addition to toxic effects.

S. DeMaria (✉)
Department of Anesthesiology, Mount Sinai School of Medicine, New York, NY, USA
e-mail: demarisa@gmail.com

E.O. Bryson and E.A.M. Frost (eds.), *Perioperative Addiction:*
Clinical Management of the Addicted Patient, DOI 10.1007/978-1-4614-0170-4_6,
© Springer Science+Business Media, LLC 2012

Table 6.1 Summary of club drugs with common names and relevant features

	MDMA	GHB	Ketamine	Flunitrazepam
Street name	Ecstasy, X, E, XTC, Adam	Liquid X, Liquid Ecstasy, Georgia Homeboy Scoop, Grievous Bodily Harm	K, Vitamin K, Special K, Kat, Cat	Rohypnol® Roofies, Rophies, Circles, Rib, Rope, R2
Duration of action (hours)	4–6	1–4	1–3	6–14
Peak effect (h)	1–3	1–3	~2	6–24
Form	Tablet or capsule, powder	Liquid	Liquid, powder	Tablet or powder
Dependence	No	Yes	No	Yes
Sought-after effects	Energy, self-confidence, well-being, heightened mood and awareness	Euphoria, decreased anxiety, relaxation	Relaxation, positive hallucinations	Euphoria, decreased anxiety, increased social comfort

Ecstasy (MDMA)

Background

An estimated 19.7 million people (or about 8.1%) over the age 12 used illicit drugs in 2005 in the US. About 500,000 of these took Ecstasy (3,4-methylenedioxymethamphetamine or MDMA) at least once during the year prior to the survey [3]. MDMA is available at approximately 70% of large dance parties, or raves, with Europe being the major origin of most of the drug trafficking [4].

MDMA is known among users as XTC, X, E, and Adam [5]. It was first patented in 1914 by Merck Pharmaceuticals as an appetite suppressant [6, 7] but given its purported effects in promoting feelings of "closeness" to others, it was later studied as a psychotherapeutic drug [8, 9]. Despite this potential application, abuse of MDMA prompted the Drug Enforcement Administration (DEA) to issue a Schedule I drug classification in the 1980s. MDMA abuse in the US has risen steadily since then.

MDMA is usually taken orally as a small pill or capsule, although it can be crushed and snorted. It may also be dissolved for injection. As it is produced illegally, the purity of MDMA is variable and contains other agents (e.g., methamphetamines and ketamine) [10]. For this reason, any acute MDMA intoxication should be approached as polysubstance intoxication. The concentration of MDMA itself may vary and accidental overdoses are not uncommon.

Mechanisms of Action

MDMA structurally resembles the hallucinogen mescaline and the stimulant amphetamine, which explains its mixture of stimulant and psychedelic effects. MDMA increases the release and decreases reuptake of serotonin and dopamine [11, 12]. Direct agonist properties at serotonergic and dopaminergic receptors as well as monoamine oxidase (MAO) inhibitor effects have also been demonstrated [13]. The drug is metabolized through the cytochrome P450 (CYP450) 2D6 enzyme [14]. 2D6 inhibitors (e.g., cocaine, methadone, haloperidol, and fluoxetine) may substantially increase side effects. Benzodiazepines are metabolized principally by the 3A4 enzyme and have limited metabolic interaction. Pro-serotonergic drugs (e.g., fluoxetine, amphetamines, St. John's wort, tramadol, and lithium) may increase the severity of side effects.

Clinical Presentation

Effects are generally felt within 20 min of ingestion and may last 6–8 h [15]. The drug produces feelings of euphoria, heightened alertness, increased emotional lability, and sexual arousal [16]. Serotonin stores are depleted by MDMA and repeated doses are associated with less euphoria but increased adverse effects. Cardiovascular activation in the form of tachycardia and hypertension is common [17]. Lethargy, fatigue, anorexia, psychosis, and mood disturbances (depression, anxiety) often follow chronic use and may persist secondary to drug-induced neuronal injury [18, 19].

The acute effects of MDMA intoxication are of greatest concern to the anesthesiologist (Table 6.2). Acute intoxication generally includes a constellation of symptoms: tachycardia, hypertension, mydriasis, bruxism, and diaphoresis with or without hyperthermia.

Hyperthermia is a major cause of MDMA-related mortality [20–22]. Temperatures as high as 42°C have been recorded [23]. The mechanism of hyperthermia is most likely serotonergic overload in the hypothalamic thermoregulatory center [24–26] but sustained muscular activity from dancing and a disregard of normal body signals, such as thirst, compound central effects [27, 28]. MDMA has been identified as a trigger of malignant hyperthermia (MH) in swine [29]. Whether this is true in humans is unclear but seems unlikely.

The clinical presentation may be confused with neuroleptic malignant syndrome or serotonin syndrome in presentation and severity [30]. The differential diagnosis includes these syndromes as well as sepsis, heat stroke, delirium tremens, and sympathomimetic or anticholinergic poisoning. Patients with neuroleptic malignant syndrome are more likely to present with extrapyramidal signs and autonomic instability and rarely present with the neuromuscular changes. Serotonin syndrome is a closer mimic and classically describes the constellation of features secondary to serotonin-selective reuptake inhibitor effects. The serotonin syndrome is most commonly seen after ingestion of two or more drugs with such actions. However, MDMA can induce such a syndrome on its own. Historical information is generally all that is necessary to determine which is occurring.

Sympathetic stimulation increases myocardial oxygen demand, leading to tachycardia, vasoconstriction, hypertension, and, in rare cases, acute myocardial infarction and dilated cardiomyopathy [31, 32]. Significant hypotension and low cardiac output may follow the hyperdynamic state due to catecholamine depletion or autonomic dysregulation [33, 34].

Many other effects can be attributed to acute MDMA intoxication. Electrolyte disturbances are common. Hyponatremia, which often results from excessive thirst, has been associated with MDMA-related seizures and altered mental status [35, 36]. Increased anti-diuretic hormone secretion may also contribute to the hyponatremia [37]. Hepatotoxicity is possible, with fulminant liver failure well documented [38–41]. Cerebrovascular events such as subarachnoid hemorrhage, cerebral infarct and venous sinus thrombosis are relatively uncommon but have been reported [42–46]. These neurological events are likely vasospastic in origin.

After MDMA use, depression, anxiety, myalgias, and fatigue may be observed [47]. These usually resolve without treatment. There is little evidence of a distinctive withdrawal syndrome which would be amenable to specific treatment.

Table 6.2 Adverse effects associated with acute MDMA intoxication

Musculoskeletal
  Rigidity and bruxism
  Rhabdomyolysis
  Extreme CPK elevations

Cardiovascular
  Hypertension
  Tachycardia
  Increased myocardial O_2 demand
  Myocardial infarction
  Cardiomyopathy
  Hypotension/cardiovascular collapse
  Disseminated intravascular coagulation

Metabolic
  Hyponatremia
  Hyperkalemia
  Hypermetabolic state

Pulmonary
  Pneumothorax
  Pneumomediastinum
  Respiratory depression

Renal
  Acute renal failure

Hepatic
  Necrosis/steatohepatits
  Fulminant hepatic failure

Neurological/Cerebrovascular
  Central thermogenesis
  Hallucinations, derealization, depersonalization
  Increased emotionality, heightened mood
  Anxiety
  Seizures
  Subarachnoid hemorrhage
  Cerebral infarction
  Venous sinus thrombosis

Management of the Patient

The MDMA-intoxicated patient may present with insult to multiple organ systems. A directed history and physical exam are important, but not always possible. As most urine toxicology screens will not detect MDMA, obtaining historical information from a patient's friends, family, or bystanders is useful. On examination, particular attention should be paid to vital signs, with suspicion heightened if the patient is hyperthermic.

If the patient is conscious and not an aspiration risk, anxiolysis with midazolam or diazepam may be useful and help raise the seizure threshold. Conversely, antipsychotics should be avoided since they may lower the seizure threshold. Perioperative management of hyperthermia, cardiovascular instability, electrolyte derangements, and renal and hepatic dysfunction is of primary concern. Core body temperature should be monitored closely. Wide swings in hemodynamics put the patient at risk for cardiomyopathy and coronary or cerebral vasospastic events [48, 49]. Blood pressure monitoring with an intra-arterial catheter is reasonable and allows for frequent sampling of electrolytes perioperatively. Hyponatremia, if corrected too aggressively, can lead to devastating neurological sequelae such as central pontine myelinolysis. Competing management strategies may be present when rhabdomyolysis (requiring generous hydration) and hyponatremia (requiring relative dehydration) are present. Acidification of urine would quicken MDMA elimination, but is contraindicated because it would increase the risk of metabolic acidosis and renal toxicity from rhabdomyolysis.

A rapid sequence induction is generally indicated for intoxicated patients presenting emergently. Propofol and thiopental are appropriate induction agents, although patients with extreme cardiovascular compromise may require ketamine. Etomidate has a stable hemodynamic profile and is probably also safe. Nondepolarizing neuromuscular blocking agents are not associated with malignant hyperthermia and may help slow down heat production in hyperthermic patients. Succinylcholine is probably safe, although the true risk of malignant hyperthermia is unknown. The serum potassium level should be checked before succinylcholine is used, as these patients are at risk for hyperkalemia when muscle breakdown is prominent. Severe hypertension and raised intracranial pressure may occur during laryngoscopy, and traditional methods used to blunt this response (e.g., intravenous lidocaine and opioids) are advisable. Volatile agents, as with succinylcholine, are likely safe for MDMA-intoxicated patients, although they are known triggers of malignant hyperthermia.

If intraoperative hypertension and tachycardia require treatment, labetalol, because of alpha- and beta-receptor antagonist effects, is a good choice. Pure beta blockade might worsen hypertension. Alternatively, nitroprusside or nitroglycerin may be useful in controlling hemodynamic instability but reflex tachycardia should be controlled with beta-blockers such as esmolol. If intraoperative hypotension is encountered, rapid infusions of crystalloid to a target of a presumed baseline pressure (presumed, since these patients may be very hypertensive on initial exam) or the use of direct alpha-1 agonists is reasonable. Since these patients are generally young, fluid overload and heart failure are seldom a reason to avoid crystalloid infusions. Indirect agonists, such as ephedrine, should be avoided to prevent the potential catastrophe generated when an already exhausted sympathetic nervous system is prompted to release catecholamines or the likelihood of an unknown intensity of endogenous catecholamine release.

Hyperthermia must be treated promptly to avoid rhabdomyolysis and disseminated intravascular coagulation (DIC) [50]. Cold fluids and active cooling are important measures. Dantrolene use is controversial as the drug inhibits the release of calcium from sarcoplasmic reticulum and MDMA-induced hyperthermia is likely a central process [51]. However, studies suggest that dantrolene may help exertional heat stroke, which is similar to MDMA-induced hyperthermia. Dantrolene raises the calcium requirements for excitation–contraction coupling and may be of some benefit, although it does not directly counteract central causes of hyperthermia.

Gamma Hydroxybutyrate

Background

Gamma hydroxybutyrate or GHB is a CNS suppressant generally used for its euphoric and sedative effects [52]. The drug is taken orally as a liquid, powder, tablet, or capsule and effects are apparent within minutes and may last up to 4 h. A salty liquid form is most common and is often mixed with alcohol as "liquid ecstasy," an ill-fitting name considering its differing effects.

GHB was introduced in the 1960s as a potential treatment for alcohol withdrawal [53]. The FDA removed it from the retail market (it had been found in health food stores) in the early 1990s [54]. Although results were encouraging, with positive studies being performed as recently as 2000 [55] and FDA approval under the trade name Xyrem® in 2002 (for cataplectic features of narcolepsy), misuse for its euphoric effects has limited the adoption of GHB by the medical community. Misuse for its purported anabolic properties by athletes and bodybuilders has also become prevalent. In 2000, 60 deaths were reported from overdose and GHB was reclassified as a schedule I controlled substance.

Restrictions on legal GHB have led to abuse of two substances that convert to GHB in the body: γ-butyrolactone (GBL), whose street names include "Lactone," "Renewtrient," "Blue Nitro," and "Verve," and 1,4-butanediol (BD), also known as "Pro-G," "Thunder," and "Pine Needle Extract." Both substances are available as industrial solvents and can be synthesized by methods easily accessed via the Internet. Seven percent of young adults in treatment for substance abuse reported use of GHB at one time [56]. A study of 450 club drug-using gay and bisexual men in New York City found that 29% used GHB in the previous 4 months [57].

Mechanisms of Action

The exact mechanism of action of GHB has yet to be fully elucidated. It is both a precursor and metabolite of gamma aminobutyric acid (GABA), and can bind to $GABA_B$ receptors, GHB receptors, or both to have central nervous system inhibitor effects [58]. An effect as an inhibitor of the dopaminergic system is suspected but still not clearly demonstrated [59].

Clinical Presentation

The sedative effects of GHB appear within 15 min of ingestion and make it popular with users seeking rapid euphoric effects or wanting to facilitate sexual assaults (i.e., a date rape drug). A "mellow" and sociable experience is reported. Severity of effects is generally related to dosage and concurrent use of other substances. Low-dose GHB may lead to drowsiness/loss of consciousness and visual disturbances. Higher doses may cause confusion, seizures, respiratory arrest and hypoxia, bradycardia, hypothermia, and coma [60]. When mixed with other sedatives such as alcohol, these effects are more pronounced and respiratory depression becomes increasingly likely. Sudden awakening and rebound agitation are characteristic of overdoses though the mechanism is unclear.

Physical dependence has been reported with GHB and its precursors and may develop rapidly in aggressive (more than four times per day) users [61]. Withdrawal from GHB is similar to that of alcohol and can last from 3 to 12 days [62, 63]. Concomitant ethanol abuse is common among users and may confound or worsen GHB withdrawal. Symptoms include tremors, insomnia anxiety, and diaphoresis. Milder symptoms occur in the first 24 h and include the tremor, anxiety, and tachycardia often seen with alcohol withdrawal. Forty eight to seventy two hours after the last GHB dose, severe symptoms can ensue such as worsening tachycardia and hypertension, hallucinations, confusion, delirium, seizures, and possibly death [64]. Adverse effects of GHB intoxication are summarized in Table 6.3.

Management of the Patient

The acutely intoxicated patient may require emergency supportive care and establishment of a definitive airway prior to the anesthesiologist's encounter with the patient (i.e., in the field). Patients known to have used GHB should be managed as if they are also intoxicated with alcohol and it is likely that MAC requirements are reduced given the mechanism of action of GHB. In patients who chronically abuse GHB, signs of withdrawal intraoperatively or postoperatively (e.g., sudden unexpected cardiovascular activation) should be treated aggressively and drugs that increase the seizure threshold (e.g., midazolam) are desirable for rapid prevention of acute withdrawal. If aspiration is suspected in the patient who presents with respiratory failure and hypoxia, intensive care and continued mechanical ventilation may be prudent postoperatively.

Table 6.3 Adverse effects associated with acute GHB intoxication

Musculoskeletal
  Hypotonia
Cardiovascular
  Hypotension
  Bradycardia
Metabolic
  Purported benefits on sleep and anabolic processes
  Hypothermia
Pulmonary
  Respiratory depression
  Cheyne-Stokes respiration
Renal
  Unknown
Hepatic
  Likely induces P450 enzymes, unknown
Neurological/Psychiatric
  Amnesia
  Somnolence/coma
  Nausea/vomiting
  Dizziness
  Confusion
  Seizures
  Withdrawal: insomnia, anxiety, tremor
  Aggression upon sudden awakening from overdose

Ketamine

Background

Ketamine is a potent anesthetic induction agent familiar to most anesthesiologists. It causes anesthesia with little respiratory or cardiovascular depression and has potent analgesic qualities. It was first used as a replacement for phencyclidine as an anesthetic in the 1960s, but like phencyclidine it also leads to vivid dreams and hallucinations, which are often unpleasant [65]. Most legal use of ketamine occurs in veterinary settings [66]. However, ketamine has reemerged as a useful drug in anesthesiology where its role as an analgesic particularly for children and at low doses makes it a useful adjunct [67]. Use in the psychiatric community for anti-depressant effects has also been reconsidered [68]. Abuse has steadily risen over the past decade and ketamine is often taken with MDMA. Effects generally last from 1 to 3 h and frequent re-dosing is common. It is available as a liquid or powder and can be abused orally, intravenously, intramuscularly, or via inhalation (smoked or snorted) [69].

Mechanisms of Action

Ketamine is an *N*-methyl-D-aspartate receptor antagonist, which causes noncompetitive antagonism of glutamate in the CNS [70]. A dual anesthetic/hallucinogenic nature comes from the composition as a chiral compound, with two enantiomers that have different effects. S-ketamine produces anesthetic effects and R-ketamine acts as a hallucinogen. In addition to its NMDA effects, ketamine causes a moderate sympathomimetic action via increased catecholamine outflow and possibly decreased reuptake [71].

Clinical Presentation

Blockade of the NMDA receptor leads to feelings of relaxation at low doses. At higher doses, users may experience dissociative or psychotic states, hallucinations, visual disturbances, and derealization or "out of body" experiences during which users are often quite still and appear to be staring off into space and drooling. This is sometimes called the "K-hole" [72]. Severe agitation and hyperexcitability may also be observed and patients may be aggressive, agitated, and uncontrollable [73]. Nystagmus is a key physical feature of intoxication which may help distinguish ketamine intoxication from use of other drugs of abuse. Table 6.4 shows some of the adverse effects of ketamine intoxication.

Management of the Patient

Management of the acutely intoxicated patient who presents for surgery is generally supportive and other measures are predicated on the degree of psychiatric impairment. Most patients are young and tolerate sympathomimetic activation of the kind induced by ketamine. Acute agitation and psychosis may make procedures such as intravenous placement, monitor placement, and awake endotracheal intubation, if needed, difficult. One or several doses of a benzodiazepine such as midazolam or diazepam are generally needed to reduce agitation and anxiety. Inclusion of antipsychotic drugs such as haloperidol is appropriate. High-dose ketamine intoxication may obtund a patient severely and aspiration precautions should be taken. Poly-drug use should be assumed, especially if symptoms and signs persist after an hour from the last ingestion. In any case, the addition of an arterial line to standard monitors allows for close hemodynamic monitoring and frequent blood sampling which may be useful should polysubstance abuse be suspected or the inciting event be a trauma.

Table 6.4 Adverse effects associated with acute ketamine intoxication

Musculoskeletal
  Occasional tonic-clonic movements

Cardiovascular
  Hypertension
  Tachycardia
  Arrhythmias

Metabolic
  None known

Pulmonary
  Hypersalivation and increased bronchial secretions
  Airway obstruction

Renal
  None known

Hepatic
  None known

Neurological/Psychological
  Hallucinations/disorientation
  Psychoses
  Dissociation/derealization
  "Near death" experiences
  Flashbacks
  Nystagmus/diplopia
  Increased intraocular pressure
  Lowered seizure threshold

Flunitrazepam

Background

Flunitrazepam is a drug abused for its sedative effects and also given as a date rape drug [74]. It was first developed by the Hoffman-LaRoche pharmaceutical company in 1975 and given its trade name Rohypnol®. Its street name, roofies, is perhaps its best-known moniker. Reports of abuse have been common in Europe since the 1970s, and in the 1990s the drug emerged in the US. Flunitrazepam is approved as a sedative/hypnotic drug in Europe, South America, Asia, and Australia where it is marketed as a sleep-aid and a preoperative anxiolytic. Most of the available street drug in the US is smuggled in from Mexico by way of mail or delivery services.

The drug is taken orally as tablets or capsules and through its benzodiazepine effects has muscle relaxant, sedative, anxiolytic, and amnestic qualities. Effects generally begin in fifteen minutes, peak within an hour of ingestion, and may last up to twelve hours. This rapid onset of action compared to other commercially available benzodiazepines makes the drug desirable for a rapid "high" and for sexual assault. The features which characterize flunitrazepam can be applied to all

Table 6.5 Adverse effects associated with acute flunitrazepam intoxication

Musculoskeletal
  Muscle relaxation
  Tremors

Cardiovascular
  Hypotension
  Bradycardia

Metabolic
  None known

Pulmonary
  Respiratory depression

Renal
  None known

Hepatic
  None known

Neurological/Cerebrovascular
  Relaxation/anxiolysis
  Drowsiness
  Anterograde amnesia
  Headaches
  Confusion
  Paradoxical excitability or aggression

benzodiazepines, with differing pharmacokinetic profiles distinguishing the various types (Table 6.5).

Mechanism of Action

A benzodiazepine, flunitrazepam, serves as a $GABA_A$-receptor agonist that increased frequency of channel opening with subsequent chloride ion flux, neuronal membrane hyperpolarization, and CNS depression.

Clinical Presentation

Adverse effects are dose-related and revolve around potent CNS depressant effects. Somnolence, confusion, stupor, and coma are all possible effects of large doses. Respiratory depression may also be present when other CNS depressants are used in conjunction such as alcohol and other benzodiazepines. Paradoxical reactions may occur with varying incidence just as with all benzodiazepines, leading to hyperexcitable states and agitation. True overdose is heralded by slurred speech, respiratory depression, bradycardia, hypotension and stupor, or coma. The withdrawal

Table 6.6 Features of common benzodiazepines

Drug	Trade name	Onset of action	Half-life (h)
Alprazolam	Xanax	Intermediate	~15
Diazepam	Valium	Rapid	20–50
Lorazepam	Ativan	Intermediate	10–24
Flunitrazepam	Xyrem	Rapid	40–120
Midazolam	Versed	Rapid	1–4

profile is not unlike that of alcohol. Adverse effects are presented below for fluni-trazepam but may be applied to all benzodiazepines (Table 6.6).

Management of the Patient

Patients acutely intoxicated by or withdrawing from flunitrazepam may be managed similarly to those who have ingested any other CNS depressant (i.e., alcohol and benzodiazepines). Reversal with flumazenil is possible but can precipitate seizures and withdrawal. A long-acting benzodiazepine taper may be required postoperatively (clonazepam is long acting and tends to be most commonly used) and any rapid changed in hemodynamic measurements intraoperatively may be due to withdrawal. In the case of young women and girls brought to the emergency room with or without signs of trauma, suspicion of rape should be entertained and appropriate consults with other health-care workers and law enforcement agencies obtained.

Conclusion

The club drugs remain an emerging problem in the US. Patients may present acutely intoxicated or withdrawing from these substances. Often patients are brought to the attention of medical personnel for reasons such as trauma related to risky behaviors while under the influence and the clouded sensorium produced either by acute intoxication with these agents or during withdrawal can make the diagnosis of underlying medical issues difficult. The management becomes difficult when presenting signs and symptoms may be due to the drug or from an injury (e.g., head trauma) secondary to injuries sustained while under the influence.

Supportive care is generally all that is needed to affect a positive outcome when these patients present to the hospital acutely intoxicated. Polysubstance abuse should be assumed when abuse of one of the drugs is suspected and while a "typical" club drug user is now very difficult to detect given their widespread use, young club goers and "ravers" remain a likely group. Alcohol is commonly used along with the club drugs and confounds or exacerbates the toxidromes of these drugs. Also, these substances are not generally detected by urine toxicology screens done in the emergency room; so, historical information and clinical signs and symptoms remain paramount in their diagnosis. Anesthesiologists should keep this in mind when taking care of intoxicated patients for emergency surgeries in their teens and early twenties and remain vigilant for rapidly evolving adverse effects intra- and postoperatively.

Spotlight on Methamphetamine

Ethan O. Bryson, MD

A synthetic derivative of amphetamine, methamphetamine is a schedule II drug with a high abuse potential, similar to that of cocaine. It has limited medical use and is currently available only through a prescription that cannot be refilled. Called *Speed*, *Meth*, *Crystal*, *Crank*, *Ice* and *Glass*, methamphetamine is a white, odorless, bitter-tasting crystalline powder that easily dissolves in water or alcohol and can be snorted, smoked, swallowed or taken intravenously. The time of onset and effects of the drug vary, depending on the route of administration, but the typical half-life is about 12 h. Once ingested, this non-catecholamine exerts its effects through sympathetic nervous system activation with both increased release of and decreased reuptake of endogenous catecholamines [75]. As a result, heart rate and blood pressure increase and appetite and fatigue are suppressed as the fight-or-flight response is activated.

Occasionally referred to as *poor man's cocaine*, *working man's cocaine* or *redneck cocaine*, presumably because it provides a "high" similar to that of cocaine though at a reduced cost, methamphetamine is abused by members of all levels of society. Though still ubiquitous, use in most segments of the population has been declining since the late 1990s. Methamphetamine is, however, considered a "drug of choice" for many gay men involved in the "club scene", where it is often mixed with methylenedioxymethamphetamine (*Party and Play*) or Viagra (*Tina*).

Toxic Effects

Once methamphetamine is ingested, a surge of dopamine is released from pre-synaptic nerve terminals. In the process these nerve terminals, as well as adjacent serotonin-releasing nerve terminals are damaged [76]. Subsequent administration cannot produce the same subjective effects experienced by the user who now has permanent change in his or her brain chemistry.

Often the addict is forever chasing that initial "high" caused by the first dopamine surge.

Vasoconstriction caused by increased levels of circulating catecholamines may damage the smaller cerebral arteries and lead to areas of focal ischemia. When this occurs in the brainstem, stereotyped and uncontrolled movements may occur and persist even when the addict is not acutely intoxicated with the drug. Imaging studies performed on the brains of human methamphetamine addicts have shown alterations in the activity of the dopamine system [77]. These physical alterations in the biochemical structure of the brain have been associated with reduced motor skills and impaired verbal learning, and may also be responsible for the emotional lability commonly seen in chronic methamphetamine abusers.

Long-term exposure to methamphetamine can lead to left ventricular hypertrophy due to increased myocyte size and increased collagen deposits. Blood pressure may be labile and difficult to control. The effected individual will likely have decreased cardiac compliance and diastolic dysfunction, and may present with heart failure [78]. While there are no documented effects of chronic methamphetamine abuse on the respiratory system, addicts who ingest methamphetamine by smoking may be at the same increased risk for intraoperative bronchospasm as the heavy tobacco smoker. The extreme weight loss associated with long-term abuse can significantly decrease levels of albumin and affect both protein binding and metabolism of many common anesthetic agents. Severe dental problems are common, including chronic infections, loose teeth, and oral abscesses that may present a significant issue with airway management. Psychiatric considerations in the acutely intoxicated individual include the development of anxiety, confusion, insomnia, mood disturbances and violent behavior. Chronic methamphetamine abusers have been known to develop psychotic features such as paranoia, visual auditory and tactile hallucinations, and delusions.

Anesthetic Considerations
It should be assumed that the chronic methamphetamine abuser will behave physiologically as a chronic, poorly controlled hypertensive. Usually these people are younger but may have the physiology of a much older patient due to the effects of chronic exposure to methamphetamines. Key anesthetic considerations include heart rate control and maintenance of blood pressure in light of what may be compromised cardiovascular function. The acutely intoxicated individual may present with tachyarrhythmias and may be acutely psychotic, requiring physical restraints. As with other "club drugs", hyperthermia may be associated with overdose. Universal precautions should be strictly observed, as chronic infection with blood borne viruses such as hepatitis B and C as well as HIV is common in addicts who administer the drug intravenously. Informed consent may be difficult to obtain.

References

1. Kelly BC, Parsons JT, Wells BE. Prevalence and predictors of club drug use among club-going young adults in New York City. J Urban Health. 2006;83(5):884–95.
2. European Monitoring Centre for Drugs and Drug addiction. The state of the drugs problem in the European Union and Norway: Annual report; 2007.
3. US Department of Heath and Human Services. National survey on drug use and health. Washington, DC: US Department of Health and Human Services; 2005.
4. National Institute on Drug Abuse. The monitoring the future national results on adolescent drug use: overview of key findings, 2001. Ann Arbor, MI: University of Michigan Institute for Social Research; 2002.
5. Teter CJ, Guthrie SK. A comprehensive review of MDMA and GHB: two common club drugs. Pharmacotherapy. 2001;21(12):1486–513.
6. Suarez RV, Riemersma R. "Ecstasy" and sudden cardiac death. Am J Forensic Med Pathol. 1988;9:339–41.
7. Shulgin AT. The background and chemistry of MDMA. J Psychoactive Drugs. 1986;18:291–304.
8. Greer GR, Tolbert R. A method of conducting therapeutic sessions with MDMA. J Psychoactive Drugs. 1998;30(4):371–9.
9. Greer G, Tolbert R. Subjective reports of the effects of MDMA in a clinical setting. J Psychoactive Drugs. 1986;18:319–27.
10. Wolff K, Hay AWM, Sherlock K, Conner M. Contents of "ecstasy". Lancet. 1995;346:1100–1.
11. Morgan MJ. Ecstasy (MDMA): a review of its possible persistent psychological effects. Psychopharmacology (Berl). 2000;152:230–48.
12. Morton J. Ecstasy: pharmacology and neurotoxicity. Curr Opin Pharmacol. 2005;5:79–86.
13. Battaglia G, Yeh SY, De Souza EB. MDMA-induced neurotoxicity: parameters of degeneration and recovery of brain serotonin neurons. Pharmacol Biochem Behav. 1988;29(2):269–74.
14. Oesterheld JR, Armstrong SC, Cozza KL. Ecstasy: pharmacodynamic and pharmacokinetic interactions. Psychosomatics. 2004;45:84–7.
15. Ferigolo M, Machado AGS, Oliveira NB, et al. Ecstasy intoxication: the toxicological basis for treatment. Rev Hosp Clin Fac Med Sao Paulo. 2003;58:332–41.
16. Cami J, Farre M, Mas M. Human pharmacology of 3,4- methylenedioxymethamphetamine ("Ecstasy"): psychomotor performance and subjective effects. J Clin Psychopharmacol. 2000;20:455–66.
17. Mas M, Farre M, de la Torre R. Cardiovascular and neuroendocrine effects and pharma-cokinetics of 3,4- methylenedioxymethamphetamine in humans. J Pharmacol Exp Ther. 1999;290:136–45.
18. Peroutka SJ. Incidence of recreational use of 3,4- methylenedioxymethamphetamine (MDMA, 'ecstasy') on an undergraduate campus. N Engl J Med. 1987;317:1542–3.
19. Cohen RS. Subjective reports on the effects of the MDMA ('Ecstasy') experience in humans. Prog Neuropsychopharmacol Biol Psychiatry. 1995;19:1137–45.
20. O'Cain PA, Hletko SB, Ogden BA, et al. Cardiovascular and sympathetic responses and reflex changes elicited by MDMA. Physiol Behav. 2000;70:141–8.
21. Walsh T, Carmichale R, Chestnut J. A hyperthermic reaction to ecstasy. Br J Hosp Med. 1994;51:476.
22. Gill JR, Hayes JA, de Souza IS, et al. Ecstasy (MDMA) deaths in New York City: a case series and review of the literature. J Forensic Sci. 2002;47:121–6.
23. Logan ASC, Stickle B, O'Keefe N, Hewitson H. Survival following 'Ecstasy' ingestion with a peak temperature of 42°C. Anaesthesia. 1993;48:1017–8.
24. Hall AP. "Ecstasy" and the anaesthetist. Br J Anaesth. 1997;79:697–8.
25. Milroy CM, Clark JC, Forrest ARW. Pathology of deaths associated with "Ecstasy" and "Eve" misuse. J Clin Pathol. 1996;49:149–53.
26. Schmidt CJ, Black CK, Abbate GM, Taylor VL. MDMA induced hyperthermia and neurotox-icity are independently mediated by 5-HT2 receptors. Brain Res. 1990;529:85–90.

27. Nimmo SM, Kennedy BW, Tullett WM, Blyth AS, Dougall JR. Drug-induced hyperthermia. Anaesthesia. 1993;48(10):892–5.
28. Benowitz NL. Amphetamines. In: Olson KR, editor. Poisoning and drug overdose. 3rd ed. Stamford, CT: Appleton & Lange; 1999. p. 68–70.
29. Fiege M, Wappler F, Weisshorn R, et al. Induction of malignant hyperthermia in susceptible swine by 3,4-methylenedioxymethamphetamine ("ecstasy"). Anesthesiology. 2003;99:1132–6.
30. Rusyniak DE, Sprague JE. Toxin-induced hyperthermic syndromes. Med Clin North Am. 2005;89(6):1277–96.
31. Ghuran A, Nolan J. Recreational drug misuse: issues for the cardiologist. Heart. 2000;83:627–33.
32. Qasim A, Townend J, Davies MK. Ecstasy induced acute myocardial infarction. Heart. 2001;85:E10.
33. Ghuran A, van Der Wieken LR, Nolan J. Cardiovascular complications of recreational drugs. BMJ. 2001;323:464–6.
34. Brody S, Krause C, Veit R, Rau H. Cardiovascular autonomic dysregulation in users of MDMA ("Ecstasy"). Psychopharmacology. 1998;136:390–3.
35. Kessel B. Hyponatraemia after ingestion of "Ecstasy". BMJ. 1994;308:414.
36. Holden R, Jackson MA. Near-fatal hyponatraemic coma due to vasopressin over-secretion after "Ecstasy" (3,4-MDMA) [letter]. Lancet. 1996;347:1052.
37. Henry JA, Fallon JK, Kicman AT. Low-dose MDMA ("Ecstasy") induces vasopressin secretion [letter]. Lancet. 1998;351:1784.
38. Khakoo SI, Coles CJ, Armstrong JS, Barry RE. Hepatotoxicity and accelerated fibrosis following 3,4-methylenedioxymetamphetamine ("Ecstasy") usage. J Clin Gastroenterol. 1995;20:244–7.
39. Brauer RB, Heidecke CD, Nathrath W, et al. Liver transplantation for the treatment of fulminant hepatic failure induced by the ingestion of ecstasy. Transpl Int. 1997;10:229–33.
40. Ellis AJ, Wendon JA, Portmann B, Williams R. Acute liver damage and ecstasy ingestion. Gut. 1996;38:454–8.
41. Jones AL, Simpson KJ. Review article: mechanisms and management of hepatotoxicity in Ecstasy (MDMA) and amphetamine intoxications. Aliment Pharmacol Ther. 1999;13:129–33.
42. Gledhill JA, Moore DF, Bell D, Henry JA. Subarachnoid haemorrhage associated with MDMA abuse. J Neurol Neurosurg Psychiatry. 1993;56(9):1036–7.
43. Manchanda S, Connolly MJ. Cerebral infarction in association with ecstasy abuse. Postgrad Med. 1993;69:874–89.
44. McEvoy AW, Kitchen ND, Thomas DG. Intracerebral haemorrhage and drug abuse in young adults. Br J Neurosurg. 2000;14:449–54.
45. McCann UD, Slate SO, Ricaurte GA. Adverse reactions with 3,4-methylenedioxymethamphetamine (MDMA; 'Ecstasy'). Drug Saf. 1996;15:107–15.
46. Ranalli E, Bouton R. Intracerebral haemorrhage associated with ingestion of "Ecstasy" [abstr]. Eur Neuropsychopharmacol. 1997;7:S263.
47. Degenhardt L, Bruno R, Topp L. Is ecstasy a drug of dependence? Drug Alcohol Depend. 2010;107(1):1–10.
48. Klein M, Kramer F. Rave drugs: pharmacological considerations. AANA J. 2004;72:61–7.
49. Reneman L, Habraken JB, Majoie CB, et al. MDMA ("Ecstasy") and its association with cerebrovascular accidents: preliminary findings. Am J Neuroradiol. 2000;21:1001–7.
50. Richards JR. Rhabdomyolisis and drugs abuse. J Emerg Med. 2000;19:51–6.
51. Singarajah C, Lavies NG. An overdose of ecstasy: a role for dantrolene. Anaesthesia. 1992;47:686–7.
52. Nicholson KL, Balster RL. GHB: a new and novel drug of abuse. Drug Alcohol Depend. 2001;63:1–22.
53. Britt GC, McCance-Katz EF. A brief overview of the clinical pharmacology of "club drugs". Subst Use Misuse. 2005;40:1189–201.
54. Okun M, Bartfield RB, Doering PL. GHB toxicity: what you need to know. Emerg Med. 2000;10–23.
55. Addolorato G, Caputo F, Capristo E, et al. Gamma-hydroxybutyric acid: efficacy, potential abuse and dependence in the treatment of alcohol addiction. Alcohol. 2000;20:217–22.

56. Halkitis PN, Palamar JJ. GHB use among gay and bisexual men. Addict Behav. 2006;31(11): 2135–9.
57. Knudsen K, Greter J, Verdicchio M, et al. A severe outburst of GHB poisonings (gamma-hydroxybutyrate, gamma-hydroxybutyric acid) on the West Coast of Sweden. Mortality numbers ahead of heroin. Clin Toxicol. 2006;44(5):637–8.
58. Tunnicliff G. Sites of action of gamma-hydroxybutyrate – a neuroactive drug with abuse potential. J Toxicol Clin Toxicol. 1997;35(6):581–90.
59. Hedou G, Chasserot-Golaz S, Kemmel V, Gobaille S, Roussel G, Artault JC, et al. Immunohistochemical studies of the localization of neurons containing the enzyme that synthesizes dopamine, GABA, or gamma-hydroxybutyrate in the rat substantia nigra and striatum. J Comp Neurol. 2000;426(4):549–60.
60. Graeme KA. New drugs of abuse. Emerg Med Clin North Am. 2000;18:625–36.
61. Galloway GP, Frederick SL, Staggers Jr F. Physical dependence on sodium oxybate. Lancet. 1994;343(8888):57.
62. Freese TE, Miotto K, Reback CJ. The effects and consequences of selected club drugs. J Subst Abuse Treat. 2002;23:151–6.
63. McDaniel CH, Miotto KA. Gamma hydroxybutyrate (GHB) and gamma butyrolactone (GBL) withdrawal: five case studies. J Psychoactive Drugs. 2001;33(2):143–9.
64. Dyer JE, Roth B, Hyma BA. Gamma-hydroxybutyrate withdrawal syndrome. Ann Emerg Med. 2001;37:147–53.
65. Green SM, Li J. Ketamine in adults: what emergency physicians need to know about patient selection and emergence reactions. Acad Emerg Med. 2000;7:278–81.
66. Rome ES. It's a rave new world: rave culture and illicit drug use in the young. Clev Clin J Med. 2001;68:541–50.
67. Berti M, Baciarello M, Troglio R, Fanelli G. Clinical uses of low-dose ketamine in patients undergoing surgery. Curr Drug Targets. 2009;10(8):707–15.
68. Skolnick P, Popik P, Trullas R. Glutamate-based antidepressants: 20 years on. Trends Pharmacol Sci. 2009;30(11):563–9.
69. Jansen KL, Darracot-Cankovic R. The nonmedical use of ketamine, part two: a review of problem use and dependence. J Psychoactive Drugs. 2001;33:151–8.
70. Kohrs R, Durieux ME. Ketamine: teaching an old drug new tricks. Anesth Analg. 1998;87:1186–93.
71. Reich DL, Silvay G. Ketamine: an update on the first twenty-five years of clinical experience. Can J Anaesth. 1989;36(2):186–97.
72. Weiner AL, Viera L, McKay CA, Bayer MJ. Ketamine abusers presenting to the emergency department: a case series. J Emerg Med. 2000;18:447–51.
73. Pal HR, Berry N, Kumar R, et al. Ketamine dependence. Anaesth Intensive Care. 2002;30:382–4.
74. Ricaurtie GA, McCann UD. Recognition and management of complications of new recreational drug use. Lancet. 2005;365:2137–45.
75. Yu Q, Montes S, Larson D, Watson RR. Effects of chronic methamphetamine exposure on heart function in uninfected and retrovirus-infected mice. Life Sci. 1995;75:29–43.
76. National Institute on Drug Abuse, Methamphetamine Abuse and addiction: what is Methamphetamine? Bethesda, MD: National Institute of Health; 1998. NIDA research report series, NIH publication 98-4210.
77. Volkow ND, Chang L, Wang GJ, et al. Association of dopamine transporter reduction with psychomotor impairment in methamphetamine abusers. Am J Psychiatry. 2001;158(3):377–82.
78. Karch SB, Stephens BG, Ho CH. Methamphetamine related deaths in San Francisco: demographic, pathologic and toxicologic profiles. J Forensic Sci. 1999;44:359–68.

Chapter 7
Anesthesia and Alcohol Addiction

Andrew Schwartz and David Knez

Introduction

Alcohol has been consumed for tens of thousands of years. Throughout history, it has held major cultural and religious significance. Some ancient cultures revered its use, while others condemned it. Despite its ubiquitous nature and important role in society and religion, drunkenness and excessive alcohol consumption have long been recognized as significant social problems. Biblical and other ancient cultural sources document a history of alcohol abuse and dependence and caution against overindulgence.

The World Health Organization (WHO) estimates that 140 million people worldwide currently suffer from dependence upon alcohol.[1] Long-term alcohol consumption and abuse lead to the loss of many life years secondary to death or disability. The public health burden from alcohol use disorder (AUD) is significant. A direct causal relationship exists between excess and prolonged alcohol consumption and a number of diseases including esophageal and liver cancers and liver cirrhosis. Alcohol consumption plays a role in a large proportion of motor vehicle accidents, homicides, and suicides. A recent epidemiologic study estimates the United States AUD prevalence to be 8.26% [1]. In 2007, the per capita adult alcohol consumption in the United States was 2.3 gallons.[2] In 2005, alcohol abuse and dependence was estimated to cost the United States economy 220 billion dollars per year, more than either cancer or obesity. Excessive alcohol consumption is the third leading risk modifiable cause of death, only behind obesity and cigarette smoking. More than 100,000 Americans die each year from alcoholism.

---

[1] www.who.int/substance_abuse/facts/alcohol (accessed 09-18-2010).
[2] www.niaaa.nih.gov/resources/databaseresources (accessed 09-18-2010).

A. Schwartz (✉)
Department of Anesthesiology, Mount Sinai School of Medicine, New York, NY, USA
e-mail: andrew.schwartz@mssm.edu

E.O. Bryson and E.A.M. Frost (eds.), *Perioperative Addiction:*
Clinical Management of the Addicted Patient, DOI 10.1007/978-1-4614-0170-4_7,
© Springer Science+Business Media, LLC 2012

In the United States, alcohol is the most common substance of abuse and dependence. Since the American Medical Association (AMA) first recognized alcoholism as a formal disease in 1956, there has been considerable research performed in the arena of alcohol and other substances of abuse and numerous theories have been proposed to explain the biologic mechanisms of addiction. Alcoholism is clearly a multifactorial disease with genetic, biochemical, psychosocial, and cultural components. Current evidence indicates that alcoholism is 50–60% genetically determined with 40–50% being environmentally based [2].

The Diagnostic and Statistical Manual Fourth Edition (DSM-IV) divides AUD into two main categories, alcohol abuse and alcohol dependence [3]. Alcohol abuse is characterized as a maladaptive use pattern with recurrent alcohol consumption resulting in failure to fulfill work or family obligations, legal problems related to consumption, use in physically risky situations (i.e., driving), and recurrent social or interpersonal problems due to alcohol consumption. Alcohol dependence contains the features of abuse with tolerance development, presence of withdrawal symptoms with an abstinent period, and a compulsive drinking pattern despite a desire to cut down or control drinking.

Mechanism of Action

Ethanol, the active ingredient in alcoholic beverages, is rapidly absorbed from the gastrointestinal tract. Peak blood levels are typically achieved within an hour after consumption. It is uniformly distributed across body fluids and readily crosses the placenta in the parturient. Alcohol is metabolized in the liver via a series of enzymatic reactions. First, ethanol is converted to acetaldehyde via alcohol dehydrogenase. Acetaldehyde is rapidly converted to acetate and eventually to carbon dioxide and water. Some alcohol is also metabolized via the P450 system in the liver, specifically cytochrome P450 2E1 (CYP2E1). This system appears to be upregulated in the chronic drinker, contributing to metabolic tolerance.

Although it has likely been in use for a longer period of time than any other substance of abuse, the mechanism of action of ethanol is less well understood than other substances of abuse. The majority of psychoactive substances have a single specific receptor target that can explain the effect of the drug. On the other hand, alcohol interacts with almost every neurochemical and endocrine system (Table 7.1). Alcohol dissolves in the lipid bilayer of cell membranes, leading to an increased fluidity, in turn leading to a modification of a vast number of ion channels and receptors. This indirect change in channel functionality has been purported as the major mechanism of action for alcohol, similar to the Meyer–Overton theory of the action of volatile anesthetics. Alcohol has been shown to increase dopamine release in the pharmacologic reward pathway. It inhibits the transport of adenosine and norepinephrine, while facilitating the transport of dopamine and serotonin, changing the extracellular concentration of these substances.

Alcohol is best understood as a multi-action central nervous system (CNS) depressant. The overall effect of consumption is an increase in the activity of inhibitory systems and a concurrent decrease in the activity of excitatory neurotransmission.

Table 7.1 Ethanol and central neurotransmitter system activity

Transmitter	Effect
Dopamine	Enhanced
Adenosine	Decreased
Norepinephrine	Decreased
Serotonin	Enhanced
GABA	Enhanced
Glycine	Enhanced
Acetylcholine	Enhanced
Glutamate	Decreased

Ethanol enhances the responses mediated by the γ-amino butyric acid a-type (GABA$_A$) receptor. It also leads to enhancement at serotonin (5-HT$_3$), glycine, and nicotinic acetylcholine receptors. The effect of the major CNS excitatory neurotransmitter, glutamate, at N-methyl-D-aspartate (NMDA) receptors is antagonized. Many of the effects of alcohol seem unlikely to involve the ligand-gated receptors listed above but may nonetheless alter synaptic transmission. Recent work indicates direct action through physical binding to a pocket on a G-protein-gated inwardly rectifying potassium (GIRK) channel [4]. Alcohol activation of this receptor dampens neuronal chemical communication.

Acute Intoxication

Acute ethanol intoxication is associated with a higher risk for trauma-related injuries, a direct result of the effects of decreased coordination and increased emotional lability. Patients under the influence of ethanol are more likely to suffer fall-related trauma, be involved in motor vehicle accidents, and be the victim of assault or homicide. Although rarely the primary reason for presentation, acute intoxication with alcohol is extremely common in patients requiring emergent care. In the United States, it is estimated that uncomplicated alcohol intoxication is responsible for upward of 600,000 emergency room visits per year [5].

A variety of signs and symptoms are associated in the patient acutely intoxicated with ethanol (Table 7.2). Common findings include nystagmus, slurred speech, unsteady gait, and inability to coordinate gross motor functions. Increased emotional lability, difficulty with memory, and impaired judgment often result in secondary injury. Altered mental status as a result of acute intoxication is a diagnosis of exclusion, however, and more serious conditions must first be ruled out, including head trauma and metabolic phenomena. Polysubstance abuse is common and intoxication with other drugs must also be considered.

Although not always correlated with the degree of intoxication, especially in chronic drinkers with increased tolerance, a blood alcohol concentration (BAC) can help in diagnosis and treatment. As blood alcohol levels rise, autonomic dysfunction

Table 7.2 Signs and symptoms of acute alcohol intoxication

Nystagmus
Slurred speech
Unsteady gait
Discoordination
Emotional labiality, aggressive behavior
Impaired judgment and memory
Hypotension
Hypothermia
Respiratory depression
Stupor, coma, death

ensues causing hypotension, hypothermia, stupor, and coma. Eventually, respiratory depression and loss of protective airway reflexes occur, which can result in significant morbidity and even death.

Treatment is mainly supportive. Blood glucose levels should be obtained and hypoglycemia treated. A thorough physical exam is essential to determine the presence of any traumatic injuries. Coma patients are administered parenteral thiamine to prevent Wernicke's encephalopathy. Intravenous hydration is often provided, as patients tend to be hypotensive and volume depleted. Serial examination of respiratory status is critical and lack of ability to protect the airway requires emergent intubation and mechanical ventilation. The acutely intoxicated patient may be confused and unable to give procedural informed consent. If possible, surgical interventions should be delayed until the patient regains baseline mentation. In emergent situations, the patient usually must be treated as lacking capacity to make decisions. The acutely intoxicated may be aggressive and violent posing a threat to the perioperative provider. In such instances, anxiolysis with a benzodiazepine or administration of a neuroleptic may prove helpful.

Chronic Alcohol Consumption

Chronic alcohol consumption can lead to a myriad of medical problems affecting almost all organ systems (Table 7.3). Up to 35% of adult patients have medical complications as a result of alcohol abuse [6]. While the pertinent and severe complications arising in the perioperative period will be discussed in detail in the following sections, a brief summary of the medical problems by organ systems is presented here. Chronic alcohol consumption leads to a variety of neurologic complications. AUD patients may have cerebellar degeneration and cerebral atrophy presenting with sensorimotor and cognitive impairments. Chronic alcohol consumption can cause neuromuscular problems related to peripheral neuropathy and myopathy. Wernicke's encephalopathy is an acute neurologic disorder in the chronic alcoholic caused by thiamine deficiency. It is manifested by the clinical triad of encephalopathy, oculomotor dysfunction, and gait ataxia. Korsakoff's syndrome is the progression of Wernicke's encephalopathy to include selective anterograde and retrograde

Table 7.3 Medical problems associated with AUD

Central nervous system
   Psychiatric disorders
   Nutritional disorders (Wernicke-Korsakoff syndrome)
   Alcohol withdrawal syndrome
   Cerbellar degeneration
   Cerebral atrophy

Cardiovascular
   Dilated cardiomyopathy
   Dysrhythmias
   Hypertension

Gastrointestinal and hepatobiliary
   Esophagitis
   Gastritis
   Pancreatitis
   Liver cirrhosis (portal hypertension manifested as esophageal varices or hemorrhoids)

Skin and musculoskeletal
   Spider angiomas
   Myopathy
   Osteoporisis

Endocrine and metabolic
   Decreased plasma testosterone
   Decreased gluconeogenesis
   Ketocacidosis
   Hypoalbuminemia
   Hypomagnesemia

Hematoligic
   Thrombocytopenia
   Leukopenia
   Anemia

This article was published in Stoetling, RK, Dierdorf, SF. Anesthesia and coexisting disease, 3rd ed. New York, NY: Churchill Livingstone; 1993: p 526

amnesia. Chronic alcoholism has vast cardiovascular effects including dilated cardiomyopathy, dysrhythmias, and hypertension. The gastrointestinal and hepatobiliary effects of alcoholism are well known (hepatic cirrhosis and its sequelae, gastritis and pancreatitis). Chronic alcohol consumption has a variety of endocrine and metabolic implications including decreased testosterone, hypoglycemia, and overall malnutrition. Pancytopenia may also occur.

Perioperative Considerations

Approximately 20% of adult patients presenting for surgery and diagnostic procedures and the critically ill have an AUD, ranging in severity from hazardous use and harmful consumption to abuse and dependence [7]. Roughly half of the patients

Table 7.4 Major perioperative complications associated with AUD

Acute alcohol withdrawal syndrome
Increased postoperative infection rates
Acute respiratory distress syndrome
Cardiovascular complications (dysrhythmia, heart failure)
Hemorrhage

Adapted from [6]

presenting for surgery with an AUD are alcohol dependent. The incidence of AUD is overrepresented in the hospitalized population. In addition to cigarette smoking, chronic alcohol abuse/dependence is the most common lifestyle risk that can influence morbidity and mortality after surgery [8]. There is a clear dose–response relationship between hazardous drinking and postoperative morbidity [9]. The complication rate is increased by 50% in patients consuming between three and four drinks per day as compared to those consuming zero to two drinks. This rate increases 200–400% in patients consuming greater than five drinks per day. The increased morbidity for AUD patients holds true over a wide range of surgical procedures. The postsurgical morbidity and mortality is 2–5 times greater in the chronic alcoholic than in the general population. AUD patients have an augmented hypothalamic–pituitary–adrenal axis (HPA axis) stress response to surgical trauma. The complications associated with AUD significantly affect postsurgical, trauma, and critical illness outcomes. The major complications associated with AUD include: alcohol withdrawal syndrome (AWS), increased postoperative infection rate, cardiovascular complications, and hemorrhage (Table 7.4) [7].

Identification of Alcohol Use Disorder in the Perioperative Period

A general lack of suspicion for an AUD exists prior to the development of complications related to alcohol consumption. It is critical that the perioperative team have a well-directed approach to screen and diagnose for AUD. The majority of pathology associated with AUD is reversible if appropriate treatment for alcohol dependency is instituted. Although these patients have an increased perioperative risk, they can be treated safely provided the proper precautions are taken.

Perioperative AUD is generally defined as daily consumption of greater than or equal to 60 g of ethanol (five drinks). Well-established diagnostic tools exist to screen for AUD. The two most common questionnaires utilized for AUD detection are the CAGE and the AUDIT (Tables 7.5 and 7.6). A recent report suggests that computerized patient self-assessment with AUDIT was more likely to establish the diagnosis of AUD than practitioner examination in the preoperative assessment clinic.

Laboratory tests can also be useful in establishing the diagnosis. Mean corpuscular volume (MCV), gamma-glutamyl transpeptidase (GGT), and carbohydrate-deficient

Table 7.5 CAGE

Have you ever felt you should *C*ut down on your drinking?

Have people *A*nnoyed you by criticizing your drinking?

Have you ever felt bad or *G*uilty about your drinking?

Have you ever felt you needed a drink first thing in the morning (*E*ye opener)
    to steady your nerves or to get rid of a hangover?

Each question is answered with a yes or no response. Each yes response received
one point while no responses receive zero points. Scores greater than or equal to
2 are considered positive

Table 7.6 AUDIT Questionnaire

1. How often did you have a drink containing alcohol in the past year?

    (0) Never

    (1) Monthly or less

    (2) 2–4 times a month

    (3) 2–3 times a week

    (4) Daily or almost daily

2. How many drinks containing alcohol did you have on a typical day when you were drinking
    in the past year?

    (0) 1 or 2

    (1) 3 or 4

    (2) 5 or 6

    (3) 7, 8 or 9

    (4) 10 or more

3. How often did you have 6 or more drinks on one occasion in the past year?

    (0) Never

    (1) Less than monthly

    (2) Monthly

    (3) Weekly

    (4) Daily or almost daily

4. How often during the last year have you found that you were not able to stop dinking once
    you had started?

    (0) Never

    (1) Less than monthly

    (2) Monthly

    (3) Weekly

    (4) Daily or almost daily

5. How often during the last you have you failed to do what was normally expected from you
    because of drinking?

    (0) Never

    (1) Less than monthly

    (2) Monthly

    (3) Weekly

    (4) Daily or almost daily

6. How often during the last year have you needed a first drink in the morning to get yourself
    going after a heavy drinking session?

    (0) Never

(continued)

Table 7.6 (continued)

(1) Less than monthly
(2) Monthly
(3) Weekly
(4) Daily or almost daily

7. How often during the last year have you had a feeling of guilt or remorse after drinking?
(0) Never
(1) less than monthly
(2) monthly
(3) weekly
(4) daily or almost daily

8. How often during the last year have you been unable to remember what happened the night before because of dinking?
(0) Never
(1) less than monthly
(2) monthly
(3) weekly
(4) daily or almost daily

9. Have you or someone else been injured as a result of your drinking?
(0) No
(2) Yes, but not in the last year
(4) Yes, during the last year

10. Has a relative or friend or doctor or other healthcare worker been concerned about your drinking or suggested you cut down?
(0) No
(2) Yes, but not in the last year
(4) Yes, during the last year

The questions sum to a total score between 0 and 40. Scores greater than 8 are considered positive for an AUD

transferrin (CDT) are commonly used biomarkers. These must be correlated with history and physical examination, as none is sufficiently sensitive to establish the diagnosis alone. Urine ethylglucuronide (EtG), a direct metabolite of alcohol, is frequently used for abstinence monitoring secondary to the extended window for assessment of drinking status (up to 5 days). A positive screening test should prompt further evaluation and referral to psychiatrists and addiction specialists. Figure 7.1 illustrates an algorithm for detection and prevention of AUD.

If an AUD is identified in the preoperative period for an elective procedure, treatment and detoxification should be considered before proceeding. A 4-week period of abstinence (with psychosocial counseling) reduced post-colorectal surgical complications from 74% to 31% [17]. If surgery cannot be postponed, stress inhibition of the AUD patient should be instituted with low-dose morphine (15 µg/kg/h) prior to induction and for 3 postoperative days or postoperative ethanol (0.5 g/kg/day) [8]. Parenteral thiamine should be administered preoperatively and maintained for 5 postoperative days to prevent Wernicke's encephalopathy and Korsakoff's syndrome.

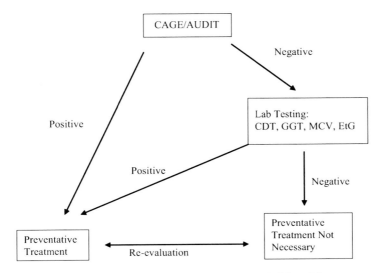

Fig. 7.1 Algorithim for detection and prevention of AUD. Modified from [6]

Early premedication with benzodiazepines should be utilized for the prevention of withdrawal delirium. Clonidine and haloperidol are recommended intraoperatively to prevent postoperative hallucinations and autonomic instability.

Rapid sequence induction is generally advised as patients commonly have delayed gastric emptying and reflux disease. Chronic alcoholics may exhibit an increased requirement for anesthetic agents secondary to cross-tolerance or metabolic tolerance (induced P-450 system). In patients with liver cirrhosis, attention needs to be paid to the increased volume of distribution for medications (secondary to hyopalbumin-emia) and the potential for exaggerated drug responses (decreased hepatic metabolism and decreased plasma protein binding). Most routine medications for the practice of general anesthesia are well tolerated.

Alcohol Withdrawal Syndrome

The development of alcohol withdrawal syndrome (AWS) is the most feared complication in the perioperative or critically ill alcohol-dependent patient. This potentially life-threatening condition occurs in upward of 25% of alcohol-dependent patients. The mortality of this condition depends significantly on proper identification and treatment (15% mortality untreated vs. 2% mortality when treated) [10].

The pathophysiology of AWS is complex and involves a variety of neurotransmitter systems. It can be thought of as the reverse of intoxication, with an increase in excitatory brain systems and a decrease in the activity of inhibitory pathways. Diagnosis of AWS is one of exclusion, requiring the ruling out of other causes of delirium.

Signs and symptoms typically develop in the alcoholic patient within 6–24 h of the last drink. This condition has a range of symptoms and severity. Autonomic hyperactivity appears early, generally peaking in the first 24–48 h. Common symptoms include tremulousness, sweating, nausea, vomiting, anxiety, and agitation. Neuronal excitation also occurs, which if left untreated can progress to grand-mal seizures.

These initial symptoms can be followed by the most serious complication of delirium tremens (DTs). When ethanol is withdrawn, a functional decrease in the inhibitory neurotransmitter GABA is seen along with a functional increase in NMDA receptor. These neurochemical changes result in the symptoms of DTs, characterized by hallucinations (auditory and visual), disorientation, and severe autonomic hyperactivity. Untreated DTs can lead to death secondary to cardiovascular and or respiratory collapse.

Perioperative treatment of AWS is critical and should not be delayed, as this may worsen symptom severity. Individualized therapy and symptom-oriented treatment should be instituted in treating the patient withdrawing from alcohol. Agitation is best treated with benzodiazepines. Benzodiazepines are also useful for seizure prophylaxis and treatment. Hallucinations are best controlled with neuroleptic medications (haloperidol, risperidone, and olanzapine). Alpha-2-agonists (clonidine and dexmedetomidine) are used to treat autonomic instability. Scoring systems exist (CIWA-Ar and the Delirium Detection Score) that can help guide treatment. Preventative treatment in surgical, trauma, and critically ill patients may avoid AWS or decrease its severity. The above medications for treatment are also appropriate for AWS prophylaxis. For an excellent in-depth review of AWS in the surgical and critically ill patient, the reader is referred to Spies and Rommelspacher (1999) [10].

Immunosuppression and the Risk for Postoperative Infections

Patients with AUDs have a three- to fivefold increased rate of infection following surgery over nonalcoholic patients [11]. The most frequent infection is nosocomial pneumonia. Thirty-eight percent of long-term alcoholics, 10% of "social drinkers," and 7% of nonalcoholic patients develop post-surgical pneumonias [12]. Alcohol leads to significant alterations in the immune system, with the most pronounced effect on the cell-mediated component. The clinical relevance of alcohol-induced immunosuppression is an increased infection rate and a theorized increased risk of malignant cell growth. Alcohol dependency is known to cause a significant decrease in delayed-type hypersensitivity (DTH), which has been linked to increased post-surgical infection rates. A decreased DTH represents a disturbance of the T helper 1 cells to T helper 2 cells ratio (Th1/Th2). Spies et al. demonstrated a significant reduction in this ratio among alcoholics and found that a low preoperative (Th1/Th2) ratio was a predictor of postoperative infection and prolonged ICU stay [13].

Chronic alcohol consumption leads to significant perturbations in both proinflammatory and anti-inflammatory cytokine levels, which may impair the immunologic response to surgical stress. Cytotoxic T-cell ratios are abnormally decreased for 5 days postoperatively in the chronic alcoholic, while these same ratios are actually increased postoperatively in the nonalcoholic [13]. This study also found a postoperative decrease in lipopolysaccharide-stimulated interferon-gamma to interleukin-10 (IFN-γ/IL-10) ratio in AUD patients, compared to an increased ratio in non-AUD patients. The decreased cytotoxic T cell 1 to cytotoxic T cell 2 ratio (Tc1/Tc2) and the decreased IFN-γ/IL-10 ratio were found to be predictive of a number of postoperative infections, particularly hospital-acquired pneumonia [14]. Spies et al. recently demonstrated that perioperative inhibition of neuroendocrine–immune regulatory pathways with low-dose ethanol, morphine, and ketoconazole in long-term alcoholic patients preserved T-cell-mediated immunity, decreased postoperative pneumonias, and reduced ICU stay. Another approach to decrease infection rates is via preoperative vaccination. HLA-DR expression is stimulated by vaccine administration and may therefore confer immunity [11].

Hemorrhage and Hematological Complications

Alcohol consumption can lead to pancytopenia. The ethanol metabolite, acetaldehyde, has direct adverse effects on hematopoiesis. Macrocytic anemia is typically present and usually multifactorial in origin (direct ethanol toxicity, iron deficiency, folate deficiency, and chronic disease). AUD patients have up to a fivefold increase in perioperative bleeding complications compared to nonalcoholics, leading to higher perioperative transfusion requirements. AUD patients are known to have prolonged bleeding times, thrombocytopenia, platelet dysfunction, and hyperfibrinolysis and can present with baseline anemia caused by folate and/or iron deficiency secondary to malnutrition. Accompanying liver disease, if severe with compromised synthetic function, can result in significant decreased coagulation factor levels. A recent report by Schoenfeld et al. [15] demonstrated significantly decreased von Willebrand factor levels among AUD patients with a concurrent increase in bleeding on postoperative day one. Although ethanol itself is an anticoagulant, its low-dose use perioperatively (for stress reduction) does not necessarily increase the risk of bleeding episodes in AUD patients. A period of abstinence results in normalization of the bleeding time in surgical patients with AUD [16].

Cardiovascular Complications

Cardiac morbidity is increased up to fivefold in the AUD patient presenting for surgery or in the trauma setting secondary to a number of cardiac complications which arise in the perioperative period. Underlying cardiac disease in this patient population may limit the ability of the heart to meet the increased demands from surgery, leading to increased dysrhythmias and acute coronary syndrome intraoperatively in the immediate postoperative period.

Chronic alcoholic patients are susceptible to a variety of cardiac rhythm disturbances including ventricular fibrillation and atrial dysrhythmias. Catecholamine levels in AUD patients are frequently elevated, and these increased levels often contribute to the development of a hyperdynamic state predisposing the patient to dysrhythmias during times of stress.

The incidence of hypertension increases significantly in the chronic alcoholic, which can lead to the development of significant perioperative complications. Chronic alcohol consumption can cause structural and functional damage of the left ventricle. These changes may increase cardiac adverse events among long-term alcoholic patients with comorbid coronary disease. Patients may be asymptomatic for cardiac disease but often show signs of concentric left ventricular hypertrophy on echocardiography [17]. Alcoholic cardiomyopathy is characterized by a dilated left ventricle and decreased ejection fraction.

Ethanol acts as a negative inotrope on the myocardium and is directly myotoxic, causing myocardial degeneration. Both diastolic and systolic dysfunction occur. The presentation of alcoholic cardiomyopathy is similar and often indistinguishable from idiopathic dilated cardiomyopathy and includes the features of decreased cardiac output. Subclinical cardiac problems are important risk factors for postoperative complications. Those involved in the perioperative care of AUD patients need to be aware of the predisposition to decreased LV function and dysrhythmia, as these conditions adversely affect morbidity and mortality.

A period of preoperative abstinence has been shown to [18] significantly reduce postoperative dysrhythmia on Holter monitoring [16]. Improved LV function and ejection fraction have been demonstrated by a period of abstinence.

Postoperative Treatment Strategies

Treatment of alcoholism requires an interdisciplinary approach. Many current models require the complete abstinence from alcohol and all other substances of abuse. Alcoholics Anonymous and other 12-step recovery programs are at the cornerstone of most recovery programs. Some pharmacologic agents can aid in the recovery process. Disulfiram is used as a deterrent secondary to the accumulation of acetaldehyde and the associated unpleasant effects with concomitant alcohol consumption. Disulfiram decreases plasma clearance of benzodiazepines, possibly leading to augmented or prolonged action. Acamprosate is another option in the treatment of alcohol dependence. It appears to act centrally helping to restore the normal balance of inhibitory and excitatory neurotransmission. Interestingly, the opioid antagonist naltrexone has been shown to substantially reduce alcohol cravings in alcohol-dependent patients. The mechanism of this action remains under investigation.

Because of the high incidence of AUD in the surgical patient population, it is assured that the perioperative healthcare practitioner will encounter patients with AUD. These patients present with a variety of morbidities related to their alcohol consumption. Multiple organ systems are affected. A variety of preoperative, intraoperative, and postoperative considerations must be used to tailor treatments of both the acutely intoxicated and the chronic alcoholic. With a multidisciplinary team approach, focused on the unique perioperative complications associated with AUD, patients can be managed safely and successfully. The perioperative diagnosis of AUD also provides the opportunity to educate and intervene, possibly beginning a patient's journey in the recovery process.

References

1. Grant BF, Dawson DA, Stinson FS, Chou SP, Dufour MC, Pickering RP. The 12-month prevalence and trends in DSM-IV alcohol abuse and dependence: United States, 1991–1992 and 2001–2002. Drug Alcohol Depend. 2004;74:223–34.
2. Dick DM, Beirut LJ. The genetics of alcohol dependence. Curr Psychiatry Rep. 2006;8:151–7.
3. American Psychiatric Association. Diagnostic and statistical manual of mental disorders. 4th ed. Washington, DC: American Psychiatric Association; 1994.
4. Aryal P, Hay D, Senyon C, Slesinger PA. A discrete alcohol pocket involved in GIRK channel activation. Nat Neurosci. 2009;12:988–96.
5. Pletcher MJ, Maselli J, Gonzales R. Uncomplicated alcohol intoxication in the emergency department; an analysis of the National Hospital Ambulatory Medical Care Survey. Am J Med. 2004;117:863.
6. Hines RL, Marschall KE. Psychiatric disease/substance abuse/drug overdose. In: Hines RL, Marschall KE, Stoetling RK, editors. Anesthesia and co-existing disease. 5th ed. Philadelphia, PA: Churchill Livingstone; 2008.
7. Kork F, Neumann T, Spies C. Perioperative managemnt of patients with alcohol, tobacco and drug dependency. Curr Opin Anaesthesiol. 2010;23:384–90.
8. Tonnesen H, Nielsen PR, Lauritzen JB, Moller AM. Smoking and alcohol intervention before surgery: evidence for best practice. Br J Anaesth. 2009;102:297–306.
9. Sorensen LT, Jorgensen T, Kirkeby LT, Skovdal J, Venntis B, Willie-Jorgensen P. Smoking and alcohol abuse are major risk factors for anastomotic leakage in colorectal surgery. Br J Surg. 1999;86:927–31.
10. Spies CD, Rommelspacher H. Alcohol withdrawal in the surgical patient: prevention and treatment. Anesth Analg. 1999;88:946–54.
11. Lau A, von Dossow V, Sander M, MacGuill M, Lanzke N, Spies C. Alcohol use disorder and perioperative immune dysfunction. Anesth Analg. 2009;108:916–20.
12. Spies CD, Nordmann A, Brummer G, Marks C, Conrad C, Berger G, et al. Intensive care unit stay is prolonged in chronic alcoholic men following tumor resection of the upper digestive tract. Acta Anaethesiol Scand. 1996;40:649–56.
13. Spies CD, von Dossow V, Eggers V, Jetschmann G, El-Hilali R, Egert J, et al. Altered cell-mediated immunity and increased postoperative infection rate in long-term alcoholic patients. Anesthesiology. 2004;100:1088–100.
14. Spies C, Eggers V, Szabo G, Lau A, von Dossow V, Schoenfeld H, et al. Intervention at the level of the neurendocrine-immune axis and postoperative pneumonia rate in long-term alcoholics. Am J Respir Crit Care Med. 2006;174:408–14.
15. Schoenfeld H, Perke C, Ziemer S, Huebner R, Schink T, Neuner B, et al. The perioperative von Willebrand Factor activity and facto VIII levels among alcohol use disorder patients undergoing total knee or hip replacement. Subst Use Misuse. 2010;45:1216–29.

16. Tonnesen H, Rosenberg J, Nielsen HJ, Rasmussen V, Hauge C, Pedersen IK, et al. Effect of preoperative abstinence on poor postoperative outcome in alcohol misusers: randomized contolled trial. Br Med J. 1999;318:1311–6.
17. Spies CD, Sander M, Stangl K, Fernandez-Sola J, Preedy V, Rubin E, et al. Effects of alcohol on the heart. Curr Opin Crit Care. 2001;7:337–43.
18. Kip MJ, Neumann T, Jugel C, Kleinwaechter R, Weiss-Gerlach E, Mac Guill M, et al. New strategies to detect alcohol use disorders in the preoperative assessment clinic of a German university hospital. Anesthesiology. 2008;109:171–9.

Chapter 8
Tobacco, the Smoking Gun?

Elizabeth A.M. Frost

Introduction

Because of its highly addictive nature and ready availability, tobacco is probably the most abused drug in our society today. Despite aggressive antismoking campaigns that have resulted in the passage of laws in many states banning smoking in public places, monumental fines against the tobacco companies, and dramatic increases in taxation, abuse of tobacco remains the primary preventable cause of morbidity and mortality in the United States [1].

The Plant, Tobacco, and Nicotine

Tobacco is an agricultural product processed from the leaves of plants in the genus *Nicotiana*, named after Jean Nicot, the French ambassador to Portugal, who in 1559 sent it as a medicine to the court of Catherine de Medici [2]. The lady became an early convert. Tobacco can be consumed, used as an organic pesticide and, in the form of nicotine tartrate, it is used in some medicines. It is most commonly used as a recreational drug and is a valuable cash crop for countries such as Cuba, China, and United States. In consumption, it is mostly smoked, chewed, snuffed, or made into a paste that can be sucked against the gum. Because of the addictive properties of nicotine, tolerance and dependence develop quickly. Absorption quantity, frequency, and speed of consumption are believed to be directly related to biological strength of nicotine dependence, addiction, and tolerance. Tobacco use is practiced by some 1.1 billion people worldwide and up to 1/3 of the adult population.

E.A.M. Frost (✉)
Department of Anesthesiology, Mount Sinai School of Medicine, New York, NY, USA
e-mail: elzfrost@aol.com

E.O. Bryson and E.A.M. Frost (eds.), *Perioperative Addiction:*
Clinical Management of the Addicted Patient, DOI 10.1007/978-1-4614-0170-4_8,
© Springer Science+Business Media, LLC 2012

The World Health Organization (WHO) reports it to be the leading preventable cause of death and estimates that it currently causes 5.4 million deaths per year [3]. Rates of smoking have leveled off or declined in developed countries; however, they continue to rise in many developing countries and especially in Middle-Eastern countries. As of 2008, approximately 1 in 5 US adults (46 million) was a regular cigarette smoker, a significant decrease from the peak in 1964 when 40% of Americans smoked and the 28% prevalence of smoking in 1988; but little changed from the figure of 21.6% quoted as a result of a survey conducted by the Center for Disease Control and Prevention in 2003 (50 million adults who smoked >100 cigarettes in their lifetime or smoked daily) [4].

Tobacco is cultivated similarly to other agricultural products. Seeds are sown in cold frames or hotbeds to prevent insect attacks, and then transplanted to fields. It is an annual crop, harvested mechanically or by hand. After harvest, tobacco is stored for curing, allowing for the slow oxidation and degradation of carotenoids, which allows the product to take on properties that are usually attributed to the "smoothness" of the smoke (Fig. 8.1). It is then packed into its various forms of consumption, such as cigars, cigarettes, chewing tobacco, and pastes.

History

The Spanish word "*tabaco*" is thought to have its origin in the Arawakan language, particularly, in the Taino language of the Caribbean [5]. In Taino, it was said to refer either to a roll of tobacco leaves (according to Bartolome de Las Casas, 1552), or to the *tabago*, a kind of Y-shaped pipe for sniffing tobacco smoke (according to Oviedo, with the leaves themselves being referred to as *cohiba*). However, similar words in Spanish and Italian were commonly used from 1410 to define medicinal herbs, originating from the Arabic *tabbaq*, a word reportedly dating to the ninth century, as a name for various herbs.

It is believed that tobacco began growing in North America about 8 millennia ago. It was thought to be a cure all and was used to dress wounds as well as a pain-killer. Chewing the leaves was said to relieve toothache. It had already long been used in the Americas when Christopher Columbus was offered dried tobacco leaves as a gift from the American Indians on October 15, 1492. These European settlers introduced the practice of smoking to Europe, where it became popular as a means to cure cancer among many other maladies. However, one of the first to note that it was difficult to stop smoking was Sir Francis Bacon in 1610. By 1632, it was declared illegal to smoke in public in Massachusetts, due more to moral beliefs than health concerns. The Pierre Lorillard Company was established in New York City to process tobacco, cigars, and snuff in 1760 and remains the oldest tobacco company in the US. Table 8.1 gives a short account of the history of tobacco.

Known to be a hallucinogen, Native Americans did not use the drug recreationally. Instead, it was often consumed as an entheogen, a sacred drug used only on designated occasions. Among some tribes, this practice meant that only experienced

Fig. 8.1 (**a**) Tobacco after it is cured and in its plant form. From http://en.wikipedia.org/wiki/File:DunhillEarly-MorningPipeMurrays.jpg. (**b**) Tobacco in its plant form. From http://en.wikipedia.org/wiki/File:Native_American_tobacco_flower.jpg

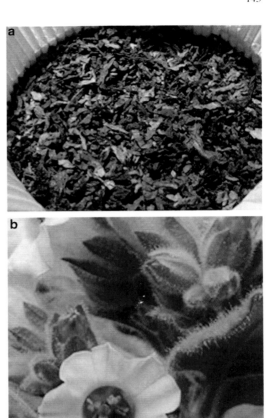

shamans or medicine men would smoke tobacco. Eastern North American tribes carried large amounts of the herb in pouches as a readily accepted trade item, and often smoked it in pipes, either in defined sacred ceremonies, or to seal a bargain [6]. They smoked at such occasions in all stages of life, even in childhood. It was believed that tobacco is a gift from the Creator and that the exhaled tobacco smoke carries one's thoughts and prayers to heaven. The European popularization (Fig. 8.2) led to the development of the southern economy of the United States until it gave way to cotton. Following the American Civil War, a change in demand and a change in labor force and the invention of an automated cigarette machine by James

Table 8.1 The history of tobacco

Year	Event	Year	Event
6000 BC	Tobacco growing in the Americas	1923	Camel controls 45% of market
1BC	American Indians use tobacco for religious and medicinal reasons	1923	Phillip Morris: Marlboro "Mild as May" for women
1492	Europeans arrive, Tobacco to Europe	1923	Lucky Strike for women
1571	Dr Nicolas Monaredes, wrote book, "Tobacco cures 36 illnesses"	1939	American Tobacco Company; Pall Mall. Largest company in USA
1588	Thomas Harriett of Virginia: daily dose of tobacco essential	1939–1945	WW II; sales at all-time high Cigarettes free to soldiers
1600s	Tobacco as money	1950s	Lung cancer?
1610	Tobacco dangerous?	1952	P Lorillard; Kent
1632	Illegal to smoke publically in MA	1953	EL Wynders; tar on mice causes tumors
1760	P. Lorillard established	1954	Salem: filter-tipped menthol cigarettes.
1776	Tobacco helps finance the Revolution	1964	Surgeon General's report, "Smoking and Health"
1826	Nicotine discovered	1965	No TV ads in the UK
1836	Samuel Green…tobacco is an insecticide	1966	Health warnings on packages
1847	Phillip Morris established	1969	Companies buy into beer and aluminum (diversification)
1849	JE Liggett established	1971	No TV ads in the US
1847	RJ Reynolds established	1977	National Great American Smokeout
1900	Cigarettes major tobacco product	1980s	Start of many lawsuits
1902	Phillip Morris established in NY, Marlboro	1982	Evidence that secondhand smoke kills
1913	RJ Reynolds, Camel	1987	No smoking on airline flights
1914–1918	WW II "The soldier's smoke"	1980s–1990s	Marketing outside the US expanded. Marlboro #1 product worldwide

Adapted from: http://academic.udayton.edu/health/syllabi/tobacco/history.htm accessed 11/09/2010

Bonsack allowed for the development of the industry. The new product quickly led to the growth of tobacco companies, until the scientific controversy of the mid-1900s.

Following the scientific revelations of the mid-1900s, tobacco became condemned as a health hazard and eventually became identified as a cause for cancer, as well as other respiratory and circulatory diseases. The Tobacco Master Settlement Agreement (MSA) settled the lawsuit in exchange for a combination of yearly payments to the states and voluntary restrictions on advertising and marketing of tobacco

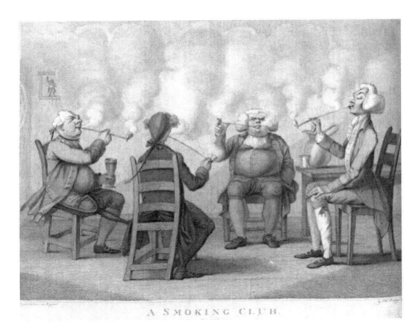

Fig. 8.2 An illustration of the important social position of tobacco use in the UK. From http://en.wikipedia.org/wiki/File:A_Smoking_Club.jpeg

products. In the 1970s, Brown and Williamson cross-bred a strain of tobacco to produce Y1. This strain of tobacco contained an unusually high amount of nicotine, nearly doubling its content from 3.2–3.5% to 6.5%. In the 1990s, the Food and Drug Administration (FDA) were prompted to use this strain as evidence that tobacco companies were intentionally manipulating the nicotine content of cigarettes.

In 2003, in response to the growth of tobacco use in developing countries, the World Health Organization (WHO) successfully rallied 168 countries to sign the Framework Convention on Tobacco Control [7]. The Convention (or Conference of the Parties) was designed to push for effective legislation and its enforcement in all countries to reduce the harmful effects of tobacco. Tobacco cessation products were developed. The Family Smoking and Prevention and Tobacco Control Act was signed in June 2009 and granted the Food and Drug Administration extensive authority to regulate tobacco products. The tobacco industry countered by filing suit in August 2009, challenging the constitutionality of the advertising and promotion restrictions of the law. Legal arguments continue as tobacco continues to wreak havoc not only on the users but on those around them by secondhand smoke [8]. The fourth session of the Conference of the Parties (now with 171 members) was held in November 2010 in Punta del Este, Uruguay.

On July 22, 2010, a law was introduced that prohibited the tobacco industry from distributing or introducing into the US market any tobacco products for which the labeling or advertising contained the descriptors "light," "low," or "mild," or any similar word, irrespective of the date of manufacture. The ruling stems from the conclusions made by the Center for Disease Control that there is no convincing evidence to indicate that low-yield cigarettes are safe. No cigarette design changes have resulted in a decrease in the diseases caused by smoking or consuming of tobacco.

Components of Tobacco

Chemical analysis of tobacco smoke has indicated some 4,000 compounds [9] including 43 proven carcinogenic compounds and 400 other toxins such as nicotine, tar, carbon monoxide, polynuclear aromatic hydrocarbons, B-naphthylanine, benzopyrene, nitrosamines, vinyl chloride, trace metals, hydrogen cyanide, arsenic, and DDT to name a few. Tumor accelerators include indole and carbazole. Ciliotoxins such as ammonia and formaldehyde are not removed by filters, which are made primarily of cellulose actate tow and do reduce the amount of tar and nicotine by 40–50% The components of mainstream cigarette smoke can be separated into two phases by passing it through a glass-fiber filter that retains nearly all particulate matter >0.1 μm in diameter. Material retained in the filter is known as the tar or particulate phase. Material that passes through the filter is referred to as the gas phase and represents about 90–95% of the total weight of mainstream smoke. Known toxins and carcinogens have been identified in both the particulate and gas phases. These components may act directly on the mucosal surfaces of the mouth, nose, pharynx, and tracheobronchial tree, or they may be absorbed to the blood stream, or dissolved in saliva and then swallowed.

Another formulation of tobacco is chewing tobacco, which is a common type of smokeless tobacco. Smokeless tobacco products consist of tobacco or a tobacco blend that can be chewed, sucked on, or sniffed, rather than smoked.

There are many types of smokeless tobacco products around the world. In the United States, the main types of smokeless tobacco include:

- Chewing tobacco: Loose tobacco leaves that are sweetened and packaged in pouches. A wad of the tobacco is placed between the cheek and gum and held there, sometimes for hours at a time. Other names include chew and chaw. Usually, the juices are spat out, but as addiction takes hold, juices are swallowed.
- Plug: Chewing tobacco is pressed into a brick shape, often with the help of syrup, such as molasses, which also sweetens the tobacco. A piece of the plug is bitten off and held it between the cheek and gum. The tobacco juices should be spat out.
- Twist: Flavored chewing tobacco is braided and twisted into rope-like strands and held between the cheek and gum.
- Snuff: Finely ground or shredded tobacco leaves are available in dry or moist forms and packaged in tins or tea bag-like pouches. A pinch of snuff is placed between the lower lip and gum or cheek and gum. Dry forms of snuff can be sniffed up the nose. Using snuff is also called dipping. Tobacco juices are spat out or swallowed.

- Snus: A smokeless, spitless tobacco product that originated in Sweden. Snus comes in a pouch that is placed between the upper lip and gum for about a half-hour and then discarded.
- Dissolvable tobacco products: Pieces of compressed powdered tobacco, similar to small hard candies, dissolve in the mouth and are also named tobacco lozenges.

While the available evidence shows that smokeless tobacco may be less dangerous than cigarettes are, long-term use of chewing tobacco and other smokeless tobacco products can cause serious health problems as they contain about 30 cancer-causing substances. Like cigarettes, smokeless tobacco also contains nicotine, which as noted is highly addictive. Indeed, more nicotine may be absorbed if juices are all swallowed and the tobacco is left for prolonged periods of time. Moreover, the addition of sugars and the increased risk of diabetes caused by nicotine lead to more complications.

Yet still other contaminants of tobacco may be harmful. Tobacco production requires the use of a large amount of pesticides. Tobacco companies recommend up to 16 separate applications of pesticides between planting the seeds in greenhouses and transplanting the young plans to the field. Pesticide use has been increased by the desire to produce larger crops in a shorter time because of the decreasing market value of tobacco. Pesticides often harm tobacco farmers, unaware of proper safety protocol for working with these chemicals. Tobacco is a crop that leeches nutrients, such as phosphorus, nitrogen, and potassium, from the soil at a rate higher than any other major crops, leading to dependence on fertilizers and environmental damage.

Both pesticides and fertilizers end up in the soil, the waterway, and subsequently the food chain. As child labor is often used in the tobacco industry, this early exposure to pesticides may increase a child's life long risk of cancer as well as cause central nervous and immune system damage.

Nicotine

Nicotine constitutes ~0.6–3.0% of the dry weight of tobacco, with biosynthesis taking place in the roots and accumulation occurring in the leaves [10]. It functions as an antiherbivore chemical with particular specificity to insects; therefore, nicotine was once used as an insecticide, and currently nicotine analogs such as imidacloprid continue to be used. Nicotine is also found in small amounts in other Solanaceae species such as eggplant and tomato.

In low concentrations (on average, cigarette yields about 1 mg of absorbed nicotine), nicotine acts as a stimulant and is the factor mainly responsible for the dependence-forming properties of tobacco smoking. According to the American Heart Association, nicotine addiction has historically been one of the hardest addictions to break, while the pharmacological and behavioral characteristics that determine tobacco addiction are similar to those that determine addiction to drugs such as heroin and cocaine. Nicotine content in cigarettes has slowly increased over the years, and one study found that there was an average increase of 1.6% per year between the years of 1998 and 2005 for all major market categories of cigarettes [11].

Nicotine crosses the blood–brain barrier about seven seconds after inhalation. The half-life of nicotine in the body is around two hours [12]. The amount of nicotine absorbed depends on many factors, including the type of tobacco, whether the smoke is inhaled, and whether a filter is used. For chewing tobacco, dipping tobacco, snus, and snuff, which are held in the mouth between the lip and gum, or taken in the nose, the amount released into the body tends to be much greater than when tobacco is smoked. Nicotine is metabolized in the liver by cytochrome P450 enzymes (mostly CYP2A6 and also by CYP2B6). A major metabolite is cotinine, which has a half-life of about 18 h. Glucuronidation and oxidative metabolism of nicotine to cotinine are both inhibited by menthol, an additive to mentholated cigarettes, thus increasing the half-life of nicotine in vivo [13]. Human CYP2B6 is found at higher levels in the brain of smokers and 7-day nicotine treatment induced rat brain CYP2B while not altering liver CYP2B. A 7-day nicotine treatment in rats resulted in an induction of CYP2B protein and in vivo activity for up to 24 h, suggesting local drug metabolism by brain CYP2B [14]. The authors surmise that humans or animals exposed to nicotine may have altered therapeutic drug response, brain levels of neurotransmitters, and/or neurotoxicity.

Pharmacodynamics

Nicotine acts on nicotinic acetylcholine receptors, specifically the ganglion-type nicotinic receptor in the adrenal medulla and other sites and also at a specific receptor within the central nervous system (CNS) to increase the levels of several neurotransmitters. Even in small concentrations, nicotine can increase the activity of these receptors. It is thought that increased levels of dopamine in the reward circuits of the brain are responsible for the euphoria and relaxation and eventual addiction caused by nicotine consumption. Nicotine has a higher affinity for acetylcholine receptors in the brain than those in skeletal muscle, though at toxic doses it can induce contractions and respiratory paralysis [15]. Nicotine's selectivity is thought to be due to a particular amino acid difference in these receptor subtypes [16].

Tobacco smoke contains the monoamine oxidase inhibitors (MAO) harman, norharman, anabasine, anatabine, and nornicotine [17]. These compounds significantly decrease MAO activity in smokers [17, 18]. MAO enzymes break down monoaminergic neurotransmitters such as dopamine, norepinephrine, and serotonin.

Chronic nicotine exposure via tobacco smoking upregulates alpha4beta2 and 8nAChR in the cerebellum and brainstem regions but not in habenulopeduncular structures [19–21]. Alpha4beta2 and alpha6beta2 receptors, present in the ventral tegmental area, play a crucial role in mediating the reinforcement effects of nicotine [22].

Nicotine also activates the sympathetic nervous system via splanchnic nerves to the adrenal medulla [23]. Acetylcholine released by preganglionic sympathetic fibers of these nerves acts on nicotinic acetylcholine receptors, causing the release of epinephrine (and norepinephrine). Nicotine also has an affinity for melanin-containing tissues due to its precursor function in melanin synthesis or its irreversible binding to melanin, which may explain the increased nicotine dependence and lower smoking cessation rates in darker pigmented individuals [24].

By binding to ganglion-type nicotinic receptors in the adrenal medulla, nicotine increases cell depolarization and an influx of calcium through voltage-gated calcium channels. Calcium triggers the exocytosis of chromaffin granules and thus the release of epinephrine (and norepinephrine). The result is tachycardia, hypertension, hyperglycemia, and hyperpnea.

Psychoactive Effects

Smokers often report that cigarettes help relieve feelings of stress. However, the stress levels of adult smokers are slightly higher than those of nonsmokers. Adolescent smokers report increasing levels of stress as they develop regular patterns of smoking, and smoking cessation reduces stress. In fact, nicotine dependency seems to exacerbate stress, confirmed in the daily mood patterns described by smokers, with normal moods during smoking and worsening moods between cigarettes. Thus, the apparent relaxant effect of smoking only reflects the reversal of the tension and irritability that develop during nicotine depletion [25].

As noted, nicotine stimulates the release of many chemical messengers including acetylcholine, norepinephrine, epinephrine, vasopressin, arginine, dopamine, autocrine agents, and beta-endorphin. Nicotine appears to enhance concentration and memory due to the increase of acetylcholine [26]. It also appears to increase alertness due to the increase of norepinephrine. Pain may be reduced by increases of acetylcholine and beta-endorphin, although a recent report indicated that smokers experienced higher levels of pain more frequently following ambulatory, surgery and a smoking history should be considered a risk factor for acute postoperative pain [27]. While this finding might be due to the requirement of smoking cessation during a hospital experience and thus sudden withdrawal of nicotine, the authors noted increased pain even after discharge when presumably smoking could be restarted. Anxiety is reduced by the increase of beta-endorphin.

At low doses (achieved by short quick puffs), nicotine potently enhances the actions of norepinephrine and dopamine, causing a stimulant effect. At higher doses (deep inhalation), nicotine enhances the effect of serotonin and opiate activity, producing a calming, pain-killing effect. Nicotine is unique in comparison to most drugs, as its profile changes from stimulant to sedative/painkiller in increasing dosages and use.

Technically, nicotine is not significantly addictive, as nicotine administered alone does not produce significant reinforcing properties [28]. However, only after coadministration with an MAOI, such as those found in tobacco, nicotine produces significant behavioral sensitization, with effects similar to amphetamine [29]. This action may explain why application of nicotine patches may help in relief of smoking addiction. Also, dopamine is one of the key neurotransmitters actively involved in the reward circuitry in the brain. Nicotine stimulates dopamine and can then become a chemical with intense addictive qualities. Like other physically addictive drugs, nicotine withdrawal causes downregulation of the production of dopamine and other stimulatory neurotransmitters. In addition, the sensitivity of nicotinic acetylcholine receptors decreases. To compensate, the brain upregulates the number of receptors, convoluting its regulatory effects with mechanisms meant to counteract other compensatory mechanisms. An example is the increase in norepinephrine, one of the successors to dopamine, which inhibit reuptake of the glutamate receptors, used for memory and cognition. The net effect is an increase in reward pathway sensitivity, opposite to other drugs of abuse such as cocaine and heroin, which reduce reward pathway sensitivity [30]. This neuronal brain alteration persists for months after administration ceases. Nicotine also has the potential to cause dependence in many animals other than humans, assuming they were to consume it. Yet another study found that nicotine exposure in adolescent mice retards the growth of the dopamine system, thus increasing the risk of substance abuse during adolescence [31].

Smoking Cessation

Several vaccination protocols have been developed. The principle is that if an antibody is attached to a nicotine molecule, it will be prevented from diffusing through the capillaries, thus making it less likely to affect the brain by binding to nicotinic acetylcholine receptors. Vaccines include attaching the nicotine molecule to a hapten such as Keyhole limpet hemocyanin or a safe modified bacterial toxin to elicit an active immune response. Often it is added with bovine serum albumin. Additionally, because of concerns with the unique immune systems of individuals being liable to produce antibodies against endogenous hormones and over-the-counter drugs, monoclonal antibodies have been developed for short-term passive immune protection [32]. Half-lives vary from hours to weeks and depend on an ability to resist degradation from pinocytosis by epithelial cells.

Other means to decrease smoking have emphasized the similar pathways to addiction shared by the opiates. The Chicago Stop Smoking Research Project at the University of Chicago studied whether naltrexone could be used as an aid to quit smoking. The researchers discovered that naltrexone improved smoking cessation rates in women by fifty percent but showed no improvement for men [33].

Noting that surgery might present a teachable moment, several studies have been undertaken to assess the benefit of referring patients preoperatively to telephone quitlines [34–36]. While many of these reports are on small groups, there is benefit in advising patients on the adverse effects of tobacco and referring them for further help, especially by facilitating referral of smokers for counseling and follow-up. Indeed, the preanesthetic assessment interview has been deemed the "teachable moment."

Systemic Effects of Tobacco

The risks associated with tobacco use include diseases affecting the heart and lungs, with smoking being a major risk factor for heart attacks, strokes, chronic obstructive pulmonary disease (COPD), emphysema, and cancer (particularly lung and cancers of the larynx and mouth). The United States Centers for Disease Control and Prevention has described tobacco use as "the single most important preventable risk to human health in developed countries and an important cause of premature death worldwide." A recent review of 635,265 patients from the American College of Surgeons National Surgical Quality Improvement Program identified 103,795 smokers [37]. Of these 82,304 were matched with nonsmoker controls. Those who smoked pipes or chewed tobacco were excluded. Smokers were 38% more likely to die than nonsmokers. They also had a significant increase in the risk of pneumonia (209%), unplanned intubation (89%) and mechanical ventilation (53%), myocardial infarction (80%), and stroke (73%).The incidence of superficial and deep infections and septic shock was also all significantly increased. Each relative 10 pack years increase was associated with increased odds of 4%, with a disproportionate increase after 10 pack years. Tobacco affects almost all systems of the body to varying degrees.

Pulmonary System

Chronic obstructive pulmonary disease is ranked as the fourth leading cause of death in the United States [38]. Only a small percentage of smokers develop COPD, but cigarette smoking remains the major cause of COPD mortality. The risk of death is directly proportional to the amount and duration of smoking [1]. The detrimental effects of tobacco on the structure and function of the lungs are summarized in Table 8.2.

Airway hyperresponsiveness is defined as the sensitivity of the bronchi and trachea to pharmacologic and physical stimuli that induce bronchoconstriction in some or all individuals. Stimuli that induce this hyperreactivity include aerosols of histamine or cholinergic agents, hyperventilation, cold or dry air, and exercise. Cigarette smoking heightens this hyperreactivity and accelerates decline in pulmonary function as measured by forced expiratory volume in 1 s (FEV_1). Possible mechanisms for the development of this effect of smoking include:

- Smoking associated reduction in prechallenge levels of pulmonary function
- Chronic airway inflammation
- Airway epithelial damage increasing epithelial permeability and impairing other epithelial functions [39]

Moreover, cigarette smoking increases protease enzyme action and decreases anti-protease activity. The numbers of macrophages and neutrophils that secrete various proteases including elastase, collagenase, and proteinase 3 in the bronchoalveolar lavage of smokers are increased [38]. These proteolytic enzymes act on connective

Table 8.2 Pathophysiologic effects of smoking

Peripheral airway	Inflammation and atrophy
	Goblet cell metaplasia and increased secretions
	Squamous metaplasia
	Smooth muscle hypertrophy
	Peribronchial hyperplasia
	Increased hyperresponsiveness
Central airway	Ciliary loss
	Mucus gland hyperplasia
	Squamous hyperplasia, carcinoma in situ, and bronchogenic permeability
Alveoli and capillaries	Distruction of peribronchial alveoli
	Loss of small arteries
	Increased macrophages and neutrophils
	Bronchoalveolar lavage fluid abnormalities
Immune function	Increased leukocyte count
	Elevation in peripheral eosinophils
	Serum IgE increased, elevated IgA and IgG
	Lower skin allergy test reactivity
	Reduced immune response to inhaled antigens

Adapted from Sherman CB. The health consequences of cigarette smoking. Pulmonary diseases. Med Clin North Am. 1992;76:357–75

tissues including collagen and elastin and are normally kept in check by antiproteases such as a_1 antitrypsin and a_2 macrogobulin. However, smoke-induced oxidants in the lungs decrease antiprotease activity leading to alveolar destruction and airflow obstruction.

Clinically, current smokers have a higher prevalence of chronic cough, phlegm production, wheeze, and dyspnea than nonsmokers have. Compounding these respiratory abnormalities is impaired clearance of secretions secondary to decreased ciliary function. Using technetium 99m-labeled macroaggregated albumin, Konrad et al. showed that during general anesthesia, smokers have a slower bronchial mucus transport than do nonsmokers, which may lead to more postoperative complications [40]. Even asymptomatic smokers with grossly normal spirometry present with abnormalities in small airway function when tested by the single-breath nitrogen test. They demonstrate increased closing volume and closing capacity and also an increase in postoperative complications such as atelectasis, hypoxic episodes, and pneumonia. Other changes include decreased diffusing capacity (6–20% lower than in age-matched nonsmokers) and altered pulmonary surfactant [38]. Also, an observational cohort study indicated increased susceptibility to influenza infection among persons exposed to tobacco smoke [41]. Live attenuated influenza virus was innoculated into the noses of active smokers, nonsmokers exposed to secondhand smoke, and unexposed controls. Measurable inflammatory and antiviral responses were found in the unexposed control group but these responses were suppressed in both of the other groups, more so in the active smokers, suggesting increased susceptibility to influenza among persons exposed to tobacco smoke.

Table 8.3 Effects of cigarette smoking on the cardiovascular system

Pathologic results	Smooth muscle cell proliferation
	Atherosclerosis progression
	Cardiomyopathy
	Intimal damage
Physiologic effects	Tachycardia, hypertension, and peripheral vasoconstriction
	Myocardial demand increased and oxygen delivery reduced
	Threshold for ventricular fibrillation decreased
	Dysrhythmias
	Impaired coronary artery flow regulation (vasoconstriction)
Hematologic consequences	Release of platelet factors that activate atherosclerosis
	Viscosity increased
	Thromboxane release and platelet aggregation
	Prostacyclin release decreased
	Red cell deformities
	Thrombosis increased
Metabolic effects	Altered metabolism of drugs
	Serum free fatty acids and LDL cholesterol increased
	Serum HDL cholesterol increased
	Growth hormone, cortisol, glucose, lactate, and pyruvate increased; estrogen decreased

Cardiovascular System

Smoking is a major cause for generalized atherosclerosis, risk factors for coronary artery disease, cerebrovascular disease, peripheral vascular disease, and aortic aneurysms. Injury to the vascular intima, probably directly caused by nicotine, can initiate the development of atherosclerosis in young people with no other risk factors. In others, smoking accelerates the progression of the disease. Carbon monoxide increases smooth muscle cell proliferation via derived platelet growth factor, released when platelets adhere to the site of intimal injury and can increase the effects of nicotine and lead to cardiomyopathy. Cigarette smoking is synergistic with other risk factors, particularly high levels of low-density lipoprotein cholesterol and low levels of low-density cholesterol [42]. Acute physiologic effects include sympathetic stimulation resulting in hypertension and tachycardia and increased carboxyhemoglobin levels. Over time, hypertension may become sustained. Contributing to the effects on the cardiovascular system are the acute and chronic effects of smoking on the hematologic and metabolic systems. Table 8.3 summarizes some of the effects of smoking on the cardiovascular system.

Atherosclerosis is a complex process involving endothelial cell injury, endothelial cell proliferation, macrophage activity, foam cell formation, lipid accumulation, and plaque formation. As can be seen from the table, the hematologic and metabolic changes caused by tobacco and nicotine all combine to accelerate the process of atherosclerosis.

While nicotine is probably the prime initiator of atherosclerosis, carbon monoxide (CO) which constitutes about 3–6% of tobacco smoke and is produced by incomplete combustion of the organic material found in cigarettes, also has a detrimental effect. The affinity of hemoglobin for CO is 200 times greater than that for oxygen. This property results in elevated levels of carboxyhemoglobin up to 15% and reduces the oxygen carrying capacity of blood. CO shifts the oxyhemoglobin dissociation curve to the left, making it more difficult for hemoglobin to release oxygen to the tissues. CO may also have weak direct negative inotropic cardiac effects. The combined effect of nicotine and CO is to increase myocardial oxygen demand and reduce oxygen delivery. Peripheral resistance is increased, including that of the coronary vessels. The imbalance thus caused may be further compounded by polycythemia and increased blood viscosity caused by chronic hypoxia.

Smoking reduces the effects of antianginal medications in patients with chronic stable angina and decreases the effects of thrombolytic therapy [43]. Moreover, angina may occur at lower work levels and be more intense after smoking in patients who already have coronary artery disease.

An association between cerebral aneurysms and smoking has long been recognized as approximately 66% of patients who present with ruptured aneurysms are presently smoking [44]. Smoking may be the most modifiable risk factor for the formation and rupture of intracranial aneurysms. Other studies have found evidence for a gene–environment interaction with smoking and aneurysm rupture [45]. The cause may be related to repeated episodes of hypoxia that weakens the cerebral vasculature, especially at junctions where aneurysms are most likely to develop.

As noted, hematologic changes are contributors to the cardiovascular changes. Smoking enhances platelet aggregation by reducing the endothelial production of prostacyclin, an inhibitor of platelet aggregation. Further, smoking also increases production of the vasoconstrictor thromboxane, a platelet agonist. Other effects that contribute to thrombus formation include increased plasma viscosity and fibrinogen levels, decreased red cell deformability and plasminogen levels, and a partial inhibition of the effects of aspirin on platelets. Postoperatively, these effects may affect the results of surgery such as revascularization procedures, as graft patency might be limited. A higher proportion of limb loss in femoral popliteal bypass has been reported in smokers; also there was a 10 times higher risk for flap necrosis after face-lift in smokers over nonsmokers [46, 47].

Drug Metabolism

Smoking can affect the pharmacokinetics and pharmacodynamics of many drugs. Some components of tobacco smoke cause hepatic enzyme induction and thus increase the metabolism of certain drugs such as pentazocine, heparin, warfarin, theophylline, and phenylbutazone, which would then have to be given in higher doses. Propranolol and pindolol are not affected by pharmacokinetics, but the direct effects of nicotine may interfere with their pharmacodynamic action. Smoking is associated with decreased absorption of subcutaneous insulin and the dose should be adjusted.

Perioperative Management

Complete abstinence from tobacco intake for several weeks prior to surgery would be ideal to allow regeneration of lung function but is rarely possible. Times required for regeneration of various functions are approximated in Table 8.4.

A carboxyhemoglobin level of 15% can reduce the availability of oxygen by up to 25%, and while this level may not be significant in asymptomatic patients, it may present a considerable risk for patients with coronary artery disease in whom a favorable myocardial balance is critical. These patients should be advised to refrain from smoking for at least 24 h prior to surgery. While pulmonary function tests are not usually helpful in predicting postoperative pulmonary events or the need for mechanical ventilation, a low preoperative oxygen room air saturation or low partial pressure of arterial oxygen may identify patients at higher risk. Other important factors in determining postoperative pulmonary complications include the site and duration of the surgical procedure and the amount of blood lost. Preoperative pulmonary therapy might be useful, if only to acquaint the patient with the several tools that may be used in the postoperative period to maintain oxygenation.

Clinical studies suggest that smoking is a risk factor in the progression of kidney disease, especially diabetic nephropathy. Nicotine promotes mesangial cell proliferation and fibronectin production and smoking may promote the progression of diabetic nephropathy by increasing the expression of profibrotic cytokines, such as transforming growth factor, and the extracellular matrix proteins fibronectin and collagen IV [48]. Thus, evaluation of kidney function and glycemic status, especially in diabetic patients is important in the smoker as is limitation of the use or doses of drugs dependent on the kidney for excretion. Also, the progression and risk of acquisition of HIV is increased by tobacco smoking [49]. HIV-infected individuals are three times more likely to smoke than the uninfected general population. There appears to be a potent enhancing effect of aqueous tobacco smoke extract on HIV infectivity that is nicotine dependent. These patients also require special perioperative consideration.

Examination of the airway is a prerequisite of all anesthetic encounters. Nicotine is a significant risk factor for the development and progression of periodontal disease [50]. The drug probably acts by decreasing gingival blood flow, increasing cytokine production, and adversely affecting the immune system to cause loosening of teeth and actual tooth loss. Chewing tobacco also causes tooth decay due to the

Table 8.4 Estimated times for return of lung function after quitting smoking

Elimination of nicotine	12 h
Elimination of carboxyhemoglobin	1–3 days
Return of ciliary function	6–7 days
Decrease of sputum production	6–8 weeks
Normalization of immune system	>8 weeks

high sugar content. Oral cancers and leukoplakia may interfere with intubation or oral airway placement due to bleeding or ulceration. Additional exposure to ethanol appears to enhance adverse changes in the buccal mucosa in vitro in more than an additive effect [51].

A hyperactive airway is a major cause of postoperative complications. Cholinergic drugs or drugs that cause histamine release may trigger bronchospasm. Even hyperventilation prior to intubation or the presence of an endotracheal tube or supraglottic airway can result in bronchospasm. Smokers, with or without a history of reactive airway disease, may be very sensitive to any airway manipulation. While some aerosols may provoke airway spasm, premedication with albuterol or with combined coricosteriods and salbutamol have been shown to reduce the possibility of intubation-evoked bronchospasm [52]. Airway reactivity may also be decreased by intravenous lidocaine (1 mg/kg).

Glycopyrrolate is probably the best choice to reduce the copious secretions associated with smoking because of its minimal cardiovascular effects. The addition of humidified fresh gas through the breathing circuit may be helpful though problems may still occur from occlusion by thick mucus secretions. High inspiratory pressures intraoperatively should raise the suspicion for a mucus plug.

The preference of anesthetic technique depends on the site of surgery and patient choice. Patients are often very anxious as nicotine levels decrease and antianxiolytics are usually indicated. If regional or neuraxial techniques are possible, they may be preferable to general anesthesia, as the risk of bronchospasm is avoided. High spinal levels (above T6), which may interfere with the ability to cough postoperatively, should also be avoided. Adequate postoperative pain therapy is critical for the patient who has undergone major surgery. While narcotics remain the mainstay for analgesia, respiratory depression is a concern, as smokers must depend on the ability to deep breathe and cough to clear secretions. Pain associated with attempts to breathe could decrease excursion and result in atelectasis and pneumonia. Chest physiotherapy must be initiated early. Epidural analgesia with local anesthetics is a good alternative to intravenous narcotics. Humidification of oxygen postoperatively is essential and ventilatory support with continuous positive pressure should be available.

Conclusion

Although smoking is declining in this country, it remains a major cause of morbidity and mortality. There are widespread physiologic and pathologic effects, especially as regards the cardiorespiratory systems. Abstinence from smoking for some days before surgery would mitigate the complications but such actions are not always obtainable. Perioperative care is determined in part by the magnitude of the alterations caused by smoking, the site and duration of surgery, and the coexistence of medical issues.

References

1. US Department of Health and Human Services. The health consequences of smoking: a report of the Surgeon General. Atlanta, GA: US Department of Health and Human Services, CDC; 2004.
2. Taylor RB. White coat tales – medicine's heroes, heritage and misadventures. New York: Springer; 2007. p. 96.
3. WHO Report on the global tobacco epidemic, 2008 (foreword and summary). World Health Organization; 2008.
4. Dube SR, Asman K, Malarcher A, et al. Cigarette smoking among adults and trends in smoking cessation. United States 2008. Centers for Disease Control and Prevention. MMWR Morb Mortal Wkly Rep. 2009;58(44):1227–32.
5. Online Etymological Dictionary. http://www.etymonline.com/index.php?term=tobacco.
6. Heckewelder JGE. History, manners and customs of the Indian nations who once inhabited Pennsylvania. Westminster MD: Heritage Books. p. 149, ISBN 1556134118.
7. WHO/WHO Framework Convention on Tobacco Control (WHO FCTC) WHO.int. http://www.who.int/fctc/en/index.html. Accessed 6 Nov 2010.
8. Bayer R, Kelly M. Tobacco control and free speech: an American Dilemma. N Engl J Med. 2010;362:281–3.
9. Adams J, O'Mara-Adams K. Hoffmann D. Toxic and carcinogenic agents in undiluted mainstream smoke and sidestream smoke of different types of cigarettes. Carcinogenesis. 1987;8:729–31.
10. Siegmund B, Leitner E, Pfannhauser W. Determination of the nicotine content of various edible nightshades (Solanaceae) and their products and estimation of the associated dietary nicotine intake. J Agric Food Chem. 1999;47(8):3113–20.
11. Connolly GN, Alpert HR, Wayne GF, Koh H. Trends in nicotine yield in smoke and its relationship with design characteristics among popular US cigarette brands, 1997–2005. Tob Control. 2007;16(5):1–5.
12. Benowitz NL, Jacob 3rd P, Jones RT, Rosenberg J. Interindividual variability in the metabolism and cardiovascular effects of nicotine in man. J Pharmacol Exp Ther. 1982;221(2):368–72.
13. Benowitz NL, Herrera B, Jacob 3rd P. Mentholated cigarette smoking inhibits nicotine metabolism. J Pharmacol Exp Ther. 2004;310(3):1208–15.
14. Khokar JY, Miksys SL. Tyndale RF Rat brain CYP2B induction by nicotine is persistent and does not involve nicotinic acetylcholine receptors. Brain Res. 2010;1348:1–9.
15. Katzung BG. Basic & clinical pharmacology (basic and clinical pharmacology). New York: McGraw-Hill Medical; 2006. p. 99–105.
16. Xiu X, Puskar NL, Shanata JAP, Lester HA, Dougherty DA. Nicotine binding to brain receptors requires a strong cation-π interaction. Nature. 2009;458:534–7.
17. Herraiz T, Chaparro C. Human monoamine oxidase is inhibited by tobacco smoke: beta-carboline alkaloids act as potent and reversible inhibitors. Biochem Biophys Res Commun. 2005;326(2):378–86.
18. Fowler JS, Volkow ND, Wang GJ, et al. Neuropharmacological actions of cigarette smoke: brain monoamine oxidase B (MAO B) inhibition. J Addict Dis. 1998;17(1):23–34.
19. Wüllner U, Gündisch D, Herzog H, et al. Smoking upregulates alpha4beta2* nicotinic acetylcholine receptors in the human brain. Neurosci Lett. 2008;430(1):34–7.
20. Walsh H, Govind AP, Mastro R, et al. Up-regulation of nicotinic receptors by nicotine varies with receptor subtype. J Biol Chem. 2008;283(10):6022–32.
21. Nguyen HN, Rasmussen BA, Perry DC. Subtype-selective up-regulation by chronic nicotine of high-affinity nicotinic receptors in rat brain demonstrated by receptor autoradiography. J Pharmacol Exp Ther. 2003;307(3):1090–7.
22. Pons S, Fattore L, Cossu G, et al. Crucial role of alpha4 and alpha6 nicotinic acetylcholine receptor subunits from ventral tegmental area in systemic nicotine self-administration. J Neurosci. 2008;28(47):12318–27.

23. Yoshida T, Sakane N, Umekawa T, Kondo M. Effect of nicotine on sympathetic nervous system activity of mice subjected to immobilization stress. Physiol Behav. 1994;55(1):53–7.

24. King G, Yerger VB, Whembolua GL, Bendel RB, Kittles R, Moolchan ET. Link between facultative melanin and tobacco use among African Americans. Pharmacol Biochem Behav. 2009;92(4):589–96.

25. Parrott AC. Does cigarette smoking cause stress? Am Psychol. 1999;54(10):817–20.

26. Rusted J, O'Connell N. Does nicotine improve cognitive function? Psychopharmacology. 1994;115:547–9.

27. YunYing S, Shilling A, Turan A, et al. Smoking as a strong risk factor for severe postopertaive pain after ambulatory surgery American Society of Anesthesiologists Annual Meeting 788 San Diego, Oct 2010.

28. Guillem K, Vouillac C, Azar MR, et al. Monoamine oxidase inhibition dramatically increases the motivation to self-administer nicotine in rats. J Neurosci. 2005;25(38):8593–600.

29. Villégier AS, Blanc G, Glowinski J, Tassin JP. Transient behavioral sensitization to nicotine becomes long-lasting with monoamine oxidases inhibitors. Pharmacol Biochem Behav. 2003;76(2):267–74.

30. Kenny PJ, Markou A. Nicotine self-administration acutely activates brain reward systems and induces a long-lasting increase in reward sensitivity. Neuropsychopharmacology. 2006;31(6): 1203–11.

31. Nolley EP, Kelley BM. Adolescent reward system perseveration due to nicotine: studies with methylphenidate. Neurotoxicol Teratol. 2007;29(1):47–56.

32. Peterson EC, Owens M. Designing immunotherapies to thwart drug abuse. Mol Interv. 2009;9(3):119–23.

33. King A, de Wit H, Riley R, Cao D, Niaura R, Hatsukami D. Efficacy of naltrexone in smoking cessation: a preliminary study and an examination of sex differences. Nicotine Tob Res. 2006;8(5):671–82.

34. Shi Y, Warner DO. Surgery as a teachable moment for smoking cessation. Anesthesiology. 2010;112(1):102–7.

35. Warner DO, Klesges RC, Dale LC, et al. Telephone quitlines to help surgical patients quit smoking and provider attitudes. Am J Prev Med. 2008;35:S486–93.

36. Warner DO, Klesges RC, Lowell C, et al. Referral of surgical patients who smoke to telephone quitlines. American Society of Anesthesiologists Annual Meeting Abstract A 975 San Diego, Oct 2010.

37. Turan A, You J, Kurz A, et al. Smoking and perioperative outcomes American Society of Anesthesiologists Annual Meeting Abstract A1189 San Diego, Oct 2010.

38. US Department of Health and Human Services National Heart, Lung and Blood Institute Chronic Obstructive Pulmonary Disease, Bethesda, MD; 2003, NIH Publication No. 03-5229.

39. O'Connor GT, Sparrow D, Weiss ST, et al. The role and nonspecific hyperresponsiveness in the pathogenesis of chronic obstructive pulmonary disease. Am Rev Respir Dis. 1989;140:225–52.

40. Konrad FX, Torsten S, Brecht-Kraus D, et al. Bronchial mucus transport in chronic smokers and non smokers during general anesthesia. J Clin Anesth. 1993;5:375–80.

41. Noah TL, Zhou H, Monaco J, et al. Tobacco smoke exposure and later nasal responses to live attenuated influenza virus. Environ Health Perspect. 2011;119(1):78–83.

42. Willet WC, Green A, Stampfer MJ, et al. Relative and absolute excess risk in coronary heart disease among women who smoke cigarettes. N Engl J Med. 1987;317:1305–9.

43. White HD, Rivers JT, Cross DB, et al. Reinfarction after thrombolytic therapy in acute myocardial infarction followed by conservative management: incidence and effect of smoking. J Am Coll Cardiol. 1990;16:340–6.

44. Sauerbeck LR, Hornung R, Moonaw CJ, et al. The effects of study participation in the familial intracranial aneurysm study on cigarette smoking. J Stroke Cerebrovasc Dis. 2008;17(6):370–2.

45. Woo D, Khoury J, Haverbusch MM, et al. Smoking and family history and risk of aneurismal subarachnoid hemorrhage. Neurology. 2009;72(1):69–72.

46. Ameli FM, Stein M, Aro L, et al. The effect of postoperative smoking on femoropopliteal bypass grafts. Ann Vasc Surg. 1989;3:20–5.

47. Silverstein D. Smoking and wound healing. Am J Med. 1992;93(Suppl A):225–45.
48. Obert DM, Hua P, Pilkerton ME, et al. Environmental tobacco smoke furthers progression of diabetic nephropathy. Am J Med Sci. 2011;341(2):126–30.
49. Zhao L, Li F, Zhang Y, et al. Mechanisms and genes involved in enhancement of HIV infectivity by tobacco smoke. Toxicology. 2010;278(2):242–8.
50. Malhotra R, Kapoor A, Grover V, et al. Nicotine and periodontal tissues. J Indian Soc Periodontol. 2010;14(1):72–9.
51. Bor-Caymaz C, Bor S, Tobey NA, et al. Effects of ethanol and extract of cigarette smoke on rabbit buccal mucosa. J Oral Pathol Med. 2011;40(1):27–32.
52. Silvanus MT, Groeben H, Peters J. Corticosteroids and inhaled salbutamol in patients with reversible airway obstruction markedly decrease the incidence of bronchospasm after tracheal intubation. Anesthesiology. 2004;100:1047–8.

Chapter 9
Marijuana, Nitrous Oxide, and Other Inhaled Drugs

Ethan O. Bryson and Elizabeth A.M. Frost

Introduction

Inhalation of many substances has been part of civilization for thousands of years, for both pleasure and medicinal reasons. Abuse of this practice has become indigenous to our society. While tobacco is probably the most abused inhalant, many other agents have been sniffed and inhaled through the respiratory tract by all segments of our population. In addition to agents produced specifically for the purpose of recreational inhalation, there exist a number of readily obtained and easily abused volatile compounds with the potential to complicate an anesthetic procedure.

Marijuana

The female plant of Cannabis sativa, specifically the dried flowers or buds, has been ingested for centuries for recreational or medicinal purposes and as part of certain religious ceremonies. Marijuana use is common in our society. As recently as 2007, it was estimated that 38.5% of students have tried the drug at least once by the time they graduate from high school, and 5% of patients between the ages of 18 and 25 regularly use the drug [1]. Although the primary psychoactive component is delta-9 tetrahydrocannabiol (THC) over 60 other compounds, some with psychoactive properties have been identified in the plant and have the potential to contribute to the adverse effects associated with acute or chronic marijuana abuse [2].

Tetrahydrocannabiol and other cannabinoids are rapidly absorbed through the lungs, producing a wide range of psychological and central nervous system (CNS)

E.O. Bryson (✉)
Department of Anesthesiology and Department of Psychiatry, Mount Sinai School of Medicine, New York, NY, USA
e-mail: ethan.bryson@mountsinai.org

E.O. Bryson and E.A.M. Frost (eds.), *Perioperative Addiction:*
Clinical Management of the Addicted Patient, DOI 10.1007/978-1-4614-0170-4_9,
© Springer Science+Business Media, LLC 2012

effects that peak in 15 min and persist for 2–4 h depending on the dose. Users report feelings of euphoria, heightened sensory perception, and a distortion of space and time. In some patients, these sensations are anxiety provoking and some have reported feelings of dysphoria. In patients with underlying psychiatric disorders, aggravation of psychotic states has been reported. Generalized CNS depression leading to drowsiness and sleep typically follows the initial psychomotor agitation. When cannabis is ingested via the oral route, the bioavailability is variable but considerably lower due to issues with adsorption and first pass metabolism by the liver. Onset of effects is slower and may persist longer [3].

Multiple attempts have been made to delineate the therapeutic uses of cannabinoids, which have been used with varying success in the treatment of spastic disorders, chronic pain, epilepsy, glaucoma, bronchial asthma, and as an anti-emetic and appetite stimulant. Beneficial effects of marijuana ingestion include mild analgesia (similar in its effectiveness to codeine), anti-emetic effects, (although tolerance does develop), and increased appetite.

Toxic Effects

Marijuana is typically ingested by inhalation, with the same symptoms of coughing, increased sputum production, and occasional wheezing associated with acute inhalation of tobacco smoke. The smoke inhaled contains several thousand compounds in both the particulate and the gas phase, many of which are the same known toxins and carcinogens found in tobacco smoke [4]. Known carcinogens in marijuana smoke include tar, the particulate matter that does not contain cannabinoids, polynuclear aromatic hydrocarbons, B-naphtylamine, benzopyrene, nitrosamines, and vinyl chloride. Tumor accelerators present in marijuana smoke include indole and carbazole. Chronic marijuana smokers, despite popular thought to the contrary, are at increased risk for the development of lung cancer. Possibly due to the practice of deeply inhaling and breath holding when smoking marijuana in order to maximize tetrahydrocannabiol (THC) absorption, patients with a history of heavy cannabis use develop cancer of the throat and lungs at a much younger age than chronic tobacco smokers [5].

Although marijuana smoke contains roughly the same amount of carbon monoxide from incomplete combustion of organic compounds as tobacco smoke, the typical marijuana smoker holds smoke in the lungs much longer, resulting in levels of carboxyhemoglobin up to five times that of the typical tobacco smoker [6]. This practice of deep inhalation and breath holding also exposes the smoker to increased levels of the same carcinogens and pulmonary toxins found in tobacco smoke and is responsible for the development of pulmonary complications in the chronic user.

Alterations in central airways that occur in the chronic marijuana smoker include loss of cilia, mucus gland hyperplasia, and an increased number of goblet cells leading to an overproduction of mucus, not easily cleared from the lungs. As a result, chronic marijuana smokers are more likely to have a chronic cough and are more prone to dyspnea with exertion. Histologically, regression of normal pseudostratified ciliated epithelium and squamous metaplasia portend the development of carcinoma in situ, eventually leading to invasive bronchogenic carcinoma.

Intoxication with marijuana decreases blood pressure due to vasodilatation and increases heart rate, leading to an increased cardiac output and myocardial demand for oxygen. Tachycardia is common in the acutely intoxicated patient; some people develop palpitations and there have been reported cases of atrial fibrillation and other tachydysrhythmias [7]. Carbon monoxide increases smooth muscle cell proliferation that can exacerbate the physiologic effects of THC on the body and chronic use may eventually lead to cardiomyopathy. These effects on the cardio-vascular system have the potential to interfere with medications administered throughout the course of an anesthetic and may cloud the interpretation of intraop-erative physiologic data. The potential for ischemic events in young healthy patients is small, although for patients at risk it is increased when anesthesia is administered to the acutely intoxicated patient [8].

Perioperative Management

Ideally, complete abstinence from smoking in the chronic marijuana smoker should be achieved prior to surgery to allow re-growth of cilia and recovery of pulmonary function. As with tobacco smoking, this abstinence requires at least 8 weeks [9]. Since the preanesthetic assessment is rarely performed more than a week prior to the scheduled date of surgery (and often only minutes prior to entering the operating room), this ideal state is rarely realized. If the preanesthetic assessment is performed the day prior to surgery, the patient should be advised to abstain for a minimum of 12 h prior to receiving anesthesia to allow for the elimination of carboxyhemo-globin. A carboxyhemoglobin level of 15% can reduce the availability of oxygen by up to 25% and it increases risk for patients with coronary artery disease. In this population, it is justifiable to postpone a case if the patient reports smoking marijuana just prior to surgery. Unfortunately, since THC is stored in adipose tissue and slowly leeches out into the central circulation, relatively steady levels of THC are present in the chronic smoker for up to 30 days.

An interaction between cannabinoids and anesthetic agents, specifically additive effects in the acutely intoxicated patient and the development of cross-tolerance in the chronic user, has long been postulated. Recently, a study examining the induction dose of propofol in chronic cannabis users and naive patients suggests that such an interaction is likely. Chronic users required clinically significant increased doses of propofol to facilitate laryngeal mask airway (LMA) placement [10]. Possible tolerance to other anesthetic agents should be considered when a history of marijuana use is elicited.

The development of hyper-reactive airways in the chronic marijuana smoker is a major cause of intraoperative complications. A case report of airway obstruction in a patient who reported smoking marijuana 4 h prior to surgery [11] underscores the necessity of eliciting a complete history of substance use during the preanesthetic interview. Chronic marijuana smokers can be exquisitely sensitive, even if they have no past medical history significant for reactive airway disease. As such, great care should be taken to avoid the use of histamine-releasing agents and the anesthesia provider should maintain a heightened awareness that bronchospasm may occur, anticipating the possibility of airway hyperreactivity in the marijuana smoker in much the same manner that such complications are anticipated in the tobacco smoker.

The addition of humidified fresh gas through the breathing circuit may reduce the potential for obstruction of the endotracheal tube, although thick mucus secretions may still develop. High on the differential diagnosis for the chronic marijuana smoker who develops high peak airway pressures during general anesthesia is the development of an obstructive mucus plug in the endotracheal tube. Often, the placement of a suction catheter down the endotracheal tube is both diagnostic and curative.

A plan for adequate postoperative pain management is of particular importance, especially for the marijuana smoker who has just undergone a large intra-abdominal procedure. Patients whose cilia have been destroyed by chronic exposure to marijuana smoke depend entirely upon their coughing mechanism to clear pulmonary secretions. The pain associated with respiratory effort could lead to atelectasis, worsening of existing shunt physiology, hypoxia, and possibly postobstructive pneumonia. If routine chest physiotherapy is ineffective and systemic opioid administration interferes with the ability to adequately clear secretions, the anesthesia team should consider placement of an epidural catheter for pain management.

Though not life threatening, the withdrawal syndrome associated with chronic marijuana use can complicate the postoperative period in the chronic user. Anxiety and agitation are common and may be misunderstood in the setting of the acute postoperative period. Rebound hyperalgesia may increase the need for postoperative pain medications, and the incidence of postoperative nausea and vomiting is increased due to rebound nausea during marijuana withdrawal.

Nitrous Oxide

Sir Humphrey Davy developed nitrous oxide in 1798 primarily as an agent for enjoyment and merriment [12]. It has since been used as an anesthetic agent, a propellant, and foaming agent in the dairy industry, and as an adjuvant in motorcar racing, but its beginnings as an agent of intoxication portend its continued diversion for illegitimate use. Nitrous oxide remained for many years an addiction mainly of dentists as the agent was considered safe, allowing sufficient analgesia for dental work but not enough for surgical procedures. As such, dentists had easier access, a situation that is still recognized [13]. Diversion of canisters of the gas intended for use in the medical or racing industry is common and nitrous oxide can be found at parties or

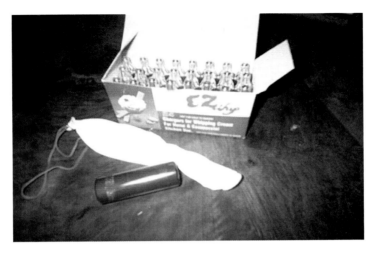

Fig. 9.1   Box of EZ Whip canisters containing nitrous oxide with balloon and aluminum cracker

concerts, dispensed in large balloons. Hospitals have been identified as a source of free inhalant drugs, for either on-site use or removal to another area [14]. There is ready, legal, and inexpensive access to nitrous oxide as it is also widely used as the propellant for whipped cream. Pre-filled pressurized cans are available for sale without restriction at grocery stores and small canisters of the gas under pressure are sold in bulk for use by professional caterers and amateur chefs. These small canisters called "whip-its" are routinely sold at "head shops" along with "crackers" or "breakers" (small metal or plastic tubes in which the canister is placed, allowing the user to "crack" or "break" the aluminum seal and access the gas) and balloons used to trap and warm the gas prior to inhalation. Because of this availability, it is likely that the abuse of nitrous oxide is wider than is believed (Fig. 9.1).

Toxic Effects

That nitrous oxide is addictive has been demonstrated for over 200 years. Pharmacologic evidence suggests that there is direct interaction with the endogenous opioid system, including a possible partial agonist effect at the mu, kappa, and sigma opioid receptors [15]. Other animal studies have shown a decrease of beta-endorphine in rat brain following nitrous oxide withdrawal, which may account for the post-anesthesia excitatory syndrome seen in man [16].

For many years, nitrous oxide was believed to have no toxicity other than that associated with its anesthetic action. However, bone marrow depression in patients administered N_2O for extended periods of time and neurological abnormalities in health-care workers who inhaled the gas recreationally have been documented [17].

Retrospective surveys of dental and medical personnel have linked occupational exposure to nitrous oxide with a number of health problems and reproductive derangements. Although the addition of scavenging systems and better ventilation of operating rooms has decreased the risk, nitrous oxide toxicity is still recognized as an occupational hazard [18]. The agent reacts with the reduced form of vitamin B12, inhibiting the action of methionine synthase, an enzyme that indirectly supports methylation reactions and nucleic acid synthesis. Many, if not all, of its nonanesthetic-related adverse effects may be ascribed to this action. Animal and human studies indicate that toxic effects are concentration- and time-dependent. A time-weighted average of no more than 100 parts per million (ppm) for an 8-h workday and/or a time-weighted average of 400 ppm per anesthetic administration should provide adequate protection of dental personnel and be achievable with existing pollution control methods.

Subacute combined degeneration of the spinal cord is the most common neurologic manifestation of vitamin B12 deficiency and is usually due to autoimmune gastritis, but may also occur in malnutrition syndrome such as is seen with chronic alcoholism, strict vegetarianism, postgastrectomy, and with nitrous oxide abuse. A clinical picture similar to acute traumatic spinal cord injury may be seen [19]. Several studies have documented damage to the nervous system of chronic nitrous oxide abusers [20]. Multimodal evoked potentials (EPs) were used to evaluate the electrophysiologic abnormalities in a man who had used four to five cans of nitrous oxide (about 2,000 ml/can) for more than 10 years. The patient complained of progressive motor disability and paresthesias in all limbs. Laboratory studies showed increased megaloblastic red blood cells and decreased vitamin B12 concentration. Subacute combined degeneration in the posterior and lateral cervical columns was seen on MRI. Multimodal EPs showed abnormal visual EPs with prolonged peak latencies, abnormal brainstem EPs with delayed wave V, and abnormal somatosensory EPs with significant decreased peak amplitudes. The authors indicated that abuse of nitrous oxide indirectly involves multiple levels of the nervous system. In another case, nitrous oxide abuse mimicked the presenting features of Guillain–Barre syndrome with motor and sensory axonal neuropathy (MSAN), creating a pattern of neurologic dysfunction almost identical to subacute combined degeneration (SCD) [21]. Several other reports have described spinal myoclonus [22], acute paralysis of the lower limbs [23], cervical myelopathy [24], and severe posterior column myelopathy identified by MRI and EPs [25]. Treatment with methionine and vitamin B12 in most cases resulted in at least partial reversal of the neurologic difficulties.

Other injuries that have been described include sudden lung collapse due to expansion of an asymptomatic pneumothorax [26]. Such a complication presents as sudden chest pain and, unless that history is elicited, the underlying problem may go undiagnosed. Exposure of the skin to nitrous oxide in abusers may cause burns and is a rare complication [27]. Since users typically inhale 100% nitrous oxide, hypoxia and anoxia are common during acute intoxication. If the user is standing up at the time of inhalation, trauma due to falling, including fractures or even head injury, may occur.

Therapeutic Effects

Throughout the centuries, abuse of one drug has been treated with attempted substitution of another agent (e.g., opioids and methadone and replacement of cocaine with morphine for Dr William Halsted). Finding that nitrous oxide inhalation reduced postwithdrawal craving in alcoholics, and aiding in their continued abstinence, rats were genetically selected as high-alcohol-drinking (HAD) and alcohol-preferring animals (P) and then exposed to ethanol 10% [28]. In both groups, exposure to nitrous oxide for 30–120 min then suppressed alcohol consumption at 1 but not 25 h. Based on these findings, psychotropic analgesic nitrous oxide (PAN) was added to a regime to treat methaqualone combined and smoked with cannabis, a combination known as "white pipe" and a major source of substance abuse in South Africa [29]. In 101 patients, the addition of PAN produced >50% improvement in withdrawal symptoms in 87 patients. Furthering the reasoning that nitrous oxide might be a valuable adjunct for relief of withdrawal symptoms in alcohol abuse, PAN was compared to carbamazepine and gabapentin [30]. Six randomized double-blind trails compared carbamazepine with drugs used in the United States and indicated efficacy, limited by drug interactions. The role of gabapentin was also unclear because of inadequate trial design. Two trials considered nitrous oxide and had conflicting results. In a Cochrane database review, five studies with 212 participants were analyzed. Use of PAN, as compared to oxygen and/or benzodiazepine regimens, showed improvement of symptoms (95% CI), decrease of amount and duration of sedative medications, and better psychomotor function [31]. No studies indicated adverse effects of PAN. However, the authors caution that the study sizes are small but results suggest that PAN may be a cost-effective means to reduce hospital admission and decrease post-admission supervision. Trials are ongoing.

Perioperative Management

In (usually young) patients presenting with abnormal neurologic symptoms for which there is no immediate, recognizable cause, the possibility of nitrous oxide abuse should be ruled out. Diagnosis is made by history of exposure, coupled with laboratory findings of megaloblastic anemia and vitamin B12 deficiency. As nitrous oxide is rarely the sole drug of abuse and is often present at "raves" and gatherings where other drugs are commonly available, the use of additional recreational drugs should be investigated. Because long-standing myelopathy has already become established, there is no evidence that the addition or avoidance of nitrous oxide during anesthesia is significant. Therapy with methionine and vitamin B12 should be started immediately and psychiatric counseling instituted. One recent study confirms what many anesthesiologists may have suspected: subjective effects of nitrous oxide are modulated by alcohol drinking status, with moderate drinkers choosing higher concentrations of nitrous oxide than light drinkers [32].

Volatile Compounds

Household items such as air freshener, nail polish remover, model glue, and even mothballs have documented abuse potential [33]. Acute intoxication with these agents can reduce anesthetic requirements and chronic abuse has been associated with organ-system damage, leading to a number of potential complications.

The recreational inhalation of volatile agents continues to be a problem in the United States, particularly among adolescents [34]. These agents are relatively easy to obtain (they are inexpensive, legal, and have legitimate use) and tend to disproportionately afflict vulnerable groups such as adolescents, low-income populations, and the mentally ill [35]. Chronic users can become dependent upon inhalants as with other drugs of abuse and exhibit tolerance, requiring greater amounts of agent to achieve the desired state of intoxication. Addicted individuals report increased levels of irritability, anxiety, and cravings that interfere with the activities of daily life [36]. Although it is not recognized by the DSM-IV, inhalant withdrawal syndrome has been reported [37].

Despite their ubiquitous nature, inhalants are the least studied of all the drugs of abuse and the mechanism of action has not yet been elucidated. Prior investigations have focused on the potential for inhaled agents to interact with gamma-aminobutyric acid (GABA)-gated chloride channels [38] and 5-hydroxytryptamine type 3 (%-HT3) receptors, [39] and have shown these agents to exhibit nonselective actions on a number of ion channels in much the same manner as volatile anesthetics [40]. Exposure to inhalants activates mesolimbic dopamine neurons, and may be the mechanism whereby the drug activates reward pathways to encourage abuse.

Patients who abuse volatile agents typically do so with the intent to quickly reach an intense level of intoxication, achieved by inhaling concentrated vapors in an enclosed space using a variety of methods. Those new to the practice, or who are experimenting, may simply inhale deeply over an open container, "sniffing" the agent in an attempt to become intoxicated. The practice of "bagging" involves placing the volatile agent into a plastic or paper bag and placing the bag over the nose and mouth while hyperventilating. Patients who abuse volatile agents in this manner may have telltale traces of the agent, i.e., paint or glue, around the mouth and nose. "Huffing" involves soaking a piece of cloth, often a sock, in the agent of choice and holding it up to the mouth so that the vapors are inhaled orally. When done alone, if the agent-soaked cloth does not fall away from the mouth once the patient becomes intoxicated, there exists a very real danger for overdose and death. Recreational use has been reported as a group activity, and the practice of holding the agent-soaked cloth over the mouth of another, forcing them to inhale the vapors, can also prove fatal. Please see the following tables for commonly abused household products (Table 9.1) and industrial agents (Table 9.2). When abused in this manner, blood levels of the volatile agent rapidly rise and create an intense feeling of euphoria, which quickly dissipates as the lipophillic agents are redistributed from the central nervous system to adipose tissue.

Table 9.1 Commonly abused household products

Cigarette lighter fluid	Butane, an aliphatic hydrocarbon
Model glues and rubber cement	Hexane, an aliphatic hydrocarbon
Mothballs	Naphthalene, an aromatic hydrocarbon
Toilet bowl freshener	An aromatic hydrocarbon
Resins and lacquers	Benzene, an aromatic hydrocarbon
Adhesives and paint thinner	Toluene, an aromatic hydrocarbon
Room air freshener	Butyl-isobutyl nitrate, an alkyl nitrate
Nail polish remover	Acetone, a ketone
Paints	Methyl n-butyl ketone
Spray paint	Methyl isobutyl ketone and toluene, an aromatic hydrocarbon

Table 9.2 Commonly abused industrial products

Bottled fuel	Propane, an aliphatic hydrocarbon
Gasoline	Octane, an aliphatic hydrocarbon and benzene, an aromatic hydrocarbon
Dry cleaning agent and spot remover	Trichloroethylene, an alkyl halide
Freon and aerosol propellants	Trichlorofluoromethane, an alkyl halide
Laboratory solvent	Diethyl ether
Anesthetic agents	Halogenated ethers
Coronary vasodilator	Amyl nitrate, an alkyl nitrate

Toxic Effects

Although the exact mechanism of action has not been determined, volatile agents are known to act as central nervous system depressants. Lipophillic and easily able to cross the blood–brain barrier, these substances have the potential to cause widespread damage throughout the central and peripheral nervous system, and chronic abusers may develop permanent neurologic damage.

Acute effects of the abused volatile agents are similar regardless of chemical structure, and depend primarily on the amount of agent inhaled. Since these agents are typically not administered under controlled circumstances, the actual blood concentration varies considerably and may even exceed what would be lethal levels of agent if maintained at that concentration for an extended period of time. At lower doses, peripheral vasodilatation occurs, with compensatory tachycardia and the potential for orthostatic hypotension. Despite the mildly increased heart rate, decreased myocardial contractility contributes to hypotension. At higher doses, bradycardia, decreased cardiac output, and sudden sniff death syndrome may occur. First reported in 1970 [41], sudden sniffing death occurs when the abuser is startled while under the influence of any number of inhalants. The hypothesized mechanism is death due to malignant arrhythmia induced by an acute catecholamine surge in a patient whose myocardium has been sensitized to epinephrine by hydrocarbon inhalation.

All of the abused inhaled agents may have the potential to be neurotoxic if present in the right concentration, a hypothesis not determined scientifically. Some specific agents are known neurotoxins, however, and chronic use can be evident in the clinical presentation of the addicted patient. Naphthalene, benzene, and toluene are all aromatic hydrocarbons found in common household items such as mothballs, toilet bowl freshener, resins, lacquers, adhesives, spray paint, and paint thinner. Of these, toluene, a typical constituent of adhesives, is thought to be the most toxic. Specific sequelae of toluene abuse include cognitive dysfunction, dementia, and encephalopathy associated with euphoria, hallucinations, and nystagmus, eventually leading to seizures and coma [34]. Cranial nerve damage, though rare, has also been associated with toluene abuse. Sensorimotor peripheral neuropathy, slurred speech, ataxia, and coma are further complications making informed consent difficult to obtain.

Direct injury to pulmonary tissues can occur as inhaled agents contact the sensitive respiratory epithelium. Patients who abuse inhalants chronically may develop a rash around the mouth and nose, and present with rhinitis or epistaxis. Inflammation of the lungs caused by chronic exposure can result in a chronic cough. In addition to the development of a chemical pneumonitis, interference with the ability of the anesthetic gas analyzer to accurately measure end-tidal anesthetic concentrations in chronic abusers of the aliphatic hydrocarbons has been reported [42]. Bronchospasm can occur in patients with a history of asthma and even in chronic abusers with no history of reactive airway disease. Inhaled vapors may displace oxygen within the alveoli, leading to asphyxiation.

Common toxic effects on the gastrointestinal system include nausea, vomiting, and diarrhea. Halogenated hydrocarbons, such as carbon tetrachloride and the anesthetic agents, are known hepatotoxins and chronic abusers have the potential to develop transaminitis and hepatitis. Renal tubular acidosis, kidney stones, and glomerulonephritis are also possible.

Perioperative Management

In order to properly care for the inhalant abuser, the anesthesia care provider should first identify the problem during the preanesthetic interview. Given the ubiquitous nature of these chemicals and the propensity of adolescents to experiment with them, it is likely that the actual number of patients in this population who routinely abuse inhalants is underreported. The anesthesia care provider should have a high index of suspicion for inhalant abuse when interviewing patients in high-risk categories, such as socially isolated, adolescent, or young adult patients with a history of polysubstance abuse or psychiatric disorders [43].

Most often these patients come to medical attention for unrelated issues and the only evidence of chronic inhalant abuse is abnormal values on routine pre-anesthetic laboratory work, a diagnostic tool now limited as evidence is overwhelming that most "routine" blood tests are unnecessary and therefore no longer performed.

Anemia, leukopenia, leukemia, and aplastic anemia, though rare, are recognized sequelae of inhalant abuse [44]. In elective cases where abnormal results on preoperative studies are obtained, it is prudent to reschedule the procedure or surgery pending further evaluation. It is also recommended that patients remain abstinent during this period of time and be referred to an appropriate addiction treatment center. Prior to receiving anesthesia, repeat laboratory tests should be performed to confirm normalization of values.

Hepatic and renal damage in chronic abusers may decrease clearance of opioids and muscle relaxants; hence, care should be taken when providing general anesthesia using these agents. Inhalants and volatile anesthetic agents may have similar mechanisms of action, so acute intoxication may decrease the minimum alveolar concentration (MAC) while chronic abuse may actually cause an increase. Acute and chronic inhalation of aliphatic and aromatic hydrocarbons may confound anesthetic gas analyzers and inhalants may cause airway irritation, leading to airway hyperreactivity. These problems are more likely to occur when the patient presents for surgery in the acutely intoxicated state.

Conclusion

The abuse of inhaled agents of any kind has the potential to damage every human organ system and put the patient at risk for death, from either disease related to chronic exposure or physiologic perturbations during acute intoxication. Trauma resulting from unsafe physical activity while under the influence may bring the patient to the attention of medical personnel, providing the opportunity for intervention before further injury occurs. The implications for the anesthesia care provider are many and proper management of these patients begins with obtaining a history of substance abuse.

Spotlight on Chemically Altered Cannabis

Ethan O. Bryson, MD

Marijuana is often chemically altered through the addition of agents designed to intensify the experience of the user. Sometimes these alterations are deliberate but occasionally these alterations are made without the knowledge of the user. Knowledge of the terminology used to describe these alterations is important so that the health-care practitioner may potentially identify the substance being abused and anticipate any complications which may arise due to acute intoxication or chronic abuse. It is important to note, however, that many terms are interchangeable and may evolve over time. In addition, it is possible that since no formal standards regarding the production of such agents exist, the name given to any chemically altered marijuana product may not correctly identify the chemical additive.

Street Terms for Altered Cannabis
A marijuana cigarette may be laced with heroin or opium (*A-bomb*, *Wack*, *Woola*), rolled with crack cocaine (*51 or 3750*, *Bazooka*, *Primo*, *Torpedo*), powder cocaine (*Candy Sticks*, *Champagne*, *Coco Puffs*, *Dirties*), phencyclidine (PCP) (*Chips*, *Dips*, *Happy Sticks*), or, most troublesome, dipped in formaldehyde or embalming fluid (*Amp*, *Clicker*, *Fry*, *Fry Stick*, *Water-water*, *Wet daddies*). The effects of such additives are variable and depend on the amount of the substance added to the marijuana, and often multiple additives are combined, confusing the picture even further.

Fry
Embalming fluid is composed of formaldehyde, methanol, ethyl alcohol, or ethanol and may also include phenol, ethylene glycol, glutaraldehyde, and other solvents. Chronic environmental exposure to this highly toxic substance is known to cause bronchitis and chronic inflammatory changes of the upper airway, impaired coordination, and nonspecific brain damage [45]. Exposure to these agents through the smoking of dipped marijuana cigarettes has been associated with hyperthermia, myocardial infarction, rhabdomyolysis, renal damage, lung damage, and brain damage, leading to seizures, coma, and death [46].

Frequently phencyclidine (PCP) is added to the product prior to dipping individual marijuana cigarettes. Previously used as an anesthetic in both humans and animals, PCP has not been available commercially since its use was discontinued in the 1970s. Despite this, it is currently available as a white powder, tablet, or capsule created illegally using unregulated processes with likely impurities. Since PCP intensifies the effects of other agents and can be ingested in any number of ways, it is commonly added to street drugs. The addition of PCP to any drug of abuse can cause hallucinations, impaired motor coordination, depression, anxiety, aggressive behavior, and a dissociative state in which the user does not experience pain and may be very difficult to subdue [47].

Spice or K2
These products, called "K2", "Spice Gold," or "herbal incense," are little more than dried vegetable matter sprayed with synthetic cannabinoids. Just like THC, the active ingredient in marijuana and other forms of cannabis, these synthetic cannabinoids stimulate the cannabinoid receptors, particularly the CB1 cannabinoid receptors concentrated in the brain. Although their effects are similar to the effects of THC, these synthetic cannabinoids are structurally different, bind to receptors with different affinities, and have not yet been tested in humans. The two most common synthetic cannabinoids found in these over-the-counter preparations are JWH 018, first synthesized in 1995 by

Clemson University researcher John W. Huffman, PhD, and a synthetic cannabinoid created by Pfizer called CP 47,497.

Because these synthetic agents bind more tightly to the endogenous cannabinoid receptors, the effects of acute intoxication mirror those of cannabis intoxication but are more pronounced and prolonged. Hypertension, tachycardia, agitation, insomnia, and other psychiatric effects can persist for days. Prolonged use has been associated with physical dependence and discontinuation with a withdrawal syndrome [48]. Nothing is known about the long-term effects these agents have on the human body but their similar structure to known carcinogens has prompted some to suspect they may turn out to be considerably more toxic than is currently thought.

References

1. Johnston LD, O'Malley PM, Bachman JG. Monitoring the future national survey results on drug use, 1975–2007: volume II, college students and adults ages 19–45 (NIH publication No. 08-6418B). Bethesda, MD: National Institute on Drug Abuse; 2008.
2. Hall W, Solowij N. Adverse effects of cannabia. Lancet. 1998;352:1611–6.
3. British Medical Association. Therapeutic uses of cannabis. London: Harwood Academic Publishers; 1997.
4. Adams J, O'Mara-Adams K, Hoffmann D. Toxic and carcinogenic agents in undiluted mainstream smoke and sidestream smoke of different types of cigarettes. Carcinogenesis. 1987;8:729–31.
5. Sridhar KS, Raub WA, Weatherby NL. Possible role of marijuana smoking as a carcinogen in the development of lung cancer at an early age. J Psychoactive Drugs. 1994;26:285–8.
6. Benson M, Bentley AM. Lung disease induced by drug addiction. Thorax. 1995;50:1125–7.
7. Korantzpoulos P, Lui T, Papaioannides D, et al. Atrial fibrillation and marijuana smoking. Int J Clin Pract. 2008;62:308–13.
8. Lawson TM, Rees A. Stroke and transient ischemic attacks in association with substance abuse in a young man. Postgrad Med. 1996;72:692–3.
9. Warner MA, Diverti MR, Tinker JH, et al. Preoperative cessation of smoking and pulmonary complications in coronary artery bypass patients. Anesthesiology. 1984;60:380–3.
10. Flisberg P, Paech MJ, Shah T, Ledowski T, Kurowski I, Parsons R. Induction dose of propofol in patients using cannabis. Eur J Anaesthesiol. 2009;26:192–5.
11. Pertwee RG. Neuropharmacology and therapeutic potential of cannabinoids. Addict Biol. 2000;5:37–46.
12. Davy H. Researches, Chemical and philosophical: chiefly concerning nitrous oxide or dephlogisticated nitrous air, and its respiration. London: Biggs and Cottle; 1800. p. 548–9.
13. Blanton A. Nitrous oxide abuse: dentistry's unique addiction. J Tenn Dent Assoc. 2006;86(4):30–1.
14. Luc MJ, Jan H. The hospital as a source of free inhalant drugs. Eur J Emerg Med. 2009; 16(3):167–8.
15. Gillman MA. Nitrous oxide, an opioid addictive agent. Review of the evidence. Am J Med. 1986;81(1):97–102.
16. Dzoljic MR, Haffmans J, Ruprehy J, et al. Decrease of beta endorphin in the brain of rats following nitrous oxide withdrawal. Drug Metabol Drug Interact. 1991;9(2):139–48.

17. Yagiela JA. Health Hazards and nitrous oxide: a time for reappraisal. Anesth Prog. 1991;38(1):1–11.
18. Merat F, Merat S. Occupational hazards related to the practice of anaesthesia. Ann Fr Anesth Reanim. 2008;27(1):63–73.
19. Reichard PI. Subacute combined degeneration mimicking traumatic spinal cord injury. Am J Forensic Med Pathol. 2009;30(1):47–8.
20. Lin CY, Guo WY, Chen JT, et al. Neurotoxicity of nitrous oxide: multimodal evoked potentials in an abuser. Clin Toxicol (Phila). 2007;45(1):67–71.
21. Tatum WO, Bui DD, Grant EG, et al. Pseudo- Guillain-barre syndrome due to "Whippet" induced myeloneuropathy. J Neuroimaging. 2009;20(4):400–1.
22. Wu MS, HSU YD, Lin JC. Spinal myoclonus in subacute combined degeneration caused by nitrous oxide intoxication. Acta Neurol Taiwan. 2007;16(2):102–5.
23. Cartner M, Sinnott M, Silburn P. Paralysis caused by "nagging". Med J Aust. 2007;187(6):366–7.
24. Waters MF, Kang GA, Mazziotta JC, et al. Nitrous oxide inhalation as a cause of cervical myelopathy. Acta Neurol Scand. 2005;12(4):270–2.
25. Butzkueven H, King JO. Nitour oxide myelopathy in an abuser of whipped cream bulbs. J Clin Neurosci. 2000;7(1):73–5.
26. Garbaz L, Mispelaere D, Boulemy M. Pneumothorax following recreational inhalation of nitrous oxide. Rev Mal Respir. 2007;24(5):622–4.
27. Hwang JC, Himel HN, Edlich RF. Frostbite of the face after recreational misuse of nitrous oxide. Burns. 1996;22(2):152–3.
28. Kosobud AE, Kebabian CE, Rebec GV. Nitrous oxide acutely suppresses ethanol consumption in HAD and P rats. Int J Neurosci. 2006;116(7):835–45.
29. Gillman MA, Harker N, Lichtigfeld FJ. Combined cannabis/methaqualone withdrawal treated with psychotropic analgesic nitrous oxide. Int J Neurosci. 2006;116(7):859–69.
30. Prince V, Turpin KR. Treatment of alcohol withdrawal syndrome with carbamazepine, gabapentin and nitrous oxide. Am J Health Syst Pharm. 2008;65(11):1039–47.
31. Gillman MA, Lichtigfeld FJ, Young TN. Psychotropic analgesic nitorus oxide for alcoholic withdrawal states. Cochrane Database Syst Rev. 2007;18(2):CD005190.
32. Zacny JP, Walker DJ, Derus LM. Choice of nitrous oxide and its subjective effects in light and moderate drinkers. Drug Alcohol Depend. 2008;98(1–2):163–8.
33. Kong JT, Schmiesing C. Concealed mothball abuse prior to anesthesia: mothballs, inhalants, and their management. Acta Anaesthesiol Scand. 2005;49:113–6.
34. Kurtzman TL, Otsuka KN, Wahl RA. Inhalant abuse by adolescents. J Adolesc Health. 2001;28:170–80.
35. Perron BE, Howard MO, Vaughn MG, Jarman CN. Inhalant withdrawal as a clinically significant feature of inhalant dependence disorder. Med Hypotheses. 2009;73:935–7.
36. Keriotis AA, Upadhyaya HP. Inhalant dependence and withdrawal symptoms. J Am Acad Child Adolesc Psychiatry. 2000;39:679–80.
37. Shen YC. Treatment of inhalant dependence with lamotrigine. Prog Neuropsychopharmacol Biol Psychiatry. 2007;31:769–71.
38. MacIver BM. Abused inhalants enhance GABA-mediated synaptic inhibition. Neuropsychopharmacology. 2009;34:2296–304.
39. Lopreato GF, Phelan R, Borghese CM, Beckstead MJ, Mihic SJ. Inhaled drugs of abuse enhance serotonin-3 receptor function. Drug Alcohol Depend. 2003;70:11–5.
40. Bieda MC, Su H, MacIver MB. Anesthetics discriminate between tonic and phasic gamma-aminobutyric acid receptors on hippocampal CA1 neurons. Anesth Analg. 2009;108:484–90.
41. Bass M. Sudden sniffing death. JAMA. 1970;212:2075–9.
42. Sicinski M, Kadam U. Monitoring of the anesthetic volatile agent may be impaired in hydrocarbon abusers. Anesthesia. 2002;57:510–1.
43. Perron BE, Howard MO. Adolescent inhalant use, abuse and dependence. Addiction. 2009;104:1185–92.
44. Broussard LA. The role of the laboratory in detecting inhalant abuse. Clin Lab Sci. 2000;13:205–9.

45. Bardana EJ, Montanaro A. Formaldehyde: an analysis of its respiratory, cutaneous, and immunologic effects. Ann Allergy. 1991;66:441–52.
46. State of Connecticut, Department of Public Health and Addiction Services. Illy contains embalming chemicals that will poison you! Brochure. Hartford, CT; 1994.
47. Yago KB, Pitts FN, Burgoyne RW, Aniline O, Yago LS, Pitts AF. The urban epidemic of phencyclidine (PCP) use: clinical and laboratory evidence from a public psychiatric hospital emergency service. J Clin Psychiatry. 1981;42:193–6.
48. Zimmermann US, Winkelmann PR, Pilhatsch M, Nees JA, Spanagel R, Schulz K. Withdrawal phenomena and dependence syndrome after the consumption of "spice gold". Dtsch Arztebl Int. 2009;106(27):464–7.

Chapter 10
Propofol Abuse

Elizabeth A.M. Frost and Ethan O. Bryson

> *One addict fell asleep at his desk so often that his lolling*
> *forehead became a permanent bruise. Another was so desperate*
> *for a fix that he started trolling through sharps bins for*
> *discarded needles and syringes with traces of drug to inject.*
> *These addicts were doctors; the drug of choice: propofol [1]*

Introduction

Propofol (2,6-diisopropylphenol), an intravenous anesthetic agent used for the rapid induction of general anesthesia and for moderate to deep sedation for painful or uncomfortable procedures, was not considered by most health-care workers as a likely drug for recreational use despite a significant potential for abuse. Nonmedical use was, at least until recently, primarily by medical professionals. It is not classified yet as a controlled substance by the United States Drug Enforcement Agency, which might suggest little potential for drug abuse although the status may change soon as the DEA is circulating a proposed rule that would classify propofol as a Schedule 1V substance putting it in the same category as the benzodiazepines and zolpidem. Fospropofol, (Lusedra®, Eisai) a drug similar to propofol was added to the Schedule in 2009. To date, (October 2010) the drug is freely available in the hospital setting, including operating and emergency rooms, critical care areas, and especially in endoscopy suites and outpatient facilities.

First synthesized in 1977, propofol has been widely used for over 20 years in the United States without significant problems of addiction and dependence surfacing. However, the tragic death of popular culture icon Michael Jackson during the summer of 2009 has brought abuse of this anesthetic agent by the layperson into the spotlight. A brief survey of medical literature immediately identified 72 articles related to propofol abuse while 250,000 sites were highlighted on a Google search [2].

E.A.M. Frost (✉)
Department of Anesthesiology, Mount Sinai School of Medicine, New York, NY, USA
e-mail: elzfrost@aol.com

E.O. Bryson and E.A.M. Frost (eds.), *Perioperative Addiction:*
Clinical Management of the Addicted Patient, DOI 10.1007/978-1-4614-0170-4_10,
© Springer Science+Business Media, LLC 2012

Propofol Overview

Propofol was initially marketed as an anesthetic but is now widely used for sedation in many settings [3]. At room temperature, it is an oil and is insoluble in water. The safety profile is remarkably good. Major side effects include dose-dependent hypotension and cardiorespiratory depression, greater with faster injection. The drug works rapidly and patients begin to lose consciousness seconds after the injection of a bolus dose. Within one circulation time the patient is entering a state of general anesthesia. Depending on the dose, patients awaken 5–10 min later as the drug redistributes from the active site in the central nervous system into the bodies lipid depots, provided, of course, any necessary supportive measures have been provided by the individual administering the medication. A short-acting agent with little or no residual effects, the patient who has received a propofol-based sedation anesthetic typically recovers feeling well and rested. Patients have reported a broad spectrum of feelings after propofol administration ranging from a general feeling of well-being to elation, euphoria, and sexual disinhibition [4].

Propofol is a global central nervous system depressant that activates the chloride current at the gamma-aminobutyric acid (GABA) type A receptor, inhibits the function of the N-methyl-D-aspartate (NMDA) receptor, and modulates calcium influx through slow calcium channel ions [5, 6]. At doses that do not produce sedation, the drug has an anxiolytic effect. It also has an immunomodulatory effect and may diminish the systemic inflammatory response responsible for organ dysfunction [3]. Some studies have suggested a neuroprotective effect in that it reduces cerebral metabolic rate of oxygen metabolism and intracranial pressure and is a potent antioxidant [3]. The brain may be protected from ischemic injury. Formulations contain disodium edentate or sodium metabisulfate, which has antifungal and antibacterial properties [3].

Because of its favorable pharmacokinetic profile, propofol has become the induction agent of choice for most general anesthetics in the United States. The extent to which this drug is used became evident when a critical shortage of the agent occurred in the fall of 2009. Suddenly faced with limited supplies of propofol due to problems with two of the three major manufacturing facilities, hospitals throughout the world quickly found out that the main alternative to a propofol induction of general anesthesia, thiopental, was also in short supply, primarily because reduced demand had significantly reduced production. These shortages have continued and may do so for some time to come. Alternatives are sought. Drug regulators took the step earlier in 2010 of importing a foreign source of propofol, Propoven®, manufactured by a sibling of a United States supplier of propofol. This drug, although almost identical, has a few key differences. The label advises not to administer the drug to patients with a known peanut allergy as it is manufactured with soy oil as some studies suggest that a cross-allergy exists. Nevertheless, the US firm importing Propoven® claims that it does not contain peanuts and to date no allergic reactions have been reported.

Fospropofol

Fospropofol (Lusedra®) may be an alternative to propofol for monitored anesthetic care [7]. It is a water-soluble, nonpyrogenic, isoosmotic pro drug sedative hypnotic agent that is metabolized to propofol and thus should have less pain on injection. It is metabolized in the liver by alkaline phosphatase to propofol. Blood levels of propofol after an equipotent injection of fospropofol reach lower peak levels and the clinical effect is longer (~1–8 min). Supplemental doses should be delayed at least 4 min to allow metabolism of the drug to release the active propofol to prevent oversedation from drug stacking. Also, a released phosphate metabolite may cause frequent but transient mild to moderate perineal paresthesias (52–74%) or pruritis (16–28%) [7]. The drug was released in November 2009. It does not provide an approved complete propofol replacement but allows clinicians to reserve the limited supplies of propofol for patients that require general anesthesia. As noted above, fospropofol has been placed by the Deputy Administrator of the Drug Enforcement Administration into Schedule 1V of the Controlled Substance act as of 2009 (Fed regist. 2009 Oct 6th 74(192): 51234–6 Schedule of controlled substances; placement of fospropofol into schedule IV. final rule). Unlike propofol, there is no shortage of fospropofol; however, the anesthetic community has less experience with this agent. Recommended dosages are 5–10 mg/kg (average 6.5 mg/kg), depending on the amount of sedation desired and the procedure to be undertaken [8–10]. It is supplied as 35 mg/ml in 30 ml vials. No formal studies of abuse potential have been conducted but euphoria was reported in patients receiving both intravenous and oral dosing. However, as the medium time to sedation is 8 min, it is conceivable that this agent may also become a drug of abuse.

Pathways to Abuse and Addiction

As with most drugs of abuse, propofol also enhances the levels of dopamine in the areas of the brain associated with reward [11]. Either through direct release of dopamine from pre-synaptic nerve terminals or through inhibition of dopamine reuptake, increased levels of dopamine in the reward circuitry of the mesocorticolimbic system serve to reinforce the behaviors associated with obtaining and injecting propofol [12]. In a more recent rat study, Xiong et al. examined the effects of propofol on the expression of a transcription factor, Delta FosB [13]. It is appreciated that drugs of abuse converge on a common circuitry, inducing addiction by modulating gene expression of Delta FosB in the nucleus accumbens (NAc), a collection of neurons in the forebrain. Propofol induced a significant Delta FosB expression, similar to that seen with nicotine and alcohol. The propofol-induced upregulation of Delta FosB was related to the dopamine D1 receptor in the NAc. Delta Fos B is unique among nuclear proteins in that, with repeated stimulation, it accumulates in the NAc and may last weeks before it disappears.

These findings raise the issue of the effects of chronic exposure in generating addiction among anesthetic care providers and others who use propofol frequently and/or on a long-term basis. The possible adverse effects of chronic exposure to propofol should particularly concern health care professionals who administer the drug on a regular basis. Several studies have found detectable amounts of propofol in the air of operating rooms – most likely exhaled from patients who had received the drug. Occupation-related secondhand exposure to intravenous drugs, especially fentanyl and propofol, has been demonstrated [14]. Aerosolized intravenous anesthetics may be an unintended source of exposure for physicians and may lead to an increased risk for developing addiction. McAuliffe et al. retrospectively reviewed the de-identified demographic information of all physicians treated for substance abuse in Florida over a 25-year period [14]. Two mass spectrometry assays were developed to detect fentanyl and propofol in was detected in cardiac rooms, and aerosolized propofol was found in the expirations of patients undergoing transurethral prostatectomies. The authors suggest that while stress may be a factor in inducing addiction, repeated use of propofol and fentanyl may be additional risk factors. Other studies have confirmed that secondhand exposure produced neurobiologic sensitization to the reinforcing effects of aerosolized intravenous agents, making later addiction more likely [15]. Secondhand exposure may occur through the skin or by inhalation. Confirmation has come from laboratory studies where it has been shown that even nanomolar amounts of propofol may stimulate glutamate transmission to dopamine neurons [16]. The authors suggest that changes induced in synaptic plasticity in the ventral tegmental areas, an addiction-related brain area, may contribute to the development of propofol abuse and the increased susceptibility to addiction of other drugs.

Abuse Prevalence

Initially, almost all cases of propofol abuse involved medical personnel with access to the agent. Follette and Farley published the first case of propofol dependence, involving an anesthesiologist who reportedly self-administered 100 mg of propofol 10–15 times per day in 1992 [17]. The frequency with which this addict was injecting this medication was such that it would be difficult to maintain such use without becoming detected if it were a controlled substance. An editorial accompanying this case report questioned whether or not propofol deserved to be included in the access-restricted system, if not advanced to controlled substance status all together [18]. Later reports noted that addicts might inject themselves 50–100 times a day to stay high [1]. Despite this early concern, many hospitals still place no more restriction on access to propofol than to other uncontrolled medications commonly found in the anesthesia carts. Free access is especially prevalent if office bases anesthetic practices.

Zacny et al. first investigated the abuse potential for propofol in 1993. They conducted a discrete-trials choice procedure [19]. Healthy volunteer subjects with some history of lifetime substance use but no history of abuse or treatment for addiction were administered propofol (0.6 mg/kg) or a similar volume of intralipid on two occasions. For the next three sessions, subjects were given a choice of which agent they would prefer to have during a subsequent session. Subjects either chose propofol because they liked the subjective effects of the drug such as feeling "spaced out" or "high" or chose the intralipid because they disliked the "dizziness" and "confusion" associated with propofol administration. The authors concluded that, for some people, propofol might be rewarding even in individuals without a history of drug abuse although further testing is needed.

Several other anecdotal reports were published over the next 15 years. In one instance, a female anesthesiologist reportedly self-administered propofol and died [20]. Analysis at the scene and toxicology reports indicated blood and liver concentrations were 2.4 ugm and 0.56 ugm, respectively, supporting the conclusion that the death was a consequence of propofol self-administration at therapeutic doses from a person who used the drug repeatedly. The first reported case of propofol dependency in a layperson was in 2002 [21]. This individual was first exposed to propofol, as treatment for tension headaches, administered by an anesthesiologist. Details as to amount, duration, and frequency were not provided, although the patient was able to identify the substance as propofol as he was subsequently able to obtain more for personal use from various veterinarians. His case came to the attention of medical professionals when his wife found him unconscious and cyanotic after an accidental overdose. Yet another recent case of a young woman found dead in her home, of apparent propofol toxicity, questioned whether her death was due to abuse or homicide. The measured blood propofol level was 4.3 µgm/ml [22]. Given there was neither history of abuse nor signs of it at autopsy, attention focused on a male nurse acquaintance that worked in a surgical intensive care unit. Another report of a middle-aged female who died of self-administered propofol intoxication measured drug levels by gas chromatography after liquid–liquid extraction [23]. The results suggested that death was not directly due to propofol but rather from respiratory failure after rapid injection, a finding that was similar to another case of a young male nurse in which propofol was also demonstrated in hair samples indicating long-term use but high postmortem levels suggested massive injection [24]. Yet another rather enterprising layman with some autodidactic medical knowledge inserted a permanent cannula into himself for repeated, daily injections of propofol, which he obtained on e bay [25]. Postmortem concentrations of propofol were 364 ng/ml in urine, 71 ng in cardiac blood, and 79 ng/ml in femoral blood. The case illustrates how job-related drug dependencies become indistinct due to information and materials freely available on the Internet.

As noted above, a recent systematic review of the literature identified 72 articles with direct relevance in 45 to evaluation of the abuse potential of propofol [2]. The articles describe the several biochemical and pharmacokinetic mechanisms of action of the agent that lend themselves to its abuse, and the physical and psychological effects that make it attractive as a recreational drug. Current evidence also supports the possibility of tolerance to and also withdrawal from propofol and its abuse potential. Based on their review and analysis, once more the authors recommend that not only the United States Drug Enforcement Administration but also other international agencies should consider regulating propofol as a controlled substance. Other reports, some more than 15 years old, of intense craving and dependency and clinical evidence supporting the abuse potential, bear out this opinion [3, 26–28].

According to a 2007 survey conducted at the University of Colorado Health Sciences Center, in Denver there has been a fivefold surge in propofol abuse over the last 10 years in academic anesthesiology programs [29]. The survey response was 100%. One or more incidents of propofol abuse or diversion in the previous 10 years were reported by 18% of departments. The observed incidence of propofol abuse was 10/10,000 anesthesia providers/decade. Of the 25 reported individuals abusing propofol, seven died as a result of the abuse (28%). There was no established system to control or monitor propofol as is done with opioids in 71% of the programs. There was no association found between the lack of control of propofol at the time of the incident or abuse. At least one case of propofol abuse or diversion was reported in 20% of the 126 academic centers in the United States. In most cases, anesthesiologists who abused propofol dropped out of the specialty, and usually of medicine entirely.

Moreover, it appears not just to be the medical community that is affected, but anesthesiologists and especially endoscopists have noted an influx of patients requesting and even scheduling unnecessary medical procedures just to receive a propofol high. After all, a feeling of euphoria with no residual "hangover" would suggest a near-perfect mind-altering drug, albeit one with a very thin window separating the dream from nonresponsive as noted by Ward [30]. If the research published in 2004 indicating that sleep deprivation can be erased by propofol can be further substantiated, the abuse potential for the drug is even higher [31, 32]. Nevertheless, the call to more regulation by Ward in his article in the Bulletin of the California Society of Anesthesiologists was met by more than one criticism by some who felt that such control would be a mistake, ineffective, and would create regulatory mechanisms for the vast majority of anesthesiologists while doing little to help the very few who are at risk [30].

Management of the Propofol Addict

Propofol is rapidly redistributed when administered as a bolus and thus the patient who has been abusing propofol and presents for surgery or a procedure requiring anesthesia will likely present no problems associated with acute intoxication. However, in cases of rapid self-administration in the absence of respiratory assistance or control of blood pressure the patient may present in cardiac arrest or with anoxic brain injury. Trauma related to falls after bolus administration may complicate the initial presentation but it is unlikely that any of the propofol administered remains in clinically relevant concentrations by the time emergency personnel arrive to administer care.

In preanesthetic assessment of the propofol abuser, as with other addicts, obtaining a history may be difficult although reasons for the presence of multiple, often infected, puncture wounds must be explored. In chronic abusers of propofol, the same issues that arise with any form of chronic intravenous drug use are applicable: infection with HIV, hepatitis C, and other blood-borne diseases (especially with bin scavengers) should be assumed until proven otherwise and standard universal precautions observed at all times. Chronic aspiration during repeated periods of apnea and loss of protected airway reflexes may lead to pneumonia or pneumonitis. Chest radiographs and room air oxygen saturation should be documented.

High doses of propofol administered in the medical setting have been associated with sudden death, a phenomenon termed propofol infusion syndrome [33]. The syndrome is characterized by the occurrence of lactic acidosis, rhabdomyolysis, and cardiovascular collapse. The mechanism is related to the production of increased serum levels of tumor necrosis factor alpha (TNF-α) and interleukin-10 (IL-10) resulting in diffuse areas of myocardial band necrosis [34]. Patients with traumatic head injury are particularly at risk of developing this complication as propofol is often used to control raised intracranial pressure [35]. At the basis of the syndrome, there appears to be an imbalance between energy utilization and cell demand resulting in cell dysfunction and ultimately necrosis or cardiac and peripheral muscle cells. A genetic susceptibility may also exist. Case report numbers are growing as propofol infusions are used widely in intensive care settings in both surgical (trauma care) and medical management (stroke). Infusion rates should not exceed 4 mg/kg/h. Malignant dysrhythmias are common, the first indicator of which may be the development of ST-segment elevation in leads V1–V3, a finding also reported in the case of a chronic propofol abuser [36]. The syndrome has also been described in a patient with respiratory failure and sepsis maintained for 7 days in an intensive care unit sedated with a propofol infusion [37]. A morbilliform rash developed on her upper body. Multiple laboratory abnormalities were found including elevated levels of alanine transferase, aspartate transaminase, amylase, lipase, creatinine kinase, and triglycerides. Electrocardiograms showed tachycardia. Computed tomography of the abdomen showed hepatomegaly, with fatty infiltration of the liver but a normal pancreas. The patient was treated with Phenobarbital maintenance therapy. Laboratory values returned to normal within 72 hours after discontinuation of propofol and the rash disappeared.

During the provision of anesthetic care to the patient known to be a chronic propofol abuser, serious consideration should be given to the use of agents, alternative to propofol for induction of general anesthesia. A preoperative ECG should be obtained regardless of age or cardiac history. Cardiac conduction disturbances and ventricular tachycardia have been described in an infant after prolonged infusion of propofol [38]. The presence of a Brugada-like pattern (Fig. 10.1) is reason enough to delay any elective case pending further cardiac evaluation (typical features in V1–3). Such a pattern, if anesthesia is induced, especially with propofol may proceed to hypotension, metabolic acidosis, prolonged QT interval, idioventricular rhythm and ventricular fibrillation, and renal failure [38–41]. In a fatal case in a young boy,

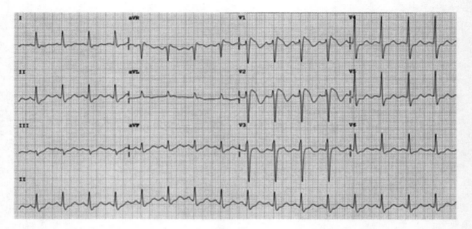

Fig. 10.1 Troublesome electrocardiographic findings suggestive of increased risk for sudden death in the chronic propofol abuser: Note the coved-type ST elevation, J-point elevation, gradually descending ST segment, and negative T-waves in the anterior pre-cordial leads. Image adapted from http://lifeinthefastlane.com/2009/09/what-is-brugada-syndrome/accessed 07/24/2010

postmortem examination revealed widespread fat accumulation in the myocardium, illustrating the proposed underlying pathophysiology of impaired muscular-free fatty acid utilization [40]. In the case of an emergent need to provide anesthesia, it is prudent to place external defibrillation pads on the chest and back prior to induction and avoid propofol altogether.

Conclusion

Propofol may well be the almost perfect drug of abuse were it not so quickly lethal. Its addictive properties are much better understood now. Anesthesiologists may be at risk for secondhand abuse, leading later to addiction or easy addiction to other substances.

Rather than surprise at the case reports of addiction to propofol, the question might be why more people are not frequent users, although only the tip of the iceberg may have been uncovered to date. Perhaps to become addicted to an anesthetic agent, the individual must have both the ability to identify the agent they received and gain access to the agent. Until last year, most patients were unable to identify the agents with which they were anesthetized and thus did not know what agent to ask for on the street or the Internet. With the publicity surrounding the death of Michael Jackson, that ignorance has gone. It would not be surprising to see a dramatic increase in the number of nonmedical personnel seeking access to and becoming addicted. Because of the evanescent nature of propofol, large amounts are required to prevent craving. Thus, abusers would have difficulty in secretive diversion.

However, because of the risk of disease transmission or bacterial growth, the manufacturer had recommended that the 20ml vial be a single patient use. As only 2–3 ml of propofol may be required per patient, large quantities may be discarded in sharps containers, ready for the scavenger. Should propofol become a controlled substance in the near future, it is likely that the public would also turn to the Internet for access, as the drug is generally available in other countries. Control of manufacture, amount of active drug, added impurities, or other drugs might then become something of a guessing game.

References

1. Marcus A. Propofol abuse growing problem for anesthesiologists. Anesthesiol News. 2007;33(5):1.
2. Wilson C, Canning P, Caravati EM. The abuse potential of propofol. Clin Toxicol (Phila). 2010;48(3):165–70.
3. Kotani Y, Shimazawa M, Yoshimura S. The experimental and clinical pharmacology of propofol, an anesthetic agent with neuroprotectice properties. CNS Neurosci Ther. 2008;14(2):95–106.
4. Brazzalotto I. Effects of propofol. Ann Fr Anesth Reanim. 1989;8:388.
5. Karowski MD, Koltchine VV, Rick CE, et al. Propofol and other intravenous anesthetics have sites of action on the gamma-aminobutyric acid type A receptor distinct from that for isoflurane. Mol Pharmacol. 1998;53:530–8.
6. Kingston S, Mao L, Yang L, et al. Propofol inhibits phosphorylation of N-methyl-D-aspartate receptor NR1 subunits in neurons. Anesthesiology. 2006;104:763–9.
7. Leslie JB. Fospropofol (Lusedra®) may be an alternative to propofol for monitored anesthetic care. APSF Newsletter Summer. 2010. www.apsf.org/newsletters/html/2010/summer/07_Fospropofol.htm. Accessed 6 Oct 2010.
8. Cohen LB, Cattau E, Goetsch A, et al. A randomized, double-blind, phase 3 study of fospropofol disodium for sedation during colonoscopy. J Clin Gastroenterol. 2010;44:345–53.
9. Silvestri GA, Vincent BD, Wahidi MM, et al. A phase 3, randomized, double-blind study to assess the efficacy and safety of fospropofol disodium injection for moderate sedation in patients undergoing flexible bronchoscopy. Chest. 2009;135:41–7.
10. Gan TJ, Berry BD, Ekman EF, et al. Safety evaluation of fospropofol for sedation during minor surgical procedures. J Clin Anesth. 2010;22:260–7.
11. Pain L, Gobaille S, Schleef C, et al. In vivo dopamine measurements in the nucleus accumbens after nonanesthetic and anesthetic doses of propofol in rats. Anesth Analg. 2002;95:191–6.
12. Keita H, Lecharny JB, Henzel D, et al. Is inhibition of dopamine uptake relevant to the hypnotic action of iv anesthetics? Br J Anaesth. 1996;77:254–6.
13. Xiong M, Zhang C. Molecular basis of propofol addiction IARS Annual Meeting 2009, San Diego, CA; 2005. (also identified in; Campton MG Anesthesiology News). Molecular basis of propofol identified. Vol 35;5;1.
14. McAuliffe PF, Gold MS, Bajpai L, et al. Second-hand exposure to aerosolized intravenous anesthetics propofol and fentanyl may cause sensitization and subsequent opiate addiction among anesthesiologists and surgeons. Med Hypotheses. 2006;68(5):874–82.
15. Merlo LJ, Goldberger BA, Kolodner D, et al. Fentanyl and propofol exposure in the operating room: sensitization hypotheses and further data. J Addict Dis. 2008;27(3):67–76.
16. Li KY, Xiao C, Xiong M, et al. Nanomolar propofol stimulates glutamate transmission to dopamine neurons: a possible mechanism of abuse potential? J Pharmacol Exp Ther. 2008;325(1):165–74.
17. Follette JW, Farley WJ. Anesthesiologist addicted to propofol. Anesthesiology. 1992;77:817–8.

18. Ward CF. Substance abuse, now and for some time to come. Anesthesiology. 1992;77:619–22.
19. Zacny JP, Lichtor JL, Thompson W, et al. Propofol at a subanesthetic dose may have abuse potential in healthy volunteers. Anesth Analg. 1993;77(3):544–52.
20. Kranioti EF, Mavroforou A, Mylonakis P, Michalodimitrakis M. Lethal self administration of propofol (Diprivan). A case report and review of the literature. Forensic Sci Int. 2007;167(1):56–8.
21. Fritz GA, Niemczyk WE. Propofol dependency in a lay person. Anesthesiology. 2002;96:505–6.
22. Kirby RR, Colaw JM, Douglas MM. Death from propofol: accident, suicide, or murder? Anesth Analg. 2009;108(4):1182–4.
23. Klausz G, Rona K, Kristof I, et al. Evaluation of a fatal propofol intoxication due to self administration. J Forensic Leg Med. 2009;16(5):287–9.
24. Iwerson-Bergmann S, Rosner P, Kohnau HC, et al. Death after excessive propofol abuse. Int J Legal Med. 2001;114(4–5):248–51.
25. Strehler M, Preuss J, Wollersen H, et al. Lethal moxed intoxication with propofol in a medical layman. Arch Kriminol. 2008;217(5–6):153–60.
26. Roussin A, Monastrue JL, Lapeyre-Mestre M. Pharmacological and clinical evidences on the potential for abuse and dependence of propofol: a review of the literature. Fuundam Clin Pharmacol. 2007;21(5):459–66.
27. Bonnet U, Harkener J, Scherbaum N. A case report of propofol dependence in a physician. J Psychactive Drugs. 2008;40(2):215–7.
28. Soyka M, Schutz CG. Propfol dependency. Addiction. 1997;92(10):1369–70.
29. Wischmeyer PE, Johnson BR, Wilson JE. A survey of propofol abuse in academic anesthesia programs. Anesth Analg. 2007;105(4):1066–71.
30. Ward CF. Propofol: Dancing with the "white rabbit". CSA Bulletin Spring. 2008;61–3.
31. Tung A, Bergman BM, Herrera S, et al. Recovery from sleep deprivation occurs during propofol anesthesia. Anesthesiology. 2004;100:1419–26.
32. Nelson LE, Franks NP, Maze M, et al. Rested and refreshed after anesthesia? Anesthesiology. 2004;100:1341–2.
33. Stelow EB, Johari VP, Smity SA, Crosson JT, Apple FS. Propofol associated rhabdomyolysis with cardiac involvement in adults: chemical and anatomic findings. Clin Chem. 2000;46:577–81.
34. Vernooy K, Delhaas T, Cremer OL, et al. Electrocardiographic changes predicting sudden death in propofol-related infusion syndrome. Heart Rhythm. 2006;3:131–7.
35. Otterspoor LC, Kalkman CJ, Cremer OL. Update on the propofol infusion syndrome in the ICU management of patients with head injury. Curr Opin Anaesthesiol. 2008;21(5):544–51.
36. Riezzo I, Centini F, Neri M, et al. Brugada-like EKG pattern and myocardial effects in a chronic propofol abuser. Clin Toxicol. 2009;47:358–63.
37. Orsini J, Ndakami A, Chen J, Cohen N. Propofol infusion syndrome: a case report and literature review. Am J Health Syst Pharm. 2009;66(10):908–15.
38. Robinson JD, Melman Y, Walsh EP. Cardiac conduction disturbances and ventricular tachycardia after prolonged propofol infusion in an infant. Pacing Clin Electrophysiol. 2008;31(8):1070–3.
39. Bebarta VS, Summera S. Predictor of mortality in suspected propofol infusion syndrome-Brugata electrocardiographic pattern. Crit Care Med. 2009;37(2):795–6.
40. Jorens PG, Van der Eynden GG. Propofol infusion syndrome with arrhythmia, myocardial fat accumulation and cardiac failure. Am J Cardiol. 2009;104(8):1160–2.
41. Riera AR, Lichida AH, Schapachnik E, et al. Propofol infusion syndrome and Brugada syndrome electrocardiographic phenocopy. Cardiol J. 2010;17(2):130–5.

Part III
Specific Populations

Chapter 11
Drugs, Alcohol, and Pregnant Women: Anesthetic Implications for Mother and Newborn

Migdalia Saloum and Jonathan N. Epstein

Introduction

The prevalence of substance abuse among young adults has increased markedly over the last 20 years. Since nearly 90% of drug-abusing women are of childbearing age, it is likely that the clinician will encounter pregnant women who abuse illicit drugs [1]. As many case reports confirm, life-threatening complications may result when the physiologic changes of pregnancy are combined with the adverse effects of drug abuse [2]. Anesthesiologists are likely to meet the drug-abusing parturient first in an acute setting either when labor analgesia is requested or in an emergency situation such as fetal distress, placental abruption, uterine rupture, or sudden onset of life-threatening maternal dysrhythmias. Risk factors suggesting drug abuse in pregnancy include lack of prenatal care, history of premature labor, and cigarette smoking [3]. The most common illicit substances encountered are alcohol, cocaine, amphetamines, opioids, marijuana, and tobacco.

Some states consider drug use during pregnancy to be a form of child abuse and neglect. When interviewed preoperatively by anesthesiologists or obstetricians, the drug-abusing parturient will most likely not be forthcoming about their addiction. Therefore, a high index of suspicion of drug abuse in pregnancy, combined with nonjudgmental questioning of every parturient is necessary. Legal actions range from charges of neglect to homicide by child abuse. In 2003, the South Carolina Supreme Court held that a pregnant woman, who smoked crack cocaine, causing her baby to die shortly after delivery, was guilty of homicide by child abuse since her unborn child was a legally protected person [4]. In 2010, a Kentucky mother faced up to ten years in prison after pleading guilty to endangering the life of her unborn baby for using cocaine while pregnant [5].

M. Saloum (✉)
Department of Anesthesiology, St. Luke's Roosevelt Hospital, New York, NY, USA
e-mail: msaloum@gmail.com

E.O. Bryson and E.A.M. Frost (eds.), *Perioperative Addiction:*
Clinical Management of the Addicted Patient, DOI 10.1007/978-1-4614-0170-4_11,
© Springer Science+Business Media, LLC 2012

The American College of Obstetricians and Gynecologists (ACOG) discourages states from pursuing criminal sanctions, and current recommendations are that the state and the caregivers should focus on prevention and, if need be, treatment [6]. ACOG makes several recommendations concerning the management of the drug-abusing parturient. First, a drug history should be taken from all patients. Second, support, aid, and counseling should be made available to all women who acknowledge substance abuse. Third, drug testing should be considered routinely to encourage abstinence in those who have a history of substance abuse. Lastly, testing the parturient and the neonate may be useful in certain clinical conditions when certain conditions such as intrauterine growth restriction (IUGR), prematurity, and placental abruption cannot be explained [6].

Alcohol

More than 15 million people in the United States are addicted to alcohol with women accounting for 25% of this number. The 2006 national survey on drug use and health found that 11.8% of pregnant women reported current alcohol use and 2.9% reported binge drinking (five drinks or greater on one occasion). Fifty-three percent of nonpregnant women of childbearing age reported current alcohol use and 23.6% reported binge drinking. Estimates from the 2002 behavioral risk factor surveillance system found that among the 7.6% of women of childbearing age not using birth control, more than half reported using alcohol [7]. Many of these women could be unaware of being pregnant and continue using alcohol. Alcohol consumption in pregnancy is considered to cause adverse fetal sequelae at any stage of development. Because alcoholism is more subtle and more difficult to diagnose than other addictions, it is frequently overlooked.

Alcohol easily crosses the placenta and is an established teratogen. No safe level of consumption has been established during pregnancy [8]. Alcohol and its metabolites (e.g., acetylaldehyde) *freely* cross the placenta. The biochemical mechanisms explaining the teratogenicity of alcohol are not fully understood. One hypothesis is cellular injury that is caused by the induction of oxidative stress. Oxidative stress leads to peroxidation of lipids (e.g., neurological tissue), nucleic acids (e.g., DNA), proteins (e.g., enzymes), and carbohydrates. Ethanol may also play a role in the production of reactive oxygen species (ROS) and in programmed cell death. It has also been postulated that alcohol mediates its neurologic effects by its actions on the central nervous system (CNS) receptors, γ-aminobutyric acid (GABA) and N-methyl D-aspartate (NMDA) [9].

The effects of alcohol on the fetus are mediated by the amount of alcohol consumption, the duration of consumption, and the developing stage of the fetus. The pattern of alcohol related birth defects is highly variable. The teratogenic insults during embryonic life may present immediately after birth, at infancy, or even later in life, especially if the damage involves the CNS [10]. It is generally recognized that in the first trimester, during organogenesis, the fetus may be more susceptible to anatomic abnormalities. In many cases, the fetus is exposed to the teratogenic effects of alcohol before pregnancy is confirmed. Sixty percent of women who drink were not aware of their pregnancy until the fourth week of conception [3]. Continued alcohol use into the later trimesters mainly affects the developing CNS, as most of the other organs have already formed. Active development of the cerebral cortex in the fetus occurs mainly in the second and third trimesters, and can consequently be a critical time period for the development of neurological impairments. Hence, the later trimester effects of alcohol may not necessarily manifest with morphological changes in the fetus but rather by neurodevelopmental disorders that may present more subtly and later in the child's development.

Spontaneous abortions, prenatal and postnatal growth restriction, low birth weight, birth defects, and neurodevelopmental deficits are all increased in pregnant women who consume alcohol. Fetal alcohol syndrome is the most commonly known disorder and it is associated with growth retardation, physical anomalies, and developmental abnormalities including mental retardation [11].

The teratogenic effects of alcohol were first reported in France in 1968 by Lemoine et al. They described a common pattern of birth defects in 127 children born to alcoholic mothers [12]. Fetal alcohol syndrome as a triad of facial dysmorphia, growth retardation, and CNS defects was first described in the United States in 1973 by Jones and Smith [13]. It is now a well-recognized disorder which consists of a characteristic facial pattern, growth retardation, and CNS neurodevelopmental abnormalities. In 2004, the National Organization of Fetal Alcohol Syndrome agreed to introduce the term fetal alcohol spectrum disorder (FASD) as an umbrella term to include other diagnostic categories in addition to FAS. The expanded criteria defined by the Institute of Medicine (IOM) describe several categories that have been recognized as a continuum of the severity of symptoms produced by alcohol on the fetus. FASD includes FAS, partial FAS, alcohol-related neurodevelopmental disorder (ARND), and alcohol-related birth defects (ARBD) (Table 11.1) [14, 15].

Several studies have described a dose/effect relationship between alcohol and fetal effects [16–18]. Fetal alcohol syndrome is associated with an exposure of approximately an average of 4 ounces of absolute alcohol per day (roughly eight drinks per day). Less recognized are the risks of prenatal exposure to moderate levels of alcohol or occasional abuse, especially binge drinking (Table 11.2).

Fetal alcohol syndrome is the leading cause of mental retardation worldwide. It is also the most preventable cause of neurobehavioral and developmental abnormalities. It is estimated that the prevalence of FAS in the United States is between 0.5 and 2 cases per 1,000 live births. FAS, ARBD, and ARND may affect at least 10 per 1,000 live births [19].

Three facial features (reduced palpebral fissure length/inner canthal distance ratio, smooth philtrum, and thin upper lip) can accurately identify individuals with FAS. Other facial features that can be present include a short upturned nose, depressed nasal bridge, hypoplastic maxilla, ear anomalies, palmar crease anomalies, and micrognathia (Figs. 11.1 and 11.2a, b). Other organ system malformations include cardiac anomalies (ASD, VSD, aberrant great vessels, and tetralogy of Fallot), skeletal changes (i.e., syndactyly), renal problems (i.e., aplastic kidneys, and ureteral duplications), and ocular, and auditory dysfunction [20]. The most obvious physical

Table 11.1 Diagnostic criteria for the fetal alcohol effects

1. Fetal alcohol syndrome (FAS)

   (a) With or without *confirmed maternal alcohol exposure*

   (b) Characteristic pattern of *facial anomalies* (midface hypoplasia; short palpebral fissures; indistinct and broad philtrum; and flattened nasal bridge)

   (c) *Growth restriction* (low birth weight for gestational age; decelerated weight gain not due to nutrition; and disproportionately low weight to height)

   (d) *CNS abnormalities* (decreased cranial size; structural abnormalities; age-appropriate neurological signs, e.g., neurosensory hearing loss or impaired motor development)

2. Partial FAS[a]

   (a) *Confirmed maternal alcohol exposure*

   (b) Some components of the *FAS face*

Either i, ii, or iii

   (i) *Growth restriction* (same as 1.c. above)

   (ii) *CNS abnormalities* (same as 1.d. above)

   (iii) Complex pattern of *behavioral or cognitive abnormalities* not explained by developmental level, family background, or environment

3. Alcohol-related neurodevelopmental disorder

   (a) *Confirmed maternal alcohol exposure*

Evidence of *CNS abnormality*, as either:

   (i) *CNS abnormalities* (same as 1.d. above)

   (ii) *Behavioral or cognitive abnormalities* (same as 2.iii. above)

4. Alcohol-related birth defects

   (a) *Confirmed maternal alcohol exposure*

   (b) Any one or more cardiac, skeletal, renal, or other congenital *malformation or dysplasia*

Reprinted with permission from: Hannigan JH, Armant DR. Alcohol in pregnancy and neonatal outcome. Semin Neonatol. 2000;5:243–254

[a]Diagnoses of partial FAS, ARND, or ARBD require *confirmed* excessive maternal alcohol intake. The diagnoses of full FAS may be made in the absence of such confirmation when all facial, growth, and CNS effects present clearly

Table 11.2 Dose and effects of fetal alcohol exposure

Feature	Amount
FAS	≥4 ounces of absolute alcohol/day
Decreased birth weight	2–3 ounces of absolute alcohol/day
Decreased I.Q. (5–7 points)	1.5 ounces of absolute alcohol/day
Spelling and reading difficulties	≥0.5 ounces of absolute alcohol/day
Functional deficits	5 drinks/occasion 1x/wk (binge drinking)
Hyperactivity, inattention	0.45 ounces of absolute alcohol/day
One standard drink = 0.48 ounces of absolute alcohol	

Reprinted with permission from: [Clarren et al. (1987), Jacobson et al. (1994), Larroque et al. (1995) and Streissguth et al. (1996, 1998)]

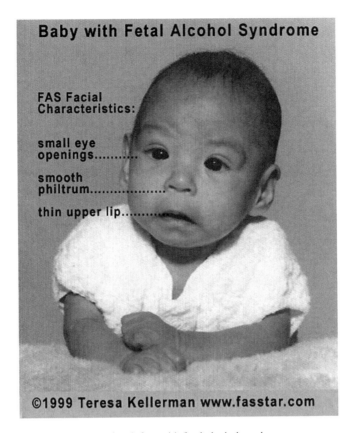

Fig. 11.1 Facial characteristics of an infant with fetal alcohol syndrome

CNS abnormality may be microcephaly. Early identification of FAS is important because early medical intervention may prevent development of secondary disabilities and can alert the physician to problem drinking in the mother. The early diagnosis of fetal alcohol syndrome or that of the lesser effects in the spectrum plays an important role in the outcome of these children. Current evidence suggests that newborns with FAS are not adequately identified in the nursery [18]. In the newborn, behavioral characteristics suggestive of FAS can include sleeping and feeding difficulties, weakness, irritability and tremulousness, excessive crying, hypersensitivity to light and sound, and failure to thrive [21].

The potential consequences to the newborn of abrupt removal from an alcohol-tolerant environment could include physical withdrawal within a day or two of birth. Because the immediate manifestations of fetal withdrawal to alcohol are subtle, immediate diagnosis is difficult. Accordingly, the severity of neonatal withdrawal to alcohol is unclear, in contrast to neonatal opiate withdrawal which is well described and clearly more profound. Symptoms manifested in the neonate with possible alcohol withdrawal include CNS hyperexcitability, seizures, tremors, irritability,

a   b

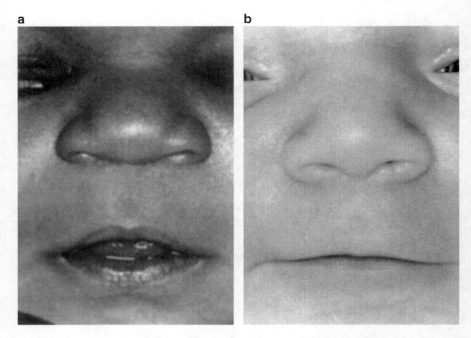

Fig. 11.2 (**a**). Infant with long upper lip, flat philtrum, thin vermilion, broad depressed nasal bridge, and anteverted nares. (**b**) Infant with depressed nasal bridge, long upper lip, flat philtrum, and thin vermilion

sweating, poor sleep patterns, excessive muscle tension, high respiratory rate, and an increased susceptibility to apnea [22].

Management of the Alcohol-Abusing Parturient

Depending on the degree of alcohol dependence and the timing of the most recent intake, patients can present in labor with a variety of clinical manifestations. Alcohol has numerous and complicated effects within the CNS and acts as both a depressant and a stimulant. Patients who are acutely intoxicated are unable to adequately protect their airways and pose a pulmonary aspiration risk. Acute alcohol intoxication increases gastric fluid acidity and gastric fluid volume. Hypoglycemia and electrolyte imbalances can result from heavy alcohol use coupled with poor food intake. Chronic alcohol use is associated with malnutrition, liver disease, altered drug metabolism, coagulopathy, pancreatitis, esophageal varices, and cardiomyopathy.

Acutely intoxicated patients may also present with the fetus in "nonreassuring" status. Regional anesthesia can be administered safely to cooperative patients. Contraindications to neuraxial anesthesia are usually encountered in chronic abusers with end-stage hepatic disease and include infection and coagulopathy. Neuropathies and pre-existing neurological impairments are relative contraindications and should be documented for medico-legal reasons. Intravascular fluid volume must be assessed in these patients who tend to be intravascularly depleted in order to avoid excessive hypotension as a consequence of sympathetic blockade.

In case of emergency delivery, or if the patient is too sedated or uncooperative to protect her airway, general anesthesia is necessary. Acute alcohol consumption is known to decrease anesthetic requirements due to the additive effects of CNS depressants. The notion that chronic alcohol abusers have a higher MAC for potent inhaled anesthetics than their nonabusing counterparts has not been substantiated. An abstract published in 1969 by Han [23] showed an increased requirement of inhaled anesthetics by chronic alcoholics in a very small study group of six. Subsequently, Swerdlow et al. [24] published a study regarding increased thiopental doses in chronic alcoholics that was inconclusive. To date, no large population studies have effectively assessed dose requirements for volatile anesthetic agents or hypnotic agents in patients who chronically abuse alcohol. Anesthesia providers should avoid arbitrarily administering high doses of inhaled anesthetics to pregnant patients with a history of chronic alcohol abuse, since these women, in addition to requiring lower MAC as a result of their pregnancy, can also be at risk for intravascular volume depletion, cardiomyopathy, and hypoalbuminenia. In addition, high concentrations of inhaled volatile anesthetics can depress uterine tone and may increase blood loss at cesarean delivery.

Acute alcohol withdrawal symptoms could be encountered 6–48 h after cessation of ethanol consumption, although delays of up to 10 days have been reported. Symptoms include nausea/vomiting, tachycardia, dysrhythmias, hypertension, delirium, hallucinations, seizures, and cardiac failure. Delirium tremens is a rare, although life-threatening, medical emergency. Symptoms of withdrawal can be treated with benzodiazepines, $\alpha 2$ adrenergic agonists (e.g., clonidine), or ethanol infusions [25].

Stigma, shame, fear of legal repercussions, and fear of mandatory placement into detoxification programs lead many pregnant alcohol users to underreport alcohol use before, during, and after pregnancy. These considerations may lead women to avoid prenatal clinics and consistent care. Simple, sensitive, and effective evidence-based screening tools have been developed to help physicians and other health-care workers detect problem drinking in pregnant women or women of childbearing age engaging in excessive drinking. There is good evidence overall for the effectiveness of screening and behavioral interventions in reducing the amount of drinking in patients [26]. Currently, screening and prevention with behavior modification are the only tools available to reduce the effects of alcohol on the mother and fetus. Various 4–5 question screening instruments have been widely validated. The TWEAK or T-ACE questionnaires are preferred because they include assessments for tolerance (how many drinks does it take to make you high?). The tolerance question assumes that there is drinking and avoids patient denial. A positive response on the tolerance question alone (i.e., two or more drinks) is a sensitive predictor of "fetal-risk" drinking (Table 11.3) [27].

Meconium, passed by newborns during their first postnatal bowel movements, can be collected for drug testing. Over the last two decades, meconium testing has been shown to be more sensitive, easier to collect, and has a larger window period for detection of the drug than other methods of testing. Meconium testing has been shown to be most sensitive in the detection of cocaine and opioids, but has a

Table 11.3 The TWEAK tool

TWEAK	Questions	Points
Tolerance	How many drinks does it take to feel the first effect? Or How many drinks does it take to get you high?	2 or more = 2 points
Worry	Have close friends worried or complained about your drinking?	Yes = 2 points
Eye-opener	Do you sometime need a drink in the morning when you first get up?	Yes = 1 point
Amnesia	Have friends or family ever told you about things you said or did while you were drinking that you could not remember?	Yes = 1 point
Kut down	Do you sometimes feel the need to cut down on your drinking?	Yes = 1 point

A total score of 7 is possible. A total score ≥2 indicates problem drinking
Reprinted with permission from: Burns E, Gray R, Smith LA. Brief screening questionnaires to identify problem drinking during pregnancy: a systematic review. Addiction. 2010;105:601–614

low sensitivity for amphetamines and cannabinoids [28]. Recently, biologic markers for detection of the presence of alcohol in the mother and fetus have been investigated. Fatty acid ethyl esters (FAEEs) are nonoxidative metabolites of alcohol that can be detected in meconium. Elevated levels of FAEEs in meconium have been shown to be effective biomarkers in detecting heavy prenatal alcohol exposure. There is promising evidence that this biomarker may be effective in prenatal screening (Fig. 11.3) [29, 30].

Cocaine

Cocaine abuse continues to be a major problem affecting society today. While it is difficult to estimate the prevalence of cocaine use in parturients, use appears to be on the rise. In 2008, 722,000 teens and adults reported first-time cocaine use [31]. The cocaine-using parturient presents unique challenges to the anesthesiologist. An understanding of maternal–fetal physiology and the effects of cocaine on this physiology is imperative to formulate any anesthetic plan.

Diagnosing the cocaine-abusing parturient presents unique challenges. The telltale tachycardia, hypertension, and dysrhythmias can all be attributed to naturally occurring labor. Further complicating matters is that denial is a frequent response to direct questioning. However, the most common cause of failure to diagnose illicit drug use is that of physician failure to ask. It is estimated that only 20% of physicians inquire about substance use when interviewing patients [32]. There are, however, certain risk factors that are associated with cocaine abuse in pregnancy, including lack of prenatal care, a history of premature labor, and cigarette smoking [33]. Even without these associated factors a high index of suspicion should accompany every preoperative evaluation. A rapid latex agglutination test detects metabolites of cocaine in

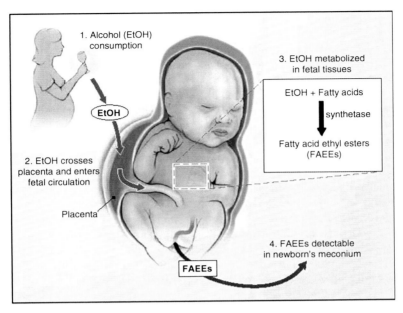

Fig. 11.3 Neonatal meconium assay for fatty acid ethyl esters (FAEEs). Most of the body's load of ethanol is eliminated after enzyme oxidation to acetaldehyde and water. However, ethanol is also esterified with fatty acids to FAEEs, which can be found in adult blood and tissue. It is now evident that FAEEs can be found in neonatal meconium and may reflect maternal drinking in pregnancy

urine within a few minutes in suspicious cases [34]. In the absence of the rapid testing, cocaine metabolites can be detected in maternal urine, meconium, and maternal hair. While maternal urine will only have detectable metabolites for up to 60 h, neonatal urine contains metabolites for up to 96 h after maternal ingestion [35].

The unique pharmacological properties of cocaine make it dangerous for the fetus. A low molecular weight and high lipophilicity, coupled with the fact that it exists primarily in its unionized form, allow cocaine to readily cross the placenta leading to rapid attainment of high levels in fetal blood and tissue [36]. In addition to the fetal anomalies associated with cocaine use early in pregnancy, including urogenital tract abnormalities, gastroschisis, microcephaly, growth restriction, CNS defects, and musculoskeletal derangements, there is also evidence that fetuses exposed to cocaine in utero have lower IQ scores and increased incidence of learning disabilities [37]. Acutely, fetal distress is more common with preterm delivery being four times more likely as compared to non-cocaine-exposed fetuses. There is also a significantly increased risk for intrauterine demise.

Complications of cocaine use in the parturient include premature rupture of membranes, placental abruption, uterine rupture, hepatic rupture, cardiac dysrhythmias and ischemia, cerebral ischemia and hemorrhage, myocardial infarction, and death [38, 39]. By increasing the three major determinants of myocardial oxygen demand, heart rate, arterial blood pressure, and left ventricular contractility, cocaine greatly increases maternal risk of myocardial ischemia and infarction. The parturient is at particular risk from cocaine as a result of the increased oxygen demand in pregnancy. Some data suggest that pregnancy may be associated with an increased sensitivity of the cardiovascular system to cocaine, secondary to either an increased sensitivity of alpha-adrenergic receptors in parturients or an increased metabolism of cocaine to the biologically active metabolite nor-cocaine, mediated by increased levels of progesterone [36].

Long-standing cocaine abuse can lead to left ventricular hypertrophy and dilated cardiomyopathy [40]. Vasoconstriction, however, is not limited to maternal circulation. While the fetus is at significant risk for uteroplacental insufficiency, hypoxia, and acidosis from the concomitant decrease in uteroplacental blood flow that accompanies maternal hypertension, animal studies have proven conclusively that the fetal blood vessels themselves are subjected to significant vasoconstriction [41]. Maternal ischemia or infarction can be the result of thrombosis, vasospasm, or direct myocardial depression. Cardiovascular complications stemming from cocaine use seem to be independent of dose. Numerous case reports have documented both morbidity and mortality resulting from "small" recreational doses [42].

Not surprisingly, the dual coronary vasoconstrictive properties of cocaine abuse combined with cigarette usage during pregnancy increase the incidence of cardiovascular complications [43]. When poly-substance abuse is an issue, the most prevalent combination seems to be that of cocaine and alcohol. Complication rates, including death, when using these drugs in tandem are statistically higher than complications associated with using either drug alone. The mechanism of action and likely cause of this higher rate of complications are related to the synergistic blockade of synaptic cleft dopamine re-uptake secondary to the actions of coca-ethylene, a metabolite of the two substances [43].

Other organ systems are affected depending on the manner in which the cocaine is ingested. Snorting the cocaine can lead to epistaxis, nasal septal injury, and oral ulcers [44]. Smoking cocaine can lead to bronchospasm, diffusion capacity abnormalities, and thermal burns in the airway if ingested as a vapor. Interstitial and alveolar hemorrhages have also been reported secondary to pulmonary and bronchial arterial vasoconstriction [45].

Management of the Cocaine-Abusing Parturient

It is generally believed that the use of neuraxial anesthesia, by reducing the levels of circulating catecholamines and diminishing the systemic effects of cocaine, benefits the cocaine-using parturient [8]. However, once cocaine use has been established, each parturient and her clinical presentation must be assessed individually for both an obstetric and anesthetic plan. The cocaine-using parturient presents unique difficulties for the anesthesiologist. Regional anesthesia has been associated with hypotension, altered pain perception, combative behavior, and cocaine-induced thrombocytopenia [46]. A well-documented phenomenon is that cocaine addicts frequently complain of pain even with a demonstrable adequate level of neuraxial anesthesia [8]. This seems to be particularly true during a cesarean section. It has been theorized that abnormalities in endorphin levels as well as chronic changes found in both mu and kappa opioid receptor densities are likely to play a role in this phenomenon [47].

When general anesthesia is indicated, it is important to remember that all volatile anesthetic agents can produce dysrhythmias in the presence of cocaine. Hypertension and myocardial ischemia have also been widely reported [48]. While the optimal induction sequence has yet to be established, ketamine should be used with caution, if at all, since its CNS-stimulating properties may potentiate the cardiac effects of cocaine by increasing catecholamine levels. Care must be taken to minimize the severe hypertension that can accompany induction and laryngoscopy. Several approaches have been suggested using drugs in our armamentarium to lower the blood pressure of the cocaine-using parturient. Labetalol, with its unique alpha- and beta-action, has been advocated by some. Others caution against using labetalol as a single agent due to its 7:1 beta predominant effect. Addressing that concern, Birnbach recommended combining labetalol with nitroglycerine as the most effective way to treat severe cocaine-induced hypertension. However, labetalol does not ameliorate cocaine-induced coronary artery vasoconstriction [42]. Hydralazine, as a direct vasodilator, will decrease systemic vascular resistance (SVR); however, the accompanying reflex tachycardia could be problematic in an already tachycardic cocaine-intoxicated parturient. Other direct vasodilators such as nitroglycerine have been demonstrated to be a safe and effective treatment of cocaine-related chest pain and myocardial ischemia/infarction.

Guidelines from the American Heart Association recommend the combination of benzodiazepines and nitroglycerine as first-line agents for cocaine-related HTN and chest discomfort [49]. Selective beta-blockade has long been discouraged as treatment of cocaine toxicity to prevent unopposed alpha-stimulation. Evidence clearly demonstrates that administration of β-blockers can worsen cardiac perfusion and/or produce paradoxical hypertension when cocaine is present. Current recommendations are that pure β-blocker medications in the setting of cocaine are not indicated [50]. Phentolamine, a selective alpha-blocker, may be used to reverse cocaine-induced vasoconstriction. Pharmacological control of the blood pressure should be obtained prior to induction. In terms of muscle relaxation, there is a theoretical concern that cocaine could alter the breakdown of succinylcholine secondary to competing metabolism of plasma cholinesterases. Although it has been rarely described, clinically, prolonged blockade does not regularly occur with standard doses of succinylcholine [51, 52].

Amphetamines

Amphetamines are a group of powerful stimulants of the CNS, with a profound ability to produce euphoria, wakefulness, alertness, and decrease appetite. They increase the release of norepinephrine, serotonin, and dopamine from presynaptic neurons and inhibit their breakdown. Amphetamines are noncatecholamine indirect-acting sympathomimetics with peripheral α- and β-adrenergic receptor activity [53]. Methamphetamine (N-methyl-1-phenyl-propan-2-amine) is methylated amphetamine, and is the most commonly abused amphetamine. Methamphetamine is more potent than amphetamine, and is the only illegal drug that can be easily produced from legally obtained ingredients such as decongestants or cold medications. Methamphetamine can exist in crystal form, or as a white odorless powder that can be inhaled, injected, swallowed, or smoked. It is has a high bioavailability and produces profound euphoria with a half-life of 9–15 h [8]. MDMA (3,4 methylene-deoxymethamphetamine), also known as ecstasy, is an analog of methamphetamine that shares properties with amphetamine and hallucinogenics [54]. Adderall, a combination of amphetamine and dextroamphetamine, is also a part of the amphetamine family that is frequently used by women of reproductive age for treatment of attention deficit/hyperactivity disorder. Fortunately, this medication is not commonly abused during pregnancy [11].

Methamphetamine accounted for 8% of admitted pregnant women with substance abuse in 1994. In 2006, the number rose to 24%. The majority of methamphetamine admissions occurred in the West (73%), among white (64%) unemployed (88%) women [55]. Since 2002, the prevalence of methamphetamine use has remained relatively stable. Many users become addicted after a single exposure as a result of the prolonged euphoria, ease of production, and relatively low cost [8]. The Infant Development, Environment And Lifestyle study (IDEAL) has estimated that 5.2% of women in particularly prevalent regions of the U.S. use methamphetamine at some point during their pregnancy [56]. The western and southwestern states have historically been the most prevalent regions for methamphetamine use. Since the 1990s methamphetamine use has been growing to include the Midwest, rocky mountain states, and Hawaii. In 2004, many state governments began to pass laws restricting the sale of the primary methamphetamine precursor, pseudoephedrine, to reduce the domestic production of methamphetamine [57].

Studies regarding methamphetamine use in pregnancy are unreliable since they mostly depend on voluntary maternal reporting and retrospective information. Frequently, amphetamine users abuse other drugs as well, making it difficult to separate out the sole effects of methamphetamine use during pregnancy and preconception [11]. There seems to be no detrimental effects associated with discontinuation of amphetamine use during pregnancy; therefore, patients who are known to abuse amphetamines should be encouraged to stop and be referred to a substance abuse program.

Amphetamines freely cross the placenta and have been found in measurable amounts in animal fetal organs, including the brain and heart. Animal studies have shown an association of methamphetamine with cleft palate, exencephaly, growth insufficiency, retinal defects, and delayed motor development. Retrospective human studies have shown significantly lower fetal gestational age, birth weight, length, and occipitofrontal circumference in comparison to control newborns [58]. Case reports suggest an association between methamphetamine use in the first trimester and congenital abnormalities such as heart defects, gastroschisis, small intestine atresia, and cleft lip/palate [59–63]. Conversely, other studies have failed to show any association between methamphetamine and congenital abnormalities [64, 65].

Overall, there is no increased incidence of birth defects associated with metham-phetamine use beyond that of the general population rate of 3%. There is no current evidence of any consistent fetal congenital syndrome resulting from methamphet-amine use in the first trimester. The most established fetal abnormality associated with methamphetamine is fetal growth insufficiency. It is unknown whether the fetal growth restriction that can result from methamphetamine exposure is related to direct vasoconstriction on the fetus or an indirect effect through nutritional deficien-cies. There have also been reports of fetal/neonatal cerebral cavitary lesions believed to be a result of hypoxia from vasoconstriction [11]. Mild neonatal withdrawal has been reported in about half of the cases of methamphetamine-addicted parturients. Symptoms described include jitteriness, drowsiness, and respiratory distress. There is an exceedingly high rate of adoption and foster care among newborns, pointing to a breakdown of the mother–infant bonding process in this population [66]. There have also been reported cases of neonatal death associated with maternal metham-phetamine use [67].

Management of the Amphetamine-Abusing Parturient

Amphetamines exert their symptoms by stimulating the release of catecholamines and inhibiting re-uptake. Hypertension, dysrhythmias, tachycardia, dilated pupils, hyperreflexia, proteinuria, and confusion all can be seen with acute amphetamine intoxication. Clinically, amphetamine intoxication is indistinguishable from cocaine. Coexistence of seizures, proteinuria, and hypertension secondary to amphetamines and cocaine has been mistaken for eclampsia. Profound thermoregulation distur-bances (heat stroke) have been known to result from MDMA intoxication. Chronic abuse of amphetamines depletes body stores of catecholamines and may manifest clinically with anxiety, somnolence, or psychosis [8].

The effect of amphetamines on the CNS may have significant anesthetic implica-tions. There is no apparent contraindication to regional anesthesia, but sympathec-tomy may precipitate hypotension that may have unpredictable responses to vasopressors. Emergent cesarean section may be needed secondary to fetal distress, placental abruption, or other obstetrical emergencies. Acute intake of amphetamines can increase the MAC of potent inhaled anesthetics [68]. In contrast, chronic inges-tion may decrease the dose requirements for general anesthetics [69]. Reports of adverse cardiac decompensation and death during cesarean section using regional or general anesthesia techniques have been described [2].

Opioids

The class of drugs known as the Opioids includes the opiates, which are natural or semi-synthetic morphine-like substances as well as the fully synthetic opioids. Opiates include morphine, codeine, hydromorphone, and heroin. Synthetic opioids include meperidine, fentanyl, and methadone. The most commonly abused opioid is heroin. Most of the information on the effects of opioids on the mother and fetus has been obtained from studies involving heroin or methadone. Recently, there has been an increase in the abuse of prescription opioids such as hydromorphone and oxycodone during pregnancy [70].

The prevalence of opioid use in pregnancy is estimated to be between 1% and 21%. The 21% in this estimate includes patients in high-risk populations [71]. It is difficult to ascertain the sole effects of heroin on the parturient and fetus because these women also tend to abuse other substances such as alcohol, tobacco, cocaine, and amphetamines. Pregnant women who use heroin can expect a sixfold increase in maternal obstetric complications such as IUGR, third trimester vaginal bleeding, malpresentation, preterm delivery, and fetal distress [72]. In addition to the chemical effects of the drug, heroin use can pose additional risks from intravenous injections. Patients who use drugs intravenously are at increased risk of developing cellulitis, endocarditis, chorioamnionitis, and HIV. There is also a higher risk of stillbirth, meconium staining, decreased head circumference, and depressed Apgar scores in the fetus [73]. Frequent testing for sexually transmitted diseases such as HIV, syphilis, gonorrhea, chlamydia, and hepatitis B and C should be included in the prenatal care for heroin-abusing patients. Patients should also be counseled regarding the benefits of a methadone-maintenance program instead of continued heroin use. Methadone is inexpensive and has been shown to dramatically reduce the incidence of criminal behavior in the mother, including prostitution, and diminish exposure to needle-borne infections [11]. Women who use methadone have decreased use of illicit drugs, better compliance with prenatal care, better obstetric outcomes, and improved infant birth weights [74]. Maintenance treatment with methadone provides a steady concentration of opiate in the pregnant women's circulation and therefore prevents acute maternal withdrawal that is associated with fetal death. Maternal methadone, however, is also associated with neonatal abstinence syndrome [74].

Methadone maintenance has been an acceptable form of therapy for opiate-addicted pregnant women since the late 1960s. Since 1995, the United States federal guidelines regarding the regulation of methadone recommends preferential admittance to pregnant women with heroin addiction into methadone-treatment programs [75]. Methadone replacement has become the "gold standard" for management of pregnant heroin users. Buprenorphine has also been administered to pregnant women dependent on opioids, and it has less placental transfer into the fetus compared to methadone, reducing the development of fetal abstinence syndrome [76]. To prevent dangerous acute withdrawal syndrome during the labor and delivery period, the pregnant opioid addict should receive methadone replacement. Patients who have previously been on methadone maintenance should be continued on their treatment regimen up until the time of delivery [8]. Infants typically show signs and symptoms of withdrawal between 8 and 48 h after the last dose of methadone [76].

All of the opioids freely cross the placenta. Within 1 h of use, heroin crosses the placenta and enters the fetal tissues [77]. Neonatal abstinence syndrome can be seen in 50–95% of infants exposed to heroin and refers to the signs and symptoms exhibited by infants undergoing withdrawal from an addictive substance [75]. Withdrawal symptoms from opioids are similar to those seen in the adult, with the addition of irritability, poorly coordinated sucking, and, in the most severe cases, seizures, and death [78]. There are no specific congenital abnormalities associated with chronic opioid abuse. Neonatal complications of opioid-abusing mothers include neonatal withdrawal syndrome, postnatal growth deficiency, microcephaly, neurobehavioral problems, and a 74-fold increase in sudden infant death syndrome (SIDS) [79, 80]. Infants born to mothers who abuse hydromorphone or oxycodone during pregnancy have also been shown to develop neonatal withdrawal syndrome.

Management of the Opioid-Abusing Parturient

Opioid-abusing parturients may present with symptoms of opioid overdose or acute opioid withdrawal. Opioid overdose can be characterized by a slow respiratory rate, increased tidal volume, and miotic pupils. Acute withdrawal syndrome is manifested by increased sympathetic nervous system activity (i.e., restlessness, insomnia, mydriasis, tachycardia, tachypnea, and hypertension). Central nervous system manifestations of acute withdrawal can range from dysphoria to unconsciousness. Craving for the drug is associated with lacrimation, rhinorrhea, yawning, and piloerection. The ability to protect the airway may be compromised and the risk of aspiration is increased. Withdrawal symptoms can occur 4–6 h following the last dose of opioid intake and can peak at 48–72 h [8]. Symptoms of withdrawal can be treated with clonidine, dyphenhydramine, or doxepin. Clonidine attenuates opioid withdrawal symptoms by replacing opioid-mediated inhibition with α-2 agonist-mediated inhibition of the central nervous system [81]. Administration of opioid antagonists or agonists–antagonists must be avoided in these patients since they can precipitate acute withdrawal syndrome. Opioid withdrawal syndrome often develops within minutes of naloxone administration [8].

Regional anesthesia may be safely administered to opioid-addicted parturients. However, increased tendency for hypotension following spinal or epidural anesthesia should be anticipated. Regional anesthesia is not contraindicated in opioid-abusing women who present with asymptomatic HIV. HIV is a neurotrophic virus and the CNS is infected early in the course of the disease process; therefore, there is no increased risk of introducing the virus into the CNS with regional anesthesia. There is a relative contraindication to neuraxial anesthesia in AIDS patients with a CNS infection or progressive demyelination [82]. An increased incidence of spinal, epidural, and disk space infections has been reported in these patients regardless of the type of anesthesia used [84]. Acute administration of opioids decreases anesthetic requirements, and may also cause respiratory depression and loss of the airway. Chronic opioid use may lead to cross-tolerance with other CNS depressants. Chronic opioid-abusing parturients have a decreased production of endogenous opioid peptides, which may be responsible for the exaggerated degree of pain they seem to experience postoperatively. Peripheral intravenous access can be difficult and central venous access may be required.

Patients frequently use opioid analgesics in the postpartum period. Opioids are excreted into breast milk in small quantities with minimal, if any, effects on the newborn. Gastrointestinal side effects, sedation, and feeding pattern changes may be seen. The postpartum period is an excellent time to re-address the possibility of gradual narcotic withdrawal and continued rehabilitation with the mother.

Marijuana

Marijuana is estimated to be used by 3–16% of parturients [79]. Similar to all other substances of abuse, statistics regarding marijuana use depend entirely on patient reporting. Marijuana is a naturally occurring substance from the plant *Cannabis sativa*. More than 60 chemicals known as cannabinoids have been identified from the cannabis plant, with delta 9-tetrahydrocannabinol (THC) being the most potent. THC is the compound most responsible for the psychoactive effects of the drug and is the most important factor in the recreational use of marijuana. Although THC is the most active ingredient, there are over 400 chemical impurities that can be found mixed into a marijuana cigarette. Cannabinoids are highly lipophilic and rapidly accumulate in adipose tissue. Complete elimination of a single dose may require up to 30 days [11].

The clinical presentation of a patient intoxicated with marijuana can include euphoria, tachycardia, conjuctival congestion, and anxiety [83]. Pharmacologic actions can be unpredictable and can resemble a mixture of alcohol, opioids, tranquilizers, and hallucinogenics. Many patients who use marijuana also abuse other illicit drugs, further complicating the clinical picture.

Even though THC readily crosses the placenta, there is no known increase in the risk of congenital abnormalities in patients who smoke marijuana in the first trimester above the background risk of 3% [79]. The exact effects of marijuana on the developing fetus are difficult to establish due to the confounding effects from frequent polysubstance abuse and poor self-reporting in the parturient. It appears that chronic use of cannabis results in decreased uteroplacental perfusion and IUGR [84]. The literature is contradictory regarding the association between marijuana use and gestational age, low birth weight (LBW), and preterm birth. Low birth weight and preterm birth have serious consequences with increased perinatal mortality and long-term morbidity and their association with marijuana use has not been validated [85]. Developmental delays have also been reported in infants born to marijuana-abusing mothers [86]. The evidence regarding fetal effects is inconclusive, and further studies are needed.

There are no established pregnancy complications in marijuana users. Data concerning the effect of marijuana on gestational length are contradictory. Some reports suggest gestational length is increased, while others suggest that it is shortened [87]. Data have described a more dysfunctional labor in parturients who smoked marijuana close to the time of delivery, but this has also not been completely collaborated [79]. Chronic marijuana use has been postulated to have a role in infertility by altering hormone production and the pituitary–adrenal axis and suppressing ovulation [88].

Management of the Marijuana-Using Parturient

Marijuana can have anesthetic implications mainly by its ability to depress the myocardium. During general anesthesia, additive effects of marijuana and potent inhaled anesthetics can result in pronounced myocardial depression. Like many other illicit substances, acute marijuana use can have additive effects with other CNS depressants. Studies have also shown cross-tolerance between cannabis and alcohol, barbiturates, opioids, benzodiazepines, and phenothiazines. Acute marijuana use can also produce tachycardia, and drugs such as ketamine, pancuronium, atropine, and epinephrine should be avoided. Lung function can also be compromised by chronic cannabis use, similar to tobacco smoking. Emphysema, bronchitis, and squamous metaplasia can all result from chronic marijuana smoking. It has been reported that airway obstruction from uvular edema and oropharyngitis can result from recent preoperative marijuana smoking [89].

Tobacco

Active and passive tobacco smoking is a major health risk. Cigarette smoking affects pulmonary function, as well as contributing to the development of various cancers and diseases. Tobacco smoke is an irritant, which decreases ciliary function, increases sputum production, and impairs gas exchange [90]. It is estimated that 21% of Americans smoke. Approximately 12–15% of all women continue to smoke during their pregnancy [91]. Among pregnant women there is an increased prevalence of smoking among the youngest (<20 years of age) and oldest (>35 years of age) patients. The lower the level of education attained, the greater is the risk of being a current smoker [92].

Nicotine, carbon monoxide, and hydrogen cyanide are the most harmful substances found in cigarettes. There are over 4,000 chemicals that are produced during smoking, and at least 43 of them are known carcinogens [93] Metabolites of the potent carcinogen 4-(methylnitrosamino)-1-(3-pyridilz)-1-butanone (NNK) have been detected in the urine in 71% of newborns of parturients who smoked during pregnancy. Nicotine has a half-life of 1–2 h and is mainly metabolized by the liver and excreted by the kidneys. Nicotine readily crosses the placenta and can result in a fetal concentration up to 88% higher than maternal plasma levels. In addition, nicotine decreases placental blood flow secondary to vasoconstriction and contributes to fetal hypoxia. Carbon monoxide also crosses the placenta and can be detected in the fetal circulation in a concentration up to 15% higher than the maternal circulation. Since carbon monoxide has 200 times the affinity for hemoglobin than oxygen, oxygen delivery to maternal and fetal tissues is decreased [94].

Tobacco use during pregnancy is associated with a higher rate of obstetric complications, and has been shown to follow a dose–response relationship [93]. In the first trimester, there is an increased risk for spontaneous abortion and ectopic pregnancy. According to several studies, ectopic pregnancy has a relative risk of

1.5–2.5, and spontaneous abortions are 20–80% higher in women who smoke during pregnancy [95]. In the second and third trimesters, there is a higher risk of placental insufficiency, low birth weight, fetal growth restriction, and preterm delivery. The relative risk of preterm delivery in smoking parturients has been reported to be 1.2 [97]. In the postpartum period, maternal smoking has been proven to be one of the most important preventable risk factors for SIDS [96].

Management of the Tobacco-Using Parturient

The anesthetic concerns regarding cigarette-smoking parturients primarily involve the function of the pulmonary system. These patients can exhibit increased sputum and secretions, decrease in ciliary motility, small airway dysfunction, and impaired gas exchange. Four to 6 weeks of abstinence from smoking is required to decrease postoperative respiratory morbidity to the level of the nonsmoker. Levels of carboxyhemoglobin in the mother can return to the levels seen in nonsmokers in as little as 48 h. Complications such as bronchospasm and postoperative respiratory dysfunction can be avoided with administration of neuraxial anesthesia.

ACOG places a strong emphasis on cessation of tobacco abuse in pregnancy. Nicotine replacement patches as well as educational and behavioral therapies are recommended. Transdermal nicotine allows pregnant women to receive nicotine while avoiding exposure to other chemicals found in cigarette smoke.

Conclusion

Substance abuse by pregnant women results in significant risks of maternal and fetal morbidity and mortality. A careful pre-anesthetic evaluation along with judgment-free questioning of possible illicit substance intake is essential. In order to optimize outcome, health-care workers must become more proactive and better at identifying drug use earlier in pregnancy and shift focus from treatment to prevention. A complete understanding of the physiology of pregnancy, pathophysiology of pregnancy-specific disorders, and anesthetic implications of drug abuse in pregnancy is of upmost importance in order to provide a safe anesthetic plan for these high-risk patients.

References

1. National Survey on Drug Use and Health. Substance abuse during pregnancy: 2002 and 2003 update. www.oas.samhsa.gov/2k5/pregnancy/pregnancy.htm. Accessed 13 Sep 2010.
2. Samuels SI, Maze A, Albright G. Cardiac arrest during cesarean section in a chronic amphetamine abuser. Anesth Analg. 1979;58:528–30.
3. Floyd RL, Decoufle P, Hungerford DW. Alcohol use prior to pregnancy recognition. Am J Prev Med. 1999;17:101–7.

4. State vs. Regina McKnight. 2003.
5. Commonwealth of Kentucky vs. Ina Cochran. case#2008-sc-000095. 2005.
6. American College of Obstetricians and Gynecologists. Committee opinion on obstetrics: Maternal and fetal medicine. Cocaine in pregnancy ACOG committee opinion No:114, Washington, DC. September 1992.
7. Kilmer G, Roberts H, Hughes E, Li Y, Valluru B, Fan A, et al. Surveillance of certain health behaviors and conditions among states and selected local areas – behavioral risk factor surveillance system, United States, 2006. MMWR Surveill Summ. 2008;57(7):1–188.
8. Kuczkowski KM. Anesthetic implications of drug abuse in pregnancy. J Clin Anesth. 2003;15:382–94.
9. Cohen-Kerem R, Koren G. Antioxidants and fetal protection against ethanol teratogenicity I. review of the experimental data and implications to humans. Neurotoxicol Teratol. 2003;25:1–9.
10. Ornoy A, Ergaz Z. Alcohol abuse in pregnant women: effects on the fetus and newborn, mode of action and maternal treatment. Int J Environ Res Public Health. 2010;7:364–79.
11. Keegan J, Parva M, Finnegan M, Gerson A, Belden M. Addiction in pregnancy. J Addict Dis. 2010;29:175–91.
12. Lemoine P, Harousseau H, Borteryu JP, Menuet JC. Children of alcoholic parents: abnormalities observed in 127 cases. Ouest Med. 1968;8:476–82.
13. Jones KL, Smith DW. Recognition of the fetal alcohol syndrome in early infancy. Lancet. 1973;2:999–1001.
14. Hannigan JH, Armant DR. Alcohol in pregnancy and neonatal outcome. Semin Neonatol. 2000;5:243–54.
15. Floyd RL, Jack BW, Cefalo R, Atrash H, Mahoney J, Herron A. The clinical content of preconception care: alcohol, tobacco, and illicit drug exposures. Am J Obstet Gynecol. 2008;199:s333–8.
16. Kesmodel U, Wisborg K, Olsen SF, Henriksen TB, Secher NJ. Moderate alcohol intake in pregnancy and the risk of spontaneous abortion. Alcohol Alcohol. 2002;37:87–92.
17. Martinez-Frias ML, Bernejo E, Rodriguez-Pinilla E, Frias JL. Risk for congenital anomalies associated with different sporadic and daily doses of alcohol consumption during pregnancy: a case control study. Birth Defects Res A Clin Mol Teratol. 2004;70:194–200.
18. Stoler JM, Holmes LB. Recognition of facial features of fetal alcohol syndrome in the newborn. Am J Med Genet. 2004;127C:21–4.
19. May PA, Gossage JP. Estimating the prevalence of fetal alcohol syndrome. A summary. Alcohol Res Health. 2005;25:159–67.
20. Hoyme HE, May PA, Kalberg WO, Kodituwakku P, Gosssage JP, Trujillo PM, et al. A practical clinical approach to diagnosis of fetal alcohol spectrum disorders: clarification of the 1996 Institute of Medicine criteria. Pediatrics. 2005;115:39–47.
21. Banakar MK, Kudlur NS, George S. Fetal alcohol spectrum disorder (FASD). Indian J Pediatr. 2009;76:1173–5.
22. Wagner CL, Katikaneni LD, Cox TH, et al. The impact of prenatal drug exposure on the neonate. Obstet Gynecol Clin North Am. 1998;25:169–94.
23. Han YH. Why do chronic alcoholics require more anesthesia? Anesthesiology. 1969;30:2.
24. Swerdlow BN, Holley FO, Maitre PO, et al. Chronic alcohol intake does not change thiopental anesthetic requirement, pharmacokinetics, or pharmacodynamics. Anesthesiology. 1990; 72:455–61.
25. Chestnut DH, Polley LS, Tsen LC, Wong CA. Obstetric anesthesia principles and practice. 4th ed. Philadelphia, PA: Mosby Elsevier; 2009. p. 1134–7.
26. Russell M, Martier S, Sokol R, Mudar P, Jacobson S, Jacobson J. Detecting risk drinking during pregnancy: a comparison of four screening questionnaires. Am J Public Health. 1996;86:1435–9.
27. Burns E, Gray R, Smith LA. Brief screening questionnaires to identify problem drinking during pregnancy: a systematic review. Addiction. 2010;105:601–14.
28. Gareri J, Klein J, Koren G. Drug of abuse testing in meconium. Clin Chim Acta. 2006; 366:101–11.

29. Ostrea Jr EM, Hernandez JD, Bielawski DM, Kan JM, et al. Fatty acid ethyl esters in meconium: are they biomarkers of fetal alcohol exposure and effect? Alcohol Clin Exp Res. 2006;30(7): 1152–9.
30. Burd L, Hofer R. Biomarkers for detection of prenatal alcohol exposure: a critical review of fatty acid ethyl esters in meconium. Birth Defects Res A Clin Mol Teratol. 2008;82(7):487–93.
31. National Institute on Drug Abuse SAaMHSA: Results from the 2008 National Survey on Drug Use and Health: National Findings. Rockville, MD: National Institute on Drug Abuse; 2009.
32. King JC. Substance abuse in pregnancy. Postgrad Med J. 1997;102:135–50.
33. McCalla S, Minkoff HL, Feldman J, et al. Predictors of cocaine use in pregnancy. Obstet Gynecol. 1992;79:641–4.
34. Birnbach DJ, Browne IM, Kim A, et al. Identification of polysubstace abuse in the parturient. Br J Anaesth. 2001;87:488–90.
35. Oyler J, Darwin WD, Preston KL, et al. Cocaine disposition in the meconium from newborns of cocaine abusing mothers and urine of adult drug users. J Anal Toxicol. 1996;20(6):453–562.
36. Plessinger MA, Woods JR. Maternal, placental and fetal pathophysiology of cocaine exposure during pregnancy. Clin Obstet Gynecol. 1993;36:267–78.
37. Andres RL. Social and illicit drug use in pregnancy. Maternal fetal med: principles and practice. 5th ed. W.B. Saunders: Philadelphia, PA; 2004. p. 55–67.
38. Buehler BA. Cocaine how dangerous is it during pregnancy? Nebr Med J. 1995;80:116–7.
39. Moen MD, Caliendo MJ, Marshall W, et al. Hepatic rupture in pregnancy associated with cocaine use. Obstet Gynecol. 1993;82:687–9.
40. Chao CR. Cardiovascular effects of cocaine during pregnancy. Semin Perinatol. 1996;20:107–14.
41. Moore TR, Sorg J, Miller L, et al. Hemodynamic effects of intravenous cocaine on the pregnant ewe and fetus. Am J Obstet Gynecol. 1986;155:883–8.
42. Schindler CW, Tella SR, Erzanki HK. Pharmacological mechanisms of cocaine's cardiovascular effects. Drug Alcohol Depend. 1995;37:183–91.
43. Lange RA, Hillis LD. Cardiovascular complications of cocaine use. N Engl J Med. 2001;345:351–8.
44. Shanti CM, Lucas CE. Cocaine and the critical care challenge. Crit Care Med. 2003;31:1851–9.
45. Restrepo CS, Carrillo JA, Martínez S, Ojeda P, Rivera AL, Hatta A. pulmonary complications from cocaine and cocaine based substances: imaging maifestations. Radiographics. 2007;27(4):941–56.
46. Kuczkowski KM, Birnbach DJ, van Zundert A. Drug Abuse in the Parturient. Semin Anesth Periop Med Pain. 2000;19:216–24.
47. Kreek MJ. Cocaine, dopamine and the endogenous opioid system. J Addict Dis. 1996;15:73–96.
48. Vertommen JD, Hughes SC, Rosen MA, et al. Hydralazine, does not restore uterine blood flow during cocaine-induced hypertension in the pregnant ewe. Anesthesiology. 1992;76:580–7.
49. Guidelines 2010 for cardiopulmonary resuscitation and emergency cardiovascular care. Circulation. 2010;122:S829–61.© 2010 American Heart Association, Inc.
50. Lange RA, Cigarroa RG, Flores ED, McBride W, Kim AS, Wells PJ, et al. Potentiation of cocaine-induced coronary vasoconstriction by beta-adrenergic blockade. Ann Intern Med. 1990;112:897–903.
51. Kain ZN, Mayes LC, Ferris CA, et al. Cocaine-abusing parturients undergoing cesarean section: a cohort study. Anesthesiology. 1996;85:1028–35.
52. Spence MR, Williams R, DiGregorio GJ, et al. The relationship between recent cocaine use and pregnancy outcome. Obstet Gynecol. 1991;78:326–9.
53. Cruickshank CC, Dyer KR. A review of the clinical pharmacology of methamphetamine. Addiction. 2009;104:1085–99.
54. Good MM, Solt I, Acuna JG, Rotsmensch S, Kim MJ. Methamphetamine use during pregnancy. Obstet Gynecol. 2010;116(2):330–4.
55. Terplan M, Smith EJ, Kozloski MJ, Pollack HA. Methamphetamine use among pregnant women. Obstet Gynecol. 2009;113:1285–91.
56. Arria AM, Derauf C, Lagasse LL, Grant P, Shah R, Smith L, et al. Methamphetamine and other substance use during pregnancy. preliminary estimates from the infant development, environment, and lifestyle (IDEAL) study. Matern Child Health J. 2006;10:293–302.

57. Gonzales R, Mooney L, Rawson AR. The methamphetamine problem in the united states. Annu Rev Public Health. 2010;31:385–98.
58. Inoue H, Nakatome M, Terada M, Mizuno M, Ono R, Iino M, et al. Maternal methamphetamine administration during pregnancy influences on fetal rat heart development. Life Sci. 2004;74:1529–40.
59. Bateman DN, McElhatton PR, Dickinson D, Wren C, Matthews JN, O'Keffe M, et al. A case control study to examine the pharmacological factors underlying ventricular septal defects in the north of England. Eur J Clin Pharmacol. 2004;60:635–41.
60. Werler MM, Sheehan JE, Mitchell AA. Association of vasoconstrictive exposures with risks of gastroschisis and small intestinal atresia. Epidemiology. 2003;14:349–54.
61. Thomas DB. Cleft palate, mortality and morbidity of infants of substance abusing mothers. J Paediatr Child Health. 1995;31:457–60.
62. Bays J. Fetal vascular disruption with prenatal exposure to cocaine or methamphetamine. Pediatrics. 1991;87:416–8.
63. Nora JJ, Vargo TA, Nora AH, Love KE, McNamara DG. Dexamphetamine: a possible environmental trigger in cardiovascular malformations. Lancet. 1970;1:1290–1.
64. Little BB, Snell LM, Gilstrap 3rd LC. Methamphetamine abuse during pregnancy: outcome and fetal effects. Obstet Gynecol. 1988;72:541–4.
65. Milkovich L, Van der Berg BJ. effects of antenatal exposure to anorectic drugs. Am J Obstet Gynecol. 1977;129:637–42.
66. Oro AS, Dixon SD. Perinatal cocaine and methamphetamine exposure: maternal and neonatal correlates. J Pediatr. 1987;111:571–8.
67. Stewart JL, Meeker JE. Fetal and infant deaths associated with maternal methamphetamine abuse. J Anal Toxicol. 1997;21:515–7.
68. Michel R, Adams AP. Acute amphetamine abuse. Problems during general anesthesia for neurosurgery. Anaesthesia. 1979;34:1016–9.
69. Johnston RR, Way WL, Miller RD. Alteration of anesthetic requirement by amphetamine. Anesthesiology. 1972;36:357–63.
70. Floyd RL, Jack BW, Cefalo R, Atrash H, Mahoney J, Herron A, et al. The clinical content of preconception care: alcohol, tobacco, and illicit drug exposures. Am J Obstet Gynecol. 2008;199:s333–9.
71. Brown HL, Britton KA, Mahaffey D, Brizendine E, Hiert AK, Turnquest MA. Methadone maintenance in pregnancy: a reappraisal. Am J Obstet Gynecol. 1998;179:459–63.
72. Minozzi S, Amato L, Vecchi S, Davoli M. Maintenance agonist treatments for opiate dependent pregnant women. Cochrane database Syst Rev. 2008;CD006318.
73. Creasy RK, Resnik R, Iams JD. Creasy and Resnik's maternal-fetal medicine: principles and practice. Philadelphia, PA: Saunders/Elsevier; 2009.
74. Lim S, Prasad MR, Samuels P, Gardner DK, Cordero L. High dose methadone in pregnant women and it's effect on duration of neonatal abstinence syndrome. Am J Obstet Gynecol. 2009;200:70el–5.
75. Rettig R. Federal regulation of methadone: table of contents and executive summary. Washington, DC: National Academy Press; 1995.
76. Rayburn W, Bogenschutz MP. Pharmacotherapy for pregnant women with addiction. Am J Obstet Gynecol. 2004;191:1885–97.
77. Briggs G, Freeman R, Yaffe J. Drugs in pregnancy and lactation. Philadelphia, PA: Lippincott Williams & Wilkins; 2008.
78. Kaltenbach K, Berghella V, Finnegan L. Opioid dependence during pregnancy: effects and management. Obstet Gynecol Clin N Am. 1998;25:139–51.
79. Fajemirokun-Odudeyi O, Sinha C, Tutty S, Pairaudeau P, Armstrong D, Phillips T, et al. Pregnancy outcomes in women who use opiates. Eur J Obstet Gynecol Reprod Biol. 2006;126(2):170–5.
80. Ludlow JP, Evans SF, Hulse G. Obstetric and perinatal outcomes in pregnancies associated with illicit substance abuse. Aust N Z J Obstet Gynaecol. 2004;44(4):301–6.

81. Gold MS, Pottash AL, Sweeney DR, Kleber HD. Opiate withdrawal using clonidine. A safe, effective, and rapid nonopiate treatment. JAMA. 1980;243:343–6.
82. Kuczkowski KM, Birnbach DDJ. The HIV infected parturient: is neuraxial anesthesia contraindicated? Curr Anesthesiol Rep. 2000;2:118–21.
83. Ashton CH. Biomedical benefits of cannnabinoids. Addict Biol. 1999;4:111–26.
84. Shiono PH, Klebanoff MA, Nugent RP, Cotch MF, Wilkins DG, Rollins DE, et al. The impact of cocaine and marijuana use on low birth weight and preterm birth: a multicenter study. Am J Obstet Gynecol. 1995;172:19–27.
85. Van Gelder M, Reefhuis J, Caton A, Werler M, Druschel C, et al. Characteristics of pregnant illicit drug users and associations between cannabis use an perinatal outcome in a population based study. Drug Alcohol Depend. 2010;109:243–7.
86. Musty RE, Reggio P, Consroe P. A review of recent advances in cannaboid research and the 1994 international symposium on cannabis and the cnnaboids. Life Sci. 1995;56:1933–40.
87. National institute on drug abuse (NIDA) research report series: Marijuana abuse. July 2005. NIH publication number 05–3859.
88. Smith CG, Asch RH. Drug abuse and reproduction. Fertil Steril. 1987;48:355–73.
89. Mallat A, Roberson J, Broch-Utne JG. Preoperative marijuana inhalation – an airway concern. Can J Anaesth. 1996;43:691–3.
90. IARC (International agency for research on cancer) working group on the evaluation of carci-nogenic risks to humans. Tobacco smoke and involuntary smoking. IARC Monogr Eval Carcinog Risks Hum. 2004;83:1–1438.
91. Goodwin RD, Keyes K, Simuro N. Mental disorders and nicotine dependence among pregnant women in the united states. Obstet Gynecol. 2007;109:875–83.
92. Kandel DB, Griesler PC, Schaffran C. Educational attainment and smoking among women: risk factors and consequences for offspring. Drug Alcohol Depend. 2009;104 Suppl 1:S24–33.
93. Thielen A, Klus H, Muller L. Tobacco smoke: unraveling a controversial subject. Exp Toxicol Pathol. 2008;60:141–56.
94. Andres RL, Day MC. Perinatal complications associated with maternal tobacco use. Semin Neonatol. 2000;5:231–41.
95. Einarson A, Riordan S. Smoking in pregnancy and lactation: a review of risks and cessation strategies. Eur J Clin Pharmacol. 2009;65:325–30.
96. MacDorman MF, Cnattingius S, Hoffman HJ, Kramer MS, Haglund B. Sudden infant death syndrome and smoking in the United states and Sweden. Am J Epidemiol. 1997;146:249–57.
97. Simmons LE, Rubens CE, Darmstadt GL, et al. Preventing preterm birth and neonatal mortality: exploring the epidemiology, causes and interventions. Semon Perinatol. 2010;34(6):408–15.

Chapter 12
Prescription Drugs: Implications for the Chronic Pain Patient

Amy S. Aloysi and Ethan O. Bryson

Introduction

Addiction is a neurobehavioral syndrome characterized by the repeated use or compulsive seeking of mood-altering substances despite the adverse psychological, physical, or social consequences associated with doing so. It is not limited to illicit substances and many prescription medications used today have the potential to cause tolerance, physical dependence, and result in withdrawal when the agent is removed. Misuse of prescription drugs has been defined by the National Institute on Drug Abuse (NIDA) as "any intentional use of a medication with intoxicating properties outside of a physician's prescription for a bona fide medical condition." There are significant issues specific to the chronic pain patient.

National epidemiologic studies conducted over the past 20 years have shown an increase in reports of nonmedical use of prescription medications, and the rates of addiction to prescription pain medication are increasing (Fig. 12.1) [1]. In 2001, there was a 117% increase in emergency room visits for opioid analgesic abuse. In at least 20 metropolitan cities, misuse of prescription opioid pain medications such as codeine, oxycodone, hydrocodone, and morphine was ranked among the top ten common causes for deaths associated with drug abuse. Accidental overdose deaths are now found more commonly from prescription medications than from illicit drugs [2].

A.S. Aloysi (✉)
Department of Psychiatry, Mount Sinai School of Medicine, New York, NY, USA
e-mail: amy.aloysi@mssm.edu

E.O. Bryson and E.A.M. Frost (eds.), *Perioperative Addiction:*
Clinical Management of the Addicted Patient, DOI 10.1007/978-1-4614-0170-4_12,
© Springer Science+Business Media, LLC 2012

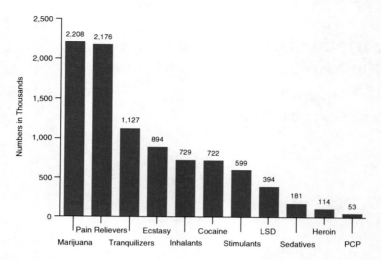

Fig. 12.1 Past Year Initiates for Specific Illicit Drugs in 2008: Note: The number of persons aged 12 or older who began misusing prescription medications is the same as those who began using marijuana during the same period and considerably higher than the number abusing all other illicit drugs. Adapted from Results from the 2008 National Survey on Drug Use and Health: National Substance Abuse and Mental Health Services Administration, 2009, (Office of Applied Studies, NSDUH Series H-36, HHS Publication No. SMA 09-4434). Rockville, MD. Used with permission

Features Unique to the Chronic Pain Patient

Chronic pain refers to pain that persists beyond the usual period of tissue healing or acute disease. Generally, this is longer than 3–6 months and often there is no identifiable pathology to explain the presence or extent of the pain. Pain is the most frequent cause of disability or suffering in patients with chronic medical conditions, and it is also the most common reason these patients seek medical help. The most common forms of chronic pain are associated with cancer, chronic visceral disorders, musculoskeletal disorders, lesions of the central nervous system, and lesions of nerve roots, peripheral nerves, or dorsal root ganglia. Not only can chronic pain significantly impair the quality of life, but 90% of chronic pain patients are also treated with opioids, which can also significantly impact day to day functioning.

Chronic pain has features unique from acute pain. Most patients have an altered neuroendocrine response and significant affective mood disorder(s). Environmental and psychological mechanisms can also play a role and there is a substantial link between psychiatric comorbidities and addiction. Studies have suggested that between 17% and 60% of patients with a drug addiction also have an anxiety or depression disorder at presentation [3]. It has been suggested that the development of addiction and psychiatric disorders in the chronic pain patient may be related to a maladaptive response to chronic stressors in the hypothalamic–pituitary–adrenal axis, though the exact mechanism is not known [4].

Hyperalgesia due to chronic opiate use may present with drug-seeking behaviors resembling addiction, and this potential adverse effect of high-dose opiate treatment needs to be managed differently [5]. Hyperalgesia or hyperesthesia is characterized by dramatically increased sensitivity to painful stimuli, thought to develop through spinal sensitization to glutamate and substance P [6]. Occasionally allodynia, which is pain elicited by a normally nonpainful stimulus, may occur. It has been postulated that these reactions may result from NMDA receptor agonist action, as NMDA antagonists have been shown to be effective in the reduction of opioid hyperalgesia [7].

Trends in Abuse Patterns

Prescription drugs abused by patients with chronic pain may include opiate analgesic medications, stimulants, sedative-hypnotics, or sedative-anxiolytics. Opioids are an established treatment of pain, both acute and chronic, and drug therapy is one of the most common modalities used to manage and treat chronic pain. However, many physicians undertreat pain and are reluctant to employ opioids due to their addictive potential. Many times an addiction begins with an appropriate opiate prescription for pain in a vulnerable patient [8]. Studies have found a variable incidence of addiction in chronic pain patients treated with opioids, with a wide range of 9–41% [9] and no significant difference in opioid abuse with patients taking short-acting hydrocodone (22%) versus long-acting methadone (24%) [10].

Factors which have been associated with an increased risk for developing addiction are sex (female patients less than 45 years of age), the presence of co-existing psychiatric illness (especially depression, bipolar disorder, panic disorder, and antisocial personality disorder), the presence of multiple painful regions of the body (especially three or more), chronic pain resulting from a motor vehicle accident, and history of prior illicit drug use. Factors that showed no significant increase in risk included the duration of pain, insurance status, workers' compensation incentives, and previous surgical history [11].

A review by Turk et al. investigating opiate misuse by chronic pain patients concluded that none of the existing questionnaires or clinical interview protocols currently employed could consistently predict opiate misuse in chronic pain patients. There is some evidence for a history of multiple substance abuse and younger age as risk factors. In general, patients without a history of psychiatric disorder, personal or family history of substance abuse, and no involvement in substance abuse subcultures are at low risk for iatrogenic addiction [12, 13].

Prescription drugs are primarily obtained from physicians who dispense them for legitimate medical reasons. When these drugs are misused, they are frequently obtained from alternate sources, most often from friends and family [2]. Frequently, these drugs are stolen; however, some patients who do not fully understand the consequences of prescription drug misuse willingly share these agents with others. Doctor shopping, theft from pharmacies, online purchases, and forged prescriptions account for only a small amount of diversion [2].

Abuse Prevention Strategies

There is a need for greater ability to quantify risk and to develop evidence-based risk-reduction interventions. Current screening instruments for addiction risk in chronic pain patients may not adequately predict patients at risk of misuse [5]. Structured interview instruments include the "Prescription Drug Use Questionnaire," the "Physician Opioid Therapy Questionnaire," and the Addiction Behaviors Checklist. Self-report questionnaires include the Screening Instrument for Substance Abuse Potential. The Current Opioid Misuse Measure (COMM) can be used to monitor for misuse in patients who are prescribed long-term opiates.

While the majority of patients with chronic pain are treated in primary care settings, less than half of practitioners implement treatment agreements and less than a third obtain urine drug tests [14]. A systematic review of the use of opioid treatment agreements and urine drug testing found only weak evidence to support the benefits of these strategies in reducing opioid misuse [14].

Appropriate screening and risk management include application of the universal protocol described by Gourlay for risk stratification of pain management patients (Table 12.1). This protocol can improve identification of high-risk patients seeking treatment for pain who will need specialty treatment centers and closely supervised care [15].

Clinical Presentation of the Patient Abusing Prescription Medications

A detailed history and physical exam are essential and physicians should maintain an appropriate index of suspicion. Table 12.2 outlines schemata for identifying addiction in the chronic pain patient. Specific information should be elicited including a complete list of medications prescribed with doses and dosing schedule and the time and amount of the last dose. Information regarding abuse of nonprescription drugs or alcohol should be obtained. In the case of the obtunded patient who cannot give a history, it is appropriate to inquire about drug use from friends or family.

Most prescription opioid-abusing patients have experienced withdrawal and are more likely to be honest regarding their drug use in order to avoid experiencing withdrawal again. Many will actually exaggerate their daily dose requirements in an attempt to receive increased medication doses. Warning signs of opioid misuse include forging prescriptions, borrowing others drugs, frequently losing prescriptions, and resisting changes to medication despite adverse effects [16].

Individuals who abuse tranquilizers and sedative-hypnotics are more likely to have anxiety symptoms, serious mental illness, a history of illicit drug use, and are at higher risk for other forms of substance abuse. These patients are more likely to have used drugs at a younger age and to have a history of intravenous drug use [17]. Prescription sedatives, particularly benzodiazepines, and alcohol are the agents most commonly abused by the geriatric population [18].

Table 12.1   Universal precautions in pain medicine

1. Make a diagnosis with appropriate differential
2. Psychological assessment including risk of addictive disorders
3. Informed consent
4. Treatment agreement
5. Pre- and post-intervention assessment of pain level and function
6. Appropriate trial of opioid therapy +/– adjunctive medication
7. Reassessment of pain score and level of function
8. Regularly assess the "four A's" of pain medicine: analgesia, activity, adverse effects, and aberrant behavior
9. Periodically review pain diagnosis and comorbid conditions, including addictive disorders
10. Documentation

Table 12.2   Schemata for identifying addiction in the chronic pain patient

Adverse consequences or harm from use
Patient appears to be intoxicated/somnolent/sedated
Declining activity
Irritable, anxious, labile mood
Increasing sleep disturbance
Increasing pain complaints
Increasing relationship dysfunction
Impaired control over use or compulsive use
Reports lost or stolen prescriptions
Frequent early renewal requests
Urgent calls or unscheduled visits
Abusing other drugs (including EtOH)
Cannot produce medications upon request
Withdrawal noted at clinic visits
Observers report overuse or sporadic use
Preoccupation of use because of craving
Frequently misses appointments unless opioid renewal expected
Does not want to try non-opioid treatments
Cannot tolerate most medications
Requests medications with high reward
No relief with anything except opioids

Adapted from Savage SR. Assessment for addiction in pain-treatment settings. Clin J Pain. 2002;18:S28–S38

Anesthetic Implications for the Prescription Drug-Abusing Patient

Tolerance is a common phenomenon associated with all chronic prescription drug use, and the prescription-abusing patient who presents for a procedure or surgery that requires sedation or anesthesia requires a greater amount of anesthetics per

Table 12.3 Conversion table for opioid medications using 10 mg intravenous morphine as the standard for comparison

Original Drug	PO (mg)	IV (mg)	Half-life (h)	Duration (h)
Morphine	30	10	2–3	2–4
Morphine CR	30		8–12	8–12
Morphine SR	30		8–12	8–12
Oxycodone	20		2–3	3–4
Oxycodone CR	20		2–3	8–12
Hydromorphone	7.5	1.5	2–3	2–4
Meperidine	300	100	2–3	2–4
Methadone	20	10	36–120	4–12
Codeine	200	100	2–3	2–4
Hydrocodone	30		2–3	3–4
Oxymorphone	10	1	2–3	2–4
Levorphanol	4	2	12–15	4–6
Fentanyl	100 mcg/h	4 mg/h	7–12	1
Fentanyl patch	100 mcg/h	4 mg/h	16–24	48–72

Calculate the 24 h dose of current drug and divide to obtain appropriate dosing interval or total dose for patients who will receive continuous infusions
Note: fentanyl patch doses are only standardized when used as directed by the manufacturer. When dissolved and injected the total dose of fentanyl is administered all at once and can be as much as 7,200 mg depending on the product used

weight than the naive patient. If the chronic prescription drug abuser has developed hyperalgesia, they may be hypersensitive to surgical and other stimuli in addition to developing tolerance and may require even higher doses of anesthetic agents than would be expected from tolerance alone.

An attempt should be made to calculate the 24-h dose of each prescription medication and convert to an oral or intravenous equivalent dose for maintenance (Table 12.3). Dividing the daily dose by 24 estimates the hourly requirement but the practitioner should assume a 20–30% increase in acute opiate requirements consistent with that required for opiate-naive patients. If the patient does not respond to the first agent administered, they might respond to an alternate opioid because of the incomplete cross-tolerance of μ-receptors across different opioid agents.

Nonopioid agents such as intravenous or oral nonsteroidal anti-inflammatory drugs (NSAIDs), the centrally acting μ-agonist tramadol, the α-2 agonist clonidine, or other adjuvant medications such as gabapentin and pregabalin may be useful (Table 12.4). Muscle relaxants such as cyclobenzaprine (Flexeril®), metaxalone (Skelaxin®), or baclofen may be used to treat postoperative splinting or spasm. The N-methyl D-aspartate (NMDA) antagonist ketamine has been shown to decrease chronic neuropathic pain and is useful in opiate-tolerant patients [19]. In refractory cases, decreasing the dose of opioid or administering a bolus or infusion of magnesium, or using transcutaneous electrical nerve stimulation (TENS) therapy, may be helpful. Acupuncture is another potentially useful adjunctive therapy and has been shown to have mild analgesic effects in a recent meta-analysis of its use in a wide variety of pain conditions [20].

Table 12.4 Suggested doses for adjuvant therapy

- Ketamine 0.1–0.5 mg/kg IV bolus pre-incision followed by 0.1–0.5 mg/kg/h infusion
- Clonidine 0.3 μ/kg IV bolus pre-incision followed by 0.3 μ/kg/h infusion
- Clonidine 1 μg/ml added to local anesthesia for epidural or peripheral nerve block
- Celecoxib (Celebrex®) 400 mg initially, followed by an additional 200 mg dose if needed on the first day. On subsequent days, the recommended dose is 200 mg twice daily as needed
- Ketorolac (Toradol®) 30 mg IV every 6 h as needed
- Acetaminophen (Tylenol®) 650 mg PO every 4–6 h as needed. Reduce dose if acetaminophen containing opioid analgesics are also administered
- Pregabalin (Lyrica®)75–150 mg PO twice daily or 50–100 mg PO three times daily

Note: The use of NSAIDs perioperatively may increase risk for bleeding and the decision to use should be made after discussion with the surgical team

Regional anesthesia targets the site of surgery and allows for the administration of lower doses of opioids. Peripheral nerve blocks (PNBs) and central (neuraxial) techniques using local anesthetics with or without opiates inhibit the conduction of pain and avoid central sensitization and remodeling (neuroplastic changes) in the dorsal horn of the spinal cord. These techniques have immediate effect as they result in less perioperative pain, as well as long-term analgesia because the risk that a chronic pain state will develop is decreased.

Side effects such as nausea and vomiting may be treated with anti-emetics. Constipation may be reduced by a peripherally acting μ-receptor antagonist such as methylnaltrexone which does not cross the blood–brain barrier and will not reduce the central analgesic effects; however, all patients receiving opioids should be given a stool softener. Postoperative ileus may respond to another peripherally acting μ-opioid receptor antagonist, alvimopam, 12 mg given preoperatively and continued for up to 7 days postoperatively. Pruritis is common and can be effectively treated with antihistamines such as diphenhydramine. Sedation is common and ventilation status (respiratory rate and oxygen saturation) should be closely monitored. A significant decrease in either signals the presence of effective levels of opioid in the patient and the clinician should decrease the opioid dose, stopping or changing the opiate altogether. If the decision is made to administer a central-acting μ-receptor antagonist, the patient should be monitored for signs of opioid withdrawal (Table 12.5) In the case of urinary retention, the bladder may need to be catheterized and an antagonist administered.

Prescription Drug Withdrawal

Clinical presentation varies by agent class, with opiate analgesic medications, stimulants, sedative-hypnotics, and sedative-anxiolytics each characterized by a discrete withdrawal syndrome.

Opiate analgesic agents rarely produce life-threatening withdrawal with reduction of dose or sudden discontinuation, but symptoms can be so physically and psychologically objectionable that avoidance of withdrawal may be the driving force behind

Table 12.5 Signs of opioid withdrawal

- Elevated resting heart rate
- Diaphoresis not accounted for by ambient temperature or activity
- Restlessness, frequent shifting or extraneous movements
- Mydriasis greater than expected given ambient light
- Bone or joint aches unrelated to injury or surgery
- Rhinorrhea or lacrimation not accounted for by cold symptoms or allergies
- Nausea, vomiting, or diarrhea
- Tremor of outstretched hands
- Yawning
- Anxiety or irritability
- Piloerection

continued abuse of these medications despite negative consequences. Common withdrawal symptoms include body aches, fatigue, chills, flu-like symptoms, nausea, vomiting, diarrhea, and autonomic hyperactivity [21]. These symptoms begin to occur depending on the half-life of the agent, with longer-acting agents typified by delayed presentations. For example, methadone, which has an extremely long half-life, has a withdrawal syndrome that begins 24–48 h after the last dose and can persist for days. Withdrawal from opioid medications is managed with re-introduction and gradual tapering of an opiate agonist such as methadone, or an agonist–antagonist such as buprenorphine. Nonopiate detoxification protocols rely on the use of clonidine, and symptomatic management of pain with NSAIDS, ketorolac, anxiety with hydroxyzine or benzodiazepines, nausea with ondansetron or phenergan, and diarrhea with loperamide.

Stimulants produce a withdrawal picture characterized by profound dysphoria, somnolence, and lethargy, occasionally with suicidal ideation. Cocaine and amphetamines are commonly abused stimulant drugs. Management is supportive, and while the depressive syndrome usually remits after several days, persistent substance-induced mood disorder or underlying major depression may require additional pharmacologic treatment or psychiatric care.

Sedative-hypnotic agents include benzodiazepines and the sleep aides including zolpidem (Ambien(R)), eszopiclone (Lunesta(R)), and others. Benzodiazepine withdrawal is a potentially life-threatening condition which may occur days or weeks after the agent has been discontinued or suddenly lowered. Diazepam has a long half-life, of 4 days, and its active metabolite may remain in the patient for up to 8 days; therefore, withdrawal symptoms may not occur until weeks later. The agent with the shortest half-life and greatest abuse potential, alprazolam, can have a more immediate withdrawal syndrome. Particular caution is needed to identify the dose and pattern of benzodiazepine usage in the weeks preceding surgery in order to avoid sudden discontinuation of these agents in the perioperative period. Symptoms of withdrawal from benzodiazepines include anxiety, tremor, autonomic hyperactivity, tachycardia, hypertension, and agitation. This can progress to acute delirium with prominent visual hallucinations, disorientation, waxing and waning of consciousness, seizures, and death [21]. Treatment includes restarting benzodiazepines, and tapering gradually, supportive care, and ensuring a safe environment for the patient.

Treatment Options and Referral Sources

Prescription drug abuse in the patient with chronic pain is a problem that needs to be addressed at several levels. First is to determine the underlying causes of pain and remedy these if possible; second, differentiation of subjective pain from malingering for secondary gain of obtaining additional medications, and identification and referral of patients with comorbid addiction issues should be undertaken. The treatment of addiction in chronic pain involves an initial phase of detoxification from the agent(s), followed by longer-term treatment with the aim of addressing pain while also preventing relapse into patterns of excess and dangerous use [22].

Close coordination between medical and addiction providers is important. National registries of controlled substance prescriptions, dispensing of short-term supplies of medications with abuse potential, treatment contracts with the provider, and routine drug screens are important components of the treatment plan. The institution of pharmacy databases to prevent multiple refills of the same medication is needed in both commercial pharmacies and veteran hospital settings in order to address the epidemic of controlled substance misuse. A high-risk population is veterans with war injuries, PTSD, and chronic pain. In addition to these external barriers to misuse, strengthening and support of internal resources of the patient are key. Identification and treatment of psychiatric disorders, psychosocial interventions, and cognitive and behavioral approaches such as 12-step programs (Narcotics Anonymous, for example) can also be helpful. Optimization of non-opiate-based pain control regimens with the use of TENS, massage, physical therapy, acupuncture, and pharmacotherapy with various nonaddictive agents may relieve symptoms of chronic pain and lessen exposure to more harmful agents.

The use of opiate agonists in a structured setting such as methadone-maintenance programs is another approach [23]. The development of new abuse-deterrent formulations such as the buprenorphine/naloxone (Suboxone(R)) combination is a trend which may lead to new agents that provide safe and effective detoxification with reduced abuse potential. Buprenorphine has been shown to reduce illicit opiate use [24]. Naltrexone can block opiate-induced euphoria and can be helpful in maintaining abstinence in patients not taking opiate regimens for pain.

NIDA is evaluating new approaches in clinical trials to address the growing problem of prescription drug misuse, and ongoing trials may provide evidence-based strategies for the management of the chronic pain patient with addiction to prescription medications.

Conclusions

The management of the prescription drug-abusing patient can present a significant challenge during the perioperative period. The anesthesiologist needs to be aware of the basic pharmacologic properties of the agents of abuse and maintain a high index of suspicion regarding misuse. The acutely intoxicated patient and the chronic prescription drug-abusing patient in withdrawal can present in ways that can mimic other organic processes and may, in fact, obscure the presentation of concurrent medical issues. Careful evaluation and supportive management are essential. The anesthesiologist can and should play an important role in the identification of opioid misuse and encourage subsequent referral for detoxification and treatment.

References

1. Gilson AM, Kreis PG. The burden of the nonmedical use of prescription opioid analgesics. Pain Med. 2009;10(2):S89–100.
2. Substance Abuse and Mental Health Services Administration. Results from the 2008 national survey on drug use and health: national findings (Office of Applied Studies, NSDUH Series H-36, HHS Publication No. SMA 09-4434). Rockville, MD; 2009.
3. Saban A, Flisher AJ. The association between psychopathology and substance use in young people: a review of the literature. J Psychoactive Drugs. 2010;42(1):37–47.
4. Ballantyne JC, LaForge KS. Opioid dependence and addiction during opioid treatment of chronic pain. Pain. 2007;129(3):235–55.
5. Turk DC, Swanson KS, Gatchel RJ. Predicting opioid misuse by chronic pain patients: a systematic review and literature synthesis. Clin J Pain. 2008;24(6):497–508.
6. Angst MS, Clark JD. Opioid-induced hyperalgesia: a qualitative systematic review. Anesthesiology. 2006;104:570–87.
7. Mizoguchi H, Watanabe C, Yonezawa A, Sakurada S. New therapy for neuropathic pain. Int Rev Neurobiol. 2009;85:249–60.
8. Mendelson J, Flower K, Pletcher MJ, Galloway GP. Addiction to prescription opioids: characteristics of the emerging epidemic and treatment with buprenorphine. Exp Clin Psychopharmacol. 2009;16(5):435–41.
9. Manchikanti L, Pampati V, Damron KS, Fellows B, Barnhill RC, Beyer CD. Prevalence of opioid abuse in interventional pain medicine practice settings: a randomized clinical evaluation. Pain Physician. 2001;4(4):358–65.
10. Manchikanti L, Manchukonda R, Pampati V, Kamron K. Evaluation of abuse of prescription and illicit drugs in chronic pain patients recieving short-acting (hydrocodone) or long-acting (methadone) opioids. Pain Physician. 2005;8(3):257–61.
11. Manchikanti L, Cash KA, Damron KS, Manchukonda R, Pampati V, McManus CD. Controlled substance abuse and illicit drug use in chronic pain patients: an evaluation of multiple variables. Pain Physician. 2006;9(3):215–25.
12. Kirsh KL, Whitcomb L, Donaghy K, Passik SD. Abuse and addiction issues in medically ill patients with pain: attempts at clarification of terms and empirical study. Clin J Pain. 2002;18:S52–60.
13. Passik SD, Kirsh KL. Opiod therapy in patients with a history of substance abuse. CNS Drugs. 2004;18(1):13–25.
14. Starrels JL, Becker WC, Alford DP, Kapoor A, Williams AR, Turner BJ. Systematic review: treatment agreements and urine drug testing to reduce opioid misuse in patients with chronic pain. Ann Intern Med. 2010;152(11):712–20.
15. Gourlay D, Heit H, Almahrezi A. Universal precautions in pain medicine: a rational approach to the treatment of chronic pain. Pain Med. 2005;6:107–12.
16. Portenoy RK. Opioid therapy for chronic nonmalignant pain: a review of the critical issues. J Pain Symptom Manage. 1996;11(4):203–17.
17. Wasan AD, Correll DJ, Kissin I, O'Shea S, Jamison RN. Iatrogenic addiction in patients treated for acute or subacute pain: a systematic review. J Opioid Manag. 2006;2:16–22.
18. Culberson JW, Ziska M. Prescription drug misuse/abuse in the elderly. Geriatrics. 2008;63(9):22–31.
19. Berti M, Baciarello M, Troglio R, Fanelli G. Clinical uses of low dose ketamine in patients undergoing surgery. Curr Drug Targets. 2009;10(8):707–15.

20. Madsen MV, Gøtzsche PC, Hróbjartsson A. Acupuncture treatment for pain: systematic review of randomised clinical trials with acupuncture, placebo acupuncture, and no acupuncture groups. BMJ. 2009;338:a3115.
21. Tetrault JM, O'Connor PG. Substance abuse and withdrawal in the critical care setting. Crit Care Clin. 2008;24(4):767–88. viii. Review. PubMed PMID: 18929942.
22. Denisco RA, Chandler RK, Compton WM. Addressing the intersecting problems of opioid misuse and chronic pain treatment. Exp Clin Psychopharmacol. 2008;16(5):417–28. Review. PubMed PMID: 18837638.
23. Kleber HD. Pharmacologic treatments for heroin and cocaine dependence. Am J Addict. 2003;12 Suppl 2:S5–18.
24. Gordon AJ, Kunins HV, Rastegar DA, et al. Update in addiction medicine for the generalist. J Gen Intern Med. 2011;26(1):77–82.

Chapter 13
The Addicted Adolescent Patient*

Corey Scher, Ethan O. Bryson, and Elizabeth A.M. Frost

Introduction

Many of us achieve insight into the expansive drug scene from blockbuster movies such as *The Hangover*, in which the main characters are given flunitrazepam (rohypnol or *roofies*) and cannot remember what happened the night before. Despite the ubiquitous nature of these drugs in popular culture, a survey of attending physicians within our department of anesthesia revealed a complete lack of knowledge of modern illicit drugs. Ecstasy (MDMA: 3,4 methylenedioxymethamphetamine), rohypnol, gamma hydroxybutyrate (GHB), and a host of other designer drugs are now a part of the adolescent social scene and the modern perioperative health-care provider must know more than just the difference between crack (the free base form of cocaine that can be smoked) and powder cocaine. The impending legalization of marijuana and the appearance of the synthetic herbal marijuana replacement known as K2 Spice (JWH-018) have left the perioperative health-care provider in a position of speculation as it concerns the real dangers of these drugs commonly used by adolescents. To underscore the dilemma, no senior member of our department knew that Spice caused "couch lock" or the inability to move, persistent body numbness, severe lung irritation, hypertension, severe and persistent headaches, blacking out, blurred vision, and extreme anxiety.

Special acknowledgment: The authors of this chapter wish to thankfully acknowledge the assistance of Dr. Jonathan H. Gardes, Department of Anesthesiology, Montefiore Medical Center's, Bronx, NY, USA, for his help in preliminary discussions about the aim and scope of this chapter.

C. Scher (✉)
New York University School of Medicine, New York, NY, USA
e-mail: coreyscher@gmail.com

E.O. Bryson and E.A.M. Frost (eds.), *Perioperative Addiction:*
Clinical Management of the Addicted Patient, DOI 10.1007/978-1-4614-0170-4_13,
© Springer Science+Business Media, LLC 2012

225

Definitions

The perioperative health-care provider should be familiar with the language attached by adolescents to these drugs to obtain an accurate drug use history. The following is by no means an exhaustive list but is designed to demonstrate the varied terms used by adolescents participating in the drug subculture. As a clinician, if one asks about drug use but does not understand an answer that includes "robo-tripping" or spending time in the "K-hole," then other questions might not receive the same honest replies.

Some examples of these terms include:

- Skin-popping: The street name for injecting drugs like heroin subcutaneously instead of intravenously. It is a high-risk behavior for abscesses and other infections.
- Foxy methoxy: The chemical name for this drug is *N,N*-diisopropyl-5-methoxy-tryptamine (5-MeO-DIPT), a short-acting psychedelic that can be swallowed, snorted, or smoked.
- Chasing the dragon: A phase that originated in Hong Kong, referring to inhalation of the fumes formed while heating heroin. It is linked to the development of toxic leukoencephalopathy, the pathophysiology of which is unknown.
- Robotripping: Refers to drinking Robitussin® or other cough syrup in volumes sufficient to achieve a hallucinogenic amount of the chemical dextromethorphan or DXM.
- K hole: A term that describes the dissociative effects of ketamine intoxication, specifically the place where one goes when high on ketamine, e.g., "I was in the K-hole for like hours at that party last night."
- Wet: There appears to be an increase in the use of substances known alternately by the slang names "embalming fluid," "fry," "formaldehyde," "wet," "water," or "amp." These drugs are sold in a variety of forms including cannabis joints or regular cigarettes dipped in liquid and cannabis leaf or tea leaves. In all of these forms, the material is then smoked.
- A-bomb: A marijuana cigarette laced with heroin or opium.
- 51 or 3,750, Bazooka, Primo, or Torpedo: A marijuana cigarette rolled with crack cocaine.
- Candy Sticks, Champagne, Coco Puffs, or Dirties: A marijuana cigarette rolled with powder cocaine.
- Chips, Dips, or Happy Sticks: A marijuana cigarette rolled with phencyclidine.
- Spice: Called "K2," "Spice Gold," or "herbal incense" these products are little more than dried vegetable matter sprayed with synthetic cannabinoids. Sold as incense, it is customized by the dealer and remains legal in most states. Just like THC, the active ingredient is marijuana and other forms of cannabis; these synthetic cannabinoids also stimulate the cannabinoid receptors, and their effects are similar to those of THC.

Some confusion can arise when nonstandard terms are used for street drugs obtained from different sources, such that often times the user is not entirely sure what drug they have ingested. For example, despite the variety of terms used to describe the drug "Wet," there is good reason to believe that these are all various preparations containing phencyclidine (PCP). In most instances, PCP is not mentioned when the substance is sold or discussed. In fact, there are constantly recirculating rumors that substances being sold by these names do not contain PCP but are instead actually the fluid (formaldehyde) used for embalming as would be used in a mortuary. But there is evidence to support that this is primarily a case of confused slang terms. "Embalming fluid" has been a common street slang term for PCP for many years. PCP can come in liquid form, so the term "fluid" is fitting. It is entirely possible (actually quite likely) that the confusion between PCP and embalming fluid (form- aldehyde) has gone so far as to cause a new trend where PCP is actually mixed with formaldehyde (or other "embalming fluids") and used as a recreational psycho- active drug. But there is little evidence that the formaldehyde itself causes any pleasant or desirable effects. Clearly, the "drug scene" is going in a direction that is not comprehended and the implications on providing safe anesthetics are obvious.

The preoperative anesthesia assessment form often appears as a checklist review of systems. Questions concerning alcohol, smoking, and drug use appear in the same area on the form. Anesthesiologists ask about alcohol and smoking but tend to skip over the "drug use" question when interrogating adult patients. There is compelling data that this question should be asked as it might significantly impact an anesthetic.

Trends in Adolescent Drug Use

The Monitoring of the Future (MTF) program consists of an ongoing series of national surveys of American adolescents and adults that addresses illegal drug, alcohol, tobacco, anabolic steroid, and psychotherapeutic drug uses [1]. Among 50-year-old high school graduates surveyed in 2008, 75% had tried marijuana and 66% had tried another illicit drug. When queried about recent use, responses sug- gested lower but still significant rates of chronic use. More respondents reported use of marijuana within the last month (7.2%) than reported other illicit drug use (5.9%). If an operating room schedule included 100 patients, six patients could have severe withdrawal effects during their time in the hospital or six untoward reactions to an anesthetic. While this chapter addresses substance use by adolescent patients, it is likely that the substance use in the 50-year-old started during adolescence.

The MTF document is a comprehensive and statistically sound compilation of surveys that clearly demonstrates that the responses of the adolescent are no less consistent than any other aged population using illicit substances. Over the decades that the MTF program has been collecting statistics, there has been substantial reduction in this country's drug use that began in the 1980s and continued into the late 1990s. Despite this overall reduction, many sobering trends remain. As of this writing, American high school students and young adults show a level of involvement with illicit drugs that is the highest among the world's industrialized nations [2]. Twenty-eight percent of 8th graders and 50% of 12th graders have tried an illicit drug. By their late 20s, the number jumps to 60% correlated with increased purchasing power. Seven percent of 12th graders have tried cocaine, a percentage that doubles in their twenties, and a startling 2.8% of high school students have tried crack which, like the use of other drugs, virtually doubles when they reach their 20s.

While parents may not easily note the use of illicit drugs including the designer drugs described above, alcohol and cigarette use is. According to the MTF, 25% of seniors in high school consumed five or more drinks in a row at least once in the 2 weeks prior to the survey. The number of "binge" drinkers escalates to almost 50% in college. There is hardly a parent who has not witnessed his or her child hunched over the toilet at 2 AM vomiting from excessive alcohol. As for cigarettes, when seniors in high school were asked about tobacco smoking, 25% reported using cigarettes within 30 days of the survey. The same survey in 2008 revealed cigarette use at 20%, which can only be viewed as a mild drop in use. The significant deceleration of cigarette smoking that began in the beginning of the decade appears to have stalled (Table 13.1 and Fig. 13.1).

Prospects for Progress

It would appear that the countless wars on drugs launched by numerous celebrities cannot be won. With new substances continuously arriving in our communities, illicit substance use can only be contained. How these drugs arrive in our communities has significantly changed since the MTF began the survey process (Table 13.2) [3]. Typing in the name of an illicit or a legitimate drug that is a controlled substance on the Internet using almost any search engine reveals an extensive list of sites on how the medication can be purchased [4]. At first glance, it appears easy to access all oral narcotics, amphetamines (such as Adderal) and benzodiazepines as these drugs are just a "click away." Is this the end of the adolescent driving himself to an unsafe part of town to purchase drugs?

The first report in the medical literature describing the purchase of an illicit drug on the Internet was in 2001. In 2005, a DEA official claimed that the Internet had become an open medicine cabinet. In 2007, former Secretary of Health, Education and Welfare Joseph A. Califano Jr. stated before a judiciary committee that the "Internet has become a pharmaceutical candy store stocked with addictive drugs, available with the click of a mouse to any kid with a credit card number" [3]. Investigators have shown that Internet pharmacy websites do indeed deliver narcotics to consumers without a prescription. Activities by local police departments, the DEA, drug task forces, and US customs do suggest that the number of websites offering illegal drugs remains high. Several studies indicate, however, that the use of the Internet to purchase addictive or illicit drugs is simply not very high. Investigations conducted by Inciardi et al. coupled with data sets from the MTF, Radars (Research Abuse Diversion), National Survey on Drug Use and Health (NSDUH), and Survey of Key Informants' Patients Program, reveal that the three most frequently accessed sources of acquiring a drug are dealers, friends or relatives (medicine cabinets), and doctors' prescriptions with dealers comprising over 60% of purchases. Internet purchases consist of a mere 3% [5].

Table 13.1 The target population is the adolescent and the price of most drugs reflects their limited funds

Web Poll	
How many grams of marijuana do you normally get for $10?	
None… I got ripped off (6,291)	13%
1 g (25,859)	53%
2 g (8,522)	18%
3 g (5,625)	12%
I don't buy weed, I grow it (2,360)	5%
48,657 total replies as of 02/19/10	

In order to better conceptualize what quantity of a drug is available to this population, the poll asks how much marijuana individuals are able to buy for $10 (http://marijuanaprices.homestead.com/~site/scripts_webpoll/webpoll.dll)

Fig. 13.1 The picture below
shows a gram of marijuana
with a quarter

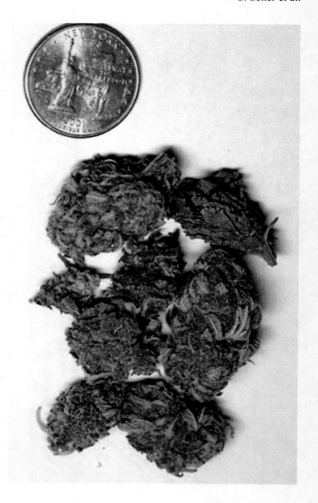

It does appear from the literature that the purchasing of drugs and illicit substances has not changed significantly over the decades. Adolescents purchase their drugs from "dealers." This does not necessarily mean that the adolescent is going to some dangerous part of town in the middle of the night to make a "score." He is simply going to one of his or her classmates who are able to obtain a supply from an older sibling or friend [6]. Access has never been easier and safer. There are even YouTube videos that explicitly give instructions on purchasing marijuana and making drugs to achieve a "high."

The "war on drugs," a term first applied by the Nixon administration began in 1971. A poll on October 2, 2008, found that three in four Americans believed that the War on Drugs was failing. The United Nations Office on Drugs and Crime (UNODC) issued a report that the global drug trade generates more than $320 billion a year in revenues. Current events in the towns along the United States

Table 13.2 Age-specific rates of emergency department visits for nonmedical use of opioid analgesics and benzodiazepines in the United States for 2004 and 2008

Characteristic	Opioid analgesics			Benzodiazepines		
	No.	Rate*	95% CI†	No.	Rate	95% CI
Total	305,900	100.6	(75.6–125.6)	271,700	89.4	(61.6–117.1)
Sex						
Male	150,800	100.6	(74.9–126.3)	119,600	79.7	(57.1–102.4)
Female	155,000	100.6	(75.1–126.1)	152,100	98.7	(64.8–132.5)
No. of drugs (including alcohol)						
One drug	116,800	38.4	(31.4–45.4)	56,900	18.7	(15.1–22.3)
Multidrug	189,000	62.2	(42.8–81.6)	214,800	70.6	(45.9–95.4)
Alcohol involvement	46,200	15.2	(10.9–19.5)	68,600	22.6	(14.6–30.6)
Admitted to hospital	72,700	23.9	(15.7–32.1)	81,300	26.8	(14.5–39.0)

*Rate is per 100,000 population

† CI = confidence interval

In 2008, ED visit rates for both types of drugs increased sharply among persons aged >18 years, peaked in the 21–24 years age group, and declined after age 54 years (Substance Abuse and Mental Health Services Administration (SAMHSA)'s Drug Abuse Warning Network (DAWN), 2004–2008. Additional information available in appendix C at http://dawninfo.samhsa.gov/files/ed2007/dawn2k7ed.pdf accessed 10/13/2010) border with Mexico where thousands of casualties have occurred in a symbiotic drug war where weapons arrive in Mexico from the United States in exchange for illegal drugs is now a regular feature on nightly newscasts [7]. The Obama administration has withdrawn the term "war on drugs" from their current initiative to control illicit substances from entering the country. As of June 2010, the CDC Morbidity and Mortality weekly report shows a dramatic increase in the misuse and abuse of prescription medications with a 111% increase in emergency department visits for nonmedical opioid analgesics and 89% increase in visits for nonmedical benzodiazepine use [8]. Between 2004 and 2008, the highest increase occurred from 2007 to 2008. Given the relative ease with which adolescents can obtain illicit substances from a friend, a dealer, the Internet, or a parent's medicine cabinet, identifying these patients preoperatively is even more essential (Table 13.3).

Risky Behaviors

While risk taking is by no means unique to the adolescent population, the combination of an unrealistic sense of invulnerability coupled with inexperience both socially and with particular drugs can lead to a host of medical complications. Binge drinking is as much a part of the adolescent social culture now as it is part of the college "experience." Once typically the result of fraternity hazing where pledges are forced to consume dangerous amounts of alcohol in a short period of time, emergency department admissions for acute alcohol poisoning more frequently include adolescent patients. Whether the result of experimentation or as part of an initiation into high-school-age fraternities or "drinking clubs," this behavior puts these young patients at risk for not only the medical consequences of toxic levels of alcohol but also the acute trauma that accompanies falls or motor vehicle accidents.

Unprotected sexual behavior while under the influence of alcohol or drugs can put the adolescent patient at risk for a number of infectious diseases as well as unintended pregnancy. The female adolescent who presents for surgery while under the influence or who reveals a recent drug history should absolutely receives a pregnancy test as part of the preanesthetic evaluation. Since the patient may not be aware of having engaged in such activity due to the amnesic effects of many of the drugs of abuse, the test should be performed even if a history of sexual activity is denied (Table 13.4).

In addition to abusing prescription drugs, alcohol, and illicit "street" drugs, adolescents are prone to experimenting with substances they may have an easier time obtaining, such as aerosol propellants or volatile solvents. In fact, the age at which inhalant use begins (16 years old) is a year younger than for any other illicit substance, likely reflecting availability and ease of abuse. Some of the more creative have experimented with producing home-made hallucinogens by combining household products or legally purchased herbs with prescription or over-the-counter medications.

Table 13.3 National estimates of Drug-related Emergency Department Visits, 2004 – 2008 drug misuse and abuse visits for individuals under 21 years of age[a]

Drugs	Weighted annual estimates				
	2004	2005	2006	2007	2008
Total ED visits	372,192	341,733	365,057	387,815	404,423
Total drug reports	533,090	503,284	550,140	580,977	612,558
Major substances of abuse	299,691	249,789	278,298	292,268	301,183
Alcohol	204,910	158,393	183,257	196,204	189,998
Alcohol-in-combination	53,922	47,794	56,553	58,835	57,156
Alcohol-alone	150,988	110,599	126,704	137,369	132,842
Non-alcohol illicits	131,588	125,805	132,165	135,893	150,057
Cocaine	30,547	29,139	38,412	32,435	21,683
Heroin	11,701	10,516	10,019	13,208	17,116
Marijuana	76,972	77,354	88,622	93,760	107,655
Stimulants	31,728	26,692	16,347	13,001	15,017
Amphetamines	8,242	7,303	6,167	3,651	4,982
Methamphetamine	24,217	20,432	10,696	9,471	10,464
MDMA (Ecstasy)	3,911	4,460	8,524	4,873	7,200
GHB	—	—	—	—	—
Flunitrazepam (Rohypnol)	—	—	—	—	—
Ketamine	—	—	—	—	—
LSD	649	551	2,120	1,382	1,425
PCP	3,765	2,131	2,961	5,153	6,563
Miscellaneous hallucinogens	2,318	2,297	2,508	3,027	2,820
Inhalants	2,687	2,073	2,497	2,714	2,865
Combinations NTA	—	—	—	—	498
Other substances	116,644	133,001	141,245	149,642	167,592

Note the significant increase in total drug-related ED visits from 2004 to 2008. The significant increase due to abuse of marijuana more than offsets the drop in the number of alcohol related admissions in this age group
[a]https://dawninfo.samhsa.gov/data/report.asp?f=Nation/AllMA/Nation_2008_AllMA_Under_21 accessed 10/13/2010

Table 13.4 Risky Behavior: trends in adolescent sexual activity 1991–2009[a]

Ever had sexual intercourse	Decreased 1991–2009
Had sexual intercourse with four or more persons (during their life)	Decreased 1991–2009
Had sexual intercourse with at least one person (during the 3 months before the survey)	Decreased 1991–2009
Used a condom during last sexual intercourse (among students who were currently sexually active)	Increased 1991–2003 No change 2003–2009
Drank alcohol or used drugs before last sexual intercourse (among students who were currently sexually active)	Increased 1991–2001 Decreased 2001–2009

Note that despite an increase in risky sexual behavior associated with drug and alcohol use observed in the 1990s, the current rate at the end of the first decade of the millennium is now back to the rate first observed in 1991

[a]The national YRBS is conducted every two years during the spring semester and provides data representative of 9th through 12th grade students in public and private schools throughout the United States. http://www.cdc.gov/HealthyYouth/yrbs/pdf/us_sexual_trend_yrbs.pdf accessed 10/13/2010

Often called *Dex*, *Robo*, *Tripple C*, *Skittles*, or *Tussin*, dextromethorphan is a cough-suppressing ingredient found in a many cold and cough medications commonly available over the counter. In high doses, dextromethorphan is a dissociative anesthetic, with effects similar to ketamine and PCP that can include hallucinations. Consuming large quantities of DXM can cause tachycardia, hypertension, hyperthermia, and, in rare cases, death. Concern over the dramatic increase in adolescent abuse of DXM led the Drug Enforcement Agency (DEA) in 2007 to petition the Federal Drug Agency (FDA) to make all DXM-containing products prescription only. In 2010, an FDA advisory committee declined to include DXM under the Controlled Substances Act, which would make it available by prescription only; however, DXM-containing cough suppressants are likely to follow pseudoephedrine behind pharmacy counters with age restrictions on its purchase.

Legal and inexpensive herbs combined in formulations designed to produce a "natural high" can be purchased over the counter in pharmacies, convenience stores, and "head shops" around the country. Marketed as *Cloud 9*, *Rave Energy*, and *Ultimate Xphoria*, Herbal Ecstasy is swallowed, snorted, or smoked to produce intense cardiovascular effects that can cause myocardial infarction and sudden death in at-risk individuals. Ephedrine, the main ingredient in Herbal Ecstasy products that stimulates the cardiovascular and central nervous system, can cause problems for people with high blood pressure, heart disease, diabetes, and other conditions. Even though the Food and Drug Administration (FDA) has banned the sale of products containing ephedrine alkaloids, this rule does not apply to drugs that contain chemically synthesized ephedrine, or to traditional Chinese herbal remedies such as Ma Huang and herbal teas. These readily available agents are often taken in conjunction with alcohol to produce hallucinations. Kava-kava, another herbal preparation, is often used during cult ceremonies when combination with alcohol has been known to cause visual hallucinations and even suicide attempts.

Preoperative Assessment

Over 80% of adult patients with chronic pain syndromes are prescribed opioids by their primary caregivers (or pain management specialists), and these long-term opioid-dependent patients provide a special challenge in the management of perioperative acute surgical pain [9]. Just like their adult equivalents, adolescents who are using these medications to get high on a regular basis need special consideration when planning an anesthetic and postoperative pain management. The first step is to identify these patients preoperatively. While the chronic pain patient is relatively identified and will likely make himself or herself known without provocation, an opioid addict and particularly an adolescent opioid addict is very reluctant to reveal his or her drug use. Establishing a good rapport between health-care professionals and these young patients is essential and must be done without a parent present if the provider is to obtain any meaningful information about drug use or dosage used. This practice should become as routine a part of the preoperative assessment as the physical examination and done with every adolescent regardless of outward appearances.

Some specific questions to ask the adolescent about drug use include the following (If the question is posed such that it is clear to the patient that these activities are assumed, they will be less likely to deny use):

- *Do you smoke? Cigarettes, marijuana, or anything else such as K2?* Clearly, it makes sense to distinguish between tobacco and marijuana, but this question is important for two other reasons: First, tobacco cigarettes are ubiquitous and, as they are legal and very much a part of our popular culture, the adolescent who smokes is more likely to admit to this activity than illicit drug use. Breaking the ice with such a question may lead to more honest answers to questions about other activities. Second, the adolescent who smokes cigarettes is eight times more likely to abuse illicit drugs than his or her peers, and activities such as this have more serious perioperative implications in this age group [10].
- *How often do you drink alcohol? What do you like to drink?* Adolescents are more likely to consume a high volume of alcohol during any period of drinking than they are to be regular drinkers, especially when peer pressure is present. Restricted access to alcohol on a regular basis and a propensity to participate in binge drinking makes it more likely that the heavy-drinking adolescent patient who presents for nonemergent, elective surgery will not be physically dependent on alcohol or in withdrawal. Even "social" drinking in this population, however, is a risk factor for other illicit drug use.
- *Do you get high? Have you ever? How? What drugs have you used? When was the last time?* The most common drug of abuse in this population is prescription opioids. Adolescents who abuse these drugs are also likely to use alcohol, marijuana, heroin, Ecstasy, cocaine, and other drugs [11].

Once these patients are identified, the health-care provider should take a multimodal approach to managing acute perioperative pain to keep the patient comfortable while also preventing opioid withdrawal syndrome. See Chap. 12 for an in-depth discussion on this multimodal approach to pain management and Chap. 16 for ways to address issues specific to the addicted adolescent patient who may benefit from in-hospital intervention.

Perioperative Management

Just as with adult chronic pain patients, whenever possible the anesthesia care provider should approximate the dose of the baseline opioid requirements. Tolerance is a common phenomenon associated with all chronic drug use, and the drug-abusing adolescent patient who presents for a procedure or surgery that requires sedation or anesthesia requires a greater amount of anesthetics per weight than the naive patient. Unlike chronic pain patients or patients enrolled in a methadone maintenance treatment program who would normally be instructed to take their regular dose prior to surgery, the adolescent patient snorting oxycontin on a daily basis cannot simply be given the medication preoperatively. An equivalent loading dose could however be administered by the anesthesia care provider intraoperatively at induction or during anesthesia to account for baseline opioid requirements, provided an accurate use history can be elicited. For chronic abusers, an attempt should be made to calculate the 24-h dose of each drug and convert to an oral or intravenous equivalent dose for maintenance. The practitioner should assume a 20–30% increase in acute opiate requirements consistent with that required for opiate-naïve patients. If the patient does not respond to the first agent administered, they might respond to an alternate opioid because of the incomplete cross-tolerance of μ-receptors across different opioid agents. Specific suggestions regarding the difficult to manage opioid-addicted patients are covered in Chap. 4.

Since the perioperative period is hardly an ideal time to detoxify a patient from these medications, the dosage of medication postoperatively must be adjusted to account for higher basal requirements. If the patient has developed hyperalgesia, they may be hypersensitive to surgical and other stimuli in addition to developing tolerance and may require even higher doses of anesthetic agents than would be expected from tolerance alone. Nonopioid pain medication adjuvants such as dexmedetomidine, gabapentin, and COX-inhibitors, and even NMDA antagonists such as dextromethorphan are excellent at lowering the postoperative opioid requirements.

The benefit of a neuraxial or regional pain management technique cannot be overemphasized in these patients because these methods can dramatically lower the total dose of analgesic medications required in the immediate postoperative period. These techniques have immediate effect as they result in less perioperative pain, as well as long-term analgesia because the risk that a chronic pain state will develop is decreased. The benefits of these techniques can readily be discussed with the adolescent patient and parent without revealing anything about chronic opioid use or abuse.

These patients would benefit even more from an intravenous patient-controlled analgesia (IV PCA) device postoperatively coupled with close monitoring by an acute pain service. Follow-up with a pain specialist to assist in medication taper postoperatively to avoid withdrawal is essential. Many of these patients may be tempted to self-medicate while an inpatient or after discharge if pain is not adequately controlled, making the therapeutic relationship between physician and patient all the more important.

Conclusion

The management of the addicted adolescent presents a significant challenge during the perioperative period. The health-care professionals involved with the care of these patients need to be aware of the potential for drug use both prior to admission and, in some cases, while an inpatient. A basic working knowledge of the current agents of abuse is essential and health-care providers must maintain a high index of suspicion regarding misuse. The chronic drug-abusing adolescent patient in withdrawal can present in ways that can mimic other organic processes and may, in fact, obscure the presentation of concurrent medical issues. Careful evaluation and supportive management are essential. The perioperative health-care provider should play an important role in the identification of drug abuse in this population and encourage subsequent referral for detoxification and treatment.

References

1. Johnson LD, O'Malley PM, Bachman JG, Schulenberg JE. Monitoring of the future-national survey on drug use 1975–2008 National Institutes of Health. US Department of Health and Human Services (NIH Publication No. 09-7401) Bethesda, MD.
2. A published report from an international collaborative study modeled largely after MTF, provides comparative data from national school surveys of 15–16 year olds that was completed in 2007 in 35 European Countries. It also includes MTF data from 10th graders in the United States. See Hibell B, Andersion B, Bjarnasson T, Ahlstrom S.
3. Inciardi JA, Surratt HL, Cicero TJ, Rosenblum A, et al. Prescription drugs purchased through the internet: Who are the end users? Drug Alcohol Depend. 2010. doi:10.1016/j.drugalcdep.2010.015.
4. Scher C, Torres A, Weider S. Internet drug access runs rampant. Anesth Anal. 2007; 105(6):1868–9.
5. Substance Abuse and Mental Health Services Administration (2009) Results from the 2008 National survey on drug use and health: national findings (Office of Applied Studies, NSDUH Series H-36, HHS Publication No. SMA 09-4434). Rockville, MD.
6. McCabe SE, Boyd CJ, Young A. Medical and nonmedical use of prescription drugs among secondary school students. J Adolesc Health. 2007;40(1):76–83.
7. Public Views Clash with U.S. Policy on Cuba, immigration, and drugs. Zogby International. http://www.zogby.com/news/readnews.cfm?ID=1568 (2008). Accessed 10 May 2010.

8. Cai R, Crane E, Poneleit K, Paulozzi L. Emergency department visits involving nonmedical use of selected prescription drugs – United States, 2004–2008. MMWR Morb Mort Wkly Rep. June 18, 2010;59(23):705–9.
9. Mitra S, Sinatra RS. Perioperative management of acute pain in the opioid-dependent patient. Anesthesiology. 2004;101(1):212–27.
10. Substance Abuse and Mental Health Services Administration and Office of Applied Studies. Substance Abuse and Mental Health Services Administration, Office of Applied Studies: Overview of Findings from the 2003 National survey on drug use and health (DHHS Publication No. SMA 04-3963), Rockville, MD: Substance Abuse and Mental Health Services Administration; 2004.
11. National Center of Addiction and Substance Abuse. National Center of Addiction and Substance Abuse, Columbia University: Under the counter: the diversion and abuse of controlled prescription drugs in the U.S. 2005. Accessed 13 Oct 2010.

Chapter 14
The Addicted Geriatric Patient

Sherry Cummings and R. Lyle Cooper

Introduction

The older population in the U.S. is growing at an unprecedented rate. At present, there are 37 million people 65 years of age and over in the United States. Due to the aging of the baby boomers, this population will expand to more than 71 million by 2030 [1]. Approximately 2.5 million older adults have substance abuse problems. This number is expected to double to 5 million by 2020 [2]. Projections indicate that increases in the number of older adults with problem substance use will increase across race, ethnicity, and gender. As the population of older substance abusers continues to grow, so too will the number of older in-patients and surgical patients with substance abuse disorders.

Prevalence

It is estimated that 1–15% of all community-dwelling older adults consume excessive amounts of alcohol [3]. This number is expected to increase dramatically by 2020. While 38.4% of adults aged 65 or older report drinking in the past month, 6.0% report binge drinking [4]. Results from national studies indicate that 9.2–10.1% of older men and 2.2–2.6% of women are heavy drinkers [5]. National data suggest that the incidence of alcohol abuse and dependence is significantly higher for men than women and significantly greater in the white than in the African American

S. Cummings (✉)
College of Social Work, University of Tennessee, Nashville, TN, USA
e-mail: scumming@utk.edu

E.O. Bryson and E.A.M. Frost (eds.), *Perioperative Addiction:*
Clinical Management of the Addicted Patient, DOI 10.1007/978-1-4614-0170-4_14,
© Springer Science+Business Media, LLC 2012

populations [6]. Marijuana is the illegal drug most frequently used by older adults, followed by cocaine. In addition, 49% of older marijuana users and 57% of cocaine users report using 30 or more times in the past year [7]. The number of marijuana users age 50 and over is expected to increase from the current 719,000 to 3.3 million by 2020, while the overall number of illicit drug users in this age group is projected to grow from 1.6 million to 3.5 million by 2020. Multi-drug use is also a growing problem among middle-aged and older adults. One national study found that over 15% have used two or more illegal drugs in the past year [7].

The projected dramatic increase in alcohol and illegal drug abuse among older adults is due to the unprecedented size of the baby boom generation combined with their higher rates of lifetime drug use. Birth cohorts that experience high rates of alcohol and drug use in youth or young adulthood have subsequently shown higher rates of use as they age, relative to other cohorts. A recent study revealed that older adults who had begun using illegal drugs by 16 years of age were four times more likely – and those who initiated drug use between the ages of 17 and 32 were three times more likely – to have a substance use disorder. As a result of the growth in the baby boomer population, the number of adults 50–59 years old with a substance use disorder is expected to increase 61%, while substance abuse among those aged 60–69 is projected to more than triple by 2020 [8].

Over 90% of older individuals use prescription and over-the-counter medications [9]. One-fourth of all prescriptions in the U.S. are written for older adults, who often have chronic conditions such as pain, insomnia, and anxiety. Thirty percent of older adults take eight or more prescribed medications each day [10]. Older individuals are also prescribed more than one-quarter of all tranquilizers and one-third of all hypnotics [11]. Consequently, it is estimated that one in four older adults use psychopharmacologic drugs with abuse potential and that the nonmedical use of such drugs will increase 190% from the current 911,000 to 2.7 million by 2020 [12]. Studies indicate that risk factors for use of multiple commonly abused prescription drugs among older adults include being white and female, having more than one limitation in activities of daily living, and experiencing comorbid medical conditions [10].

The most often abused psychoactive drugs are benzodiazepines and opioid analgesics [13, 14]. In recent years, an opiate (hydrocodone/acetaminophen) has been cited as the most prescribed drug, while benzodiazepines are the seventh-most prescribed [15]. These medications are often prescribed for the treatment of pain, sleep disorders, and anxiety, which are common in older adults. In a study on the inappropriate use of prescription drugs by older adults, Hanlon, Schmader, Boult et al. [16] found that the drug class with the most problems was benzodiazepines. While some older adults unintentionally misuse prescription drugs, others intentionally abuse psychotropic medications by taking higher dosages than prescribed, securing multiple medications from various physicians, and obtaining medications that have been prescribed to another person. Older adults who have previous or current alcohol/drug histories and those with mental illnesses are at heightened risk for prescription drug abuse.

Substance Use and Aging

Substance abuse among older adults is associated with increased physical and psychological morbidity and mortality. Because of reduced body mass and water, slowed metabolism, and decreased absorption rate in the gastrointestinal system, drugs remain in the bodies of older persons for longer periods of time and at higher rates of concentration. As a result of altered pharmacokinetics, older adults have an increased sensitivity to alcohol and other drugs and are more vulnerable to the effects of drugs than are younger persons. Drinking levels that are acceptable for younger adults become hazardous to the health of older individuals. In recognition of this reality, the National Institute on Alcoholism and Alcohol Abuse has published specialized drinking standards for older adults [17]. These standards indicate that older adults should consume no more than one drink per day or seven drinks per week, and no more than two drinks on any drinking day. Likewise, it is generally recommended that medications be prescribed to older adults at lower dosages. While benzodiazepines can be very useful in the treatment of anxiety, the prescription of this class of drugs to older adults, even at modest dosages, can increase the risk of harmful consequences (e.g., hip fracture). Meanwhile, benzodiazepines with shorter half-lives may not be safer than their counterparts with longer half-life [18].

Research indicates that substance misuse by older adults can affect cognitive and motor functioning necessary for both complex and simple daily tasks such as driving, bill paying, meal preparation, and ambulation. Alcohol and illicit drugs can interact with prescribed medications, causing unanticipated and harmful consequences [14]. Older drinkers suffer from increased rates of cancer of the head, neck, liver, and esophagus, cardiovascular disease, malnutrition, and chronic diarrhea [19]. Health outcomes related to illicit drug use by older adults include myocardial infarction, seizures, stroke, HIV, hepatitis, pulmonary hemorrhage, pneumonia, chronic obstructive lung disease (COPD), and endocarditis [20]. Data indicate that negative medication reactions occur 3–7 times more often for older adults [21]. Psychotropic drugs are often used by older adults for insomnia, chronic pain, anxiety, and depression. Studies show that older adults using certain classes of psychotherapeutic drugs, such as benzodiazepines, have a significantly greater risk of falling, car accidents and injury, and experience functional impairment to the same extent as do older persons with several chronic medical conditions [19]. Use of alcohol and other drugs can also have negative effects on perioperative outcomes. Older surgical patients with a history of alcohol abuse and regular use of psychotropic drugs before admission have a greater risk of postoperative delirium. Alcohol abuse has also been identified as a preoperative risk factor for infection following spinal surgery [22, 23]. Because of this, research on the impact of inclusion of substance abuse screening in the perioperative management of older patients has been recommended [24].

Comorbidity

Older adults who abuse drugs and alcohol also suffer from high rates of psychiatric illness, including depression and anxiety [21]. Studies indicate that 20% of older adults with depression have a co-occurring alcohol use disorder and that 37.6% of older psychiatric in-patients have co-occurring psychiatric and substance use disorders. Both alcohol abuse and affective disorders correlate highly with lifetime drug abuse [13, 25]. Increased rates of dementia are also associated with heavy drinking in the older population [26]. Additionally, combining prescription or over-the-counter medications with alcohol and other drugs can lead to decreased cognition, impairment of memory and attention, and increased falls [21].

The high rates of medical and psychiatric disorders among older substance abusers present a substantial public health burden. A history of drug and/or alcohol use in older adults is linked to high rates of medical treatment and longer hospitalizations. It has been estimated that alcohol abuse alone is responsible for over $184 billion in costs in the U.S [27]. Research indicates that 25% of hospitalized older adults suffer from alcohol abuse [28]. Substance abuse is a leading risk factor for trauma-related (e.g., motor vehicle accidents, falls) hospitalizations among older adults. In addition, the presence of a secondary alcohol-related diagnosis significantly increases length of stay and charges for older patients seen in the emergency room [29]. Co-occurring substance misuse and mental health disorders are associated with poor health outcomes and higher health-care utilization.

Substance abuse among older adults is currently under-diagnosed, under-treated, and has been called an "invisible epidemic." [30] Health-care providers tend to overlook substance misuse among older people, mistaking the symptoms for those of dementia, depression, or other problems common to older adults [30]. They are often unaware of the special physiological vulnerabilities of older adults and the resultant reduced substance use guidelines established for older adults [3]. One study, investigating primary care physicians' ability to screen substance abuse in older adults, revealed that only 1% accurately recognized the symptoms [13]. Another study examining the referral of older in-patients for substance abuse consultation found that, while 30% of older patients were estimated to have substance abuse problems, only 1% received a substance abuse referral [31]. Health-care professionals also often overlook prescription drug abuse. Poor communication among prescribing physicians [21], lack of physician inquiry concerning older patients' medication concerns [32], and medical professionals' failure to determine whether an older patient uses alcohol or other substances with abuse potential [13] all contribute to the inappropriate and hazardous use of prescription drugs by older adults.

Older adults themselves often do not recognize the signs of addiction. Older persons who have "successfully" been consuming alcohol and drugs for many years can have difficulty recognizing the increasing negative effects of their use. They may also perceive the negative effects of substance use as natural consequences of aging [21]. Physiological changes in older adults lead to increased negative side effects from smaller dosages of alcohol and other drugs. Therefore, older adults may find it difficult to identify their own risky drinking and drug use. Prescription drug abuse in the older population is often unintentional. Older adults may engage in dangerous behavior such as borrowing medication from a friend, taking medications for other than approved purposes, and taking higher than prescribed doses, without realizing the potentially dangerous effects of such behavior [13]. Therefore, older adults who misuse substances often continue this behavior until a severe or life-threatening crisis occurs, such as an acute medical condition, a fall, depressive episode, or suicide attempt.

Screening for Substance Use Disorders in Older Adults

Of central importance in working with persons with substance use disorders is accurate identification. Screening for alcohol and drug abuse generally involves either lab tests or self-report instruments that are based on population norms that can identify patients' likelihood of having an alcohol or drug problem. Findings from a screening do not definitively identify the presence of a disorder; rather, they provide a likelihood and, thus, indicate the need for further assessment. Screening can be a process that takes no more than five minutes, be administered by medical support staff, and, in some cases, be done using a self-administered questionnaire. There are a great number of alcohol-screening tools and a few drug-abuse-screening tools available. We describe several of the instruments currently in use with older adults along with their validity and reliability and recommendations for implementation.

Two tools have shown particular utility in identifying alcohol use disorders in older adults: the CAGE and the MAST-G. The CAGE, as noted in chapter 7, is one of the most well-known and simplest screening tools. It consists of four questions: (a) Have you ever felt you should CUT DOWN on your drinking? (b) Have people ANNOYED you by criticizing your drinking? (c) Have you ever felt bad or GUILTY about your drinking? (d) Have you ever had a drink first thing in the morning (EYE OPENER) to steady your nerves or get over a hangover? [33] These questions can be administered both through an interview with a doctor or nurse, or they can be added to intake paper work, making addition of this protocol time efficient. Further, this tool has demonstrated utility with the geriatric population [34, 35]. Conigliaro and colleagues [35] suggest a lower cut point (one affirmative answer as opposed to two) for the use of the CAGE with older adults, to account for the more deleterious effects of alcohol consumption on older adults.

By far, more studies of the CAGE have been conducted than for any other screening tool for older adult alcohol misuse. Sensitivity and specificity for this instrument vary quite widely, with sensitivity ranging from a low of 15% with randomly selected emergency room patients [36] to a high in the 90% range when applied with Veterans Administration patients [37, 38]. Specificity also varies significantly with the CAGE from 48% [39] to a high of 90% [40].

The MAST-G is a modification of the Michigan Alcoholism Screening Test [34] (Moore, 1972) that includes items specific to older adult alcohol misuse consequences

(Table 14.1). The MAST-G is a longer screening tool with 24 questions, and in order to be included as an at-risk drinker, respondents must give five affirmative answers. Sensitivity and specificity also range with this instrument depending upon the population to which it is applied. Morton and colleagues [41] found in their study of male Veterans Administration outpatients that the MAST-G yielded a 86% sensitivity rate and a 61% specificity rate when five is used as the cut point and 70% and 81% respectively when the cut point was dropped to three.

Both screening tools described above have demonstrated utility with older adults. Implementation considerations for these screens include the prevalence and consequences of alcohol misuse among the geriatric sub-population predominantly served. For instance, if in a practice more patients are expected to have an alcohol problem, or if the consequences of alcohol use could be more severe, then a more sensitive screen should be used, or the cut point used to identify an at-risk drinker should be set lower.

Self-report screening instruments for illicit drug abuse are not as prevalent as alcohol screens for the overall population. To date, no studies have examined the applicability of current drug abuse screens with older adults. Screening for illicit drug abuse in a perioperative setting may best be conducted through laboratory tests. One area of drug abuse screening is prescription drug misuse. Two tools that demonstrate promise in prescription drug abuse screening with older adults are described below.

The Current Opiod Misuse Measure (COMM) is a relatively new screening tool designed to identify misuse of prescription opioid pain-relieving drugs. [42] It is a 17-item questionnaire covering six domains:

1. Poor response to medication
2. Evidence of lying and drug use
3. Medication misuse
4. Appointment patterns cancellation or change
5. Emotional problems and
6. Signs and symptoms of drug use

The measure focuses on the past 30 days and contains questions such as "How often have you had to go to someone other than your prescribing physician to get sufficient pain relief from medications?," "How often have you needed to take pain medications belonging to someone else?," "How often have you had trouble with thinking clearly or had memory problems?," "How often have you had to visit the Emergency Room?," "How often have you had trouble controlling your anger," and "How often have you been worried about how you're handling medications?". Butler et al. [42] found that with a cutoff point of 9, the receiver operating characteristic (ROC) curve analysis indicated the COMM provides significantly more information about opioid misuse than chance when comparing it to the Aberrant Drug Behavior Index (ABDI) (95% confidence interval 0.74–0.86; standard error=0.031; $p<0.001$; $n=227$).

Cuevas et al. [43] modified the Severity of Dependence Scale (SDS) to screen for benzodiazepine dependence. The SDS is a four-question, self-report instrument that

Table 14.1 Michigan alcohol screening test – geriatric version (MAST-G)

	No	Yes
1. After drinking have you ever noticed and increase in your heart rate or beating in your chest?		
2. When talking with others do you ever underestimate how much you actually drink?		
3. Does alcohol make you sleepy so that you often fall asleep in your chair?		
4. After a few drinks, have you sometimes not eaten, or skipped a meal because you didn't feel hungry?		
5. Does having a few drinks help decrease your shakiness or tremors?		
6. Does alcohol sometimes make it hard for you to remember parts of the day or night?		
7. Do you have rules for yourself that you won't drink before a certain time of the day?		
8. Have you lost interest in hobbies or activities that you used to enjoy?		
9. When you wake up in the morning do you ever have trouble remembering parts of the night before?		
10. Does a drink help you sleep?		
11. Do you hide your alcohol bottles from family members?		
12. After a social gathering have you ever felt embarrassed because you drank too much?		
13. Have you ever been concerned that drinking might be harmful to your health?		
14. Do you like to end the evening with a night cap?		
15. Did you find that your drinking increased after someone close to you died?		
16. In general, would you prefer to have a few drinks at home rather than go out to social events?		
17. Are you drinking more now than in the past?		
18. Do you usually take a drink to relax or calm your nerves?		
19. Do you drink to take your mind off of your problems?		
20. Have you ever increased your drinking after experiencing a loss in your life?		
21. Do you sometimes drive when you have had too much to drink?		
22. Has a doctor or nurse ever said they were worried or concerned about your drinking?		
23. Have you ever made rules to manage your drinking?		
24. When you feel lonely does having a drink help?		

Scoring – 5 or more "yes" responses is indicative of an alcohol problem

inquires about the patient's need for and control of benzodiazepine use (Table 14.2). Compared to the Composite International Diagnostic Interview (CIDI), the SDS had a positive predictive value of 94% and a negative predictive value of 98% with a cut point of ≥6. While to date studies of these tools have not focused on the older adult population, the large number of older adults being prescribed both pain relievers and benzodiazepines make screening for their abuse among the elderly crucial.

The tools described above are indicated for patients who are prescribed opioids and benzodiazepines. If a patient does not have a prescription for these classes of drugs, these screens are not needed. If an older adult is using these drugs without a prescription, then abuse or dependence is likely. Additionally, some older adults

Table 14.2 Severity of dependence scale (SDS)

	Never/almost never	Sometimes	Often	Always/nearly always
Do you think your use of (insert benzo being used) was out of control?	0	1	2	3
Did the prospect of missing a dose make you anxious or worried?	0	1	2	3
Did you worry about your use of (insert benzo being used)?	0	1	2	3
Did you wish you could stop?	0	1	2	3
	Not difficult	Quite difficult	Very difficult	Impossible
How difficult do you find it to stop or go without (insert benzo being used)?	0	1	2	3

SDS total: _____

may not indicate a problem with prescription drugs alone but may be drinking alcohol along with taking prescription medications. In such cases, a review of the patient's current medications, coupled with the administration of one of the alcohol screens described above, can provide information for the determination of the need for further substance use assessment.

Review of Studies on Older-Adult-Specific Substance Use Disorder Treatment

Cummings et al. [44] note in their review of interventions for older adult substance abuse that interventions for this population are sparse and that age-specific interventions, while sparse, do produce improved outcomes. Many of the interventions available cannot be delivered in perioperative settings due to the time and space needed for their delivery. Cummings et al. [45] reviewed substance abuse interventions for older adults, drawing on motivational interviewing, and found two that had favorable results and are likely applicable to perioperative settings due to their brevity and flexibility. The studies of motivational interventions that can be applied in general medical settings are reviewed below, as are studies comparing age-specific and mixed-age interventions.

Brief Substance Abuse Interventions

Perhaps one of the most important questions regarding how to intervene with an older adult substance misuser who presents as a perioperative patient is, in what intervention will they engage? As a part of the PRISM-E study, [46] researchers sought to answer whether patients were better retained in substance abuse treatment in integrated medical, substance abuse, and mental health care or through an enhanced referral process. This study found that 71% of the integrated group engaged in treatment versus only 49% of the enhanced referral group. Thus, when available, integrated approaches are superior. However, integrated approaches are not always offered, and in such cases referral to age-specific treatment is the best option, as indicated in the comparative studies below.

While it is not likely that integrated mental and behavioral health programs will be located within a perioperative setting, they may be available through the hospital in which the patient is being treated or through a primary care clinic where patients already receive health care. Below, two studies on brief interventions for drug and alcohol abuse among older adults are summarized. These interventions are brief and offer multiple delivery options (e.g., phone delivery, implementation by para-professionals), making integration into existing medical practices a possibility.

Gordon et al. [47] compared Motivational Enhancement (ME), Brief Advice (BA), and Treatment as Usual (TAU) to determine which had the greatest impact on alcohol use reduction among the older (65 years+) population. Screenings occurred in primary care offices and participants were randomly assigned to the ME ($n = 18$), BA ($n = 12$), and TAU ($n = 12$) groups. The ME intervention focused on feedback, consequences of drinking, and goal setting. ME consisted of a 45–60-min session with two 10–15-min follow-up sessions conducted at 2 and 6 weeks after the initial session. The BA intervention was one, 10–15-min session that focused on feedback from a drinking assessment questionnaire dealing with the social and health implications of drinking and on advice about how to stop or reduce alcoholic consumption. Results indicated that there was a statistically significant decrease in alcohol consumption for those in the ME and BA conditions as compared to those receiving TAU. No difference in effectiveness was found between BA and ME.

The Florida Brief Intervention and Treatment for Elders (BRITE) utilized a screening and brief intervention and referral to treatment (SBIRT) approach to address substance abuse and mental health problems simultaneously [48]. SBIRT is an intervention often delivered in health-care settings that utilizes screening procedures coupled with feedback in a motivational interviewing style and referral to substance abuse treatment. A single group pretest–posttest design with follow-up was used to evaluate the effectiveness of the BRITE intervention. Older adults who screened positive for prescription medication problems, alcohol misuse, or illegal drug use were referred for intervention. Of those completing the intervention with prescription drug problems ($n = 187$), 60 indicated improvement at discharge, and the remaining 127 did not. The participants referred for alcohol misuse ($n = 109$) decreased use significantly at discharge, and the 60 participants who completed a follow-up interview 30 days after discharge continued to show significantly decreased alcohol use. Only 12 illicit drug users completed the treatment and, of those, nine indicated abstinence from these substances at discharge.

Age-Specific Versus Mixed-Age Interventions

A retrospective, nonrandomized study conducted by Kofoed et al. [49] compared a sample of 24 older alcoholics treated in traditional mixed-age outpatient groups with a sample of 25 older alcoholics treated in older adult peer groups. The traditional groups, which usually contained one to two older adults in each group of six to ten people, emphasized expression of feelings and contained frequent peer and staff confrontation. The age-specific groups emphasized socialization and support, progressed at a slower pace, and contained less confrontation than the traditional groups. Patients could participate in both treatment conditions for up to 1 year. Results indicated that older patients treated in the age-specific groups had better attendance rates and completed one year of treatment at a rate four times higher than older patients in the mixed-age groups.

Kashner et al. [50] in a randomized controlled study of 137 male alcoholic patients aged 45 and older, compared an age-specific treatment program to a traditional, mixed-age treatment program. Both treatment groups received 2–7 days of inpatient detoxification, 3–4 weeks of inpatient treatment, and 1 year of outpatient aftercare. Individual and group counseling were provided in both conditions. The mixed-age program included problem solving, vocational development, and life change, and a more confrontational counseling approach was employed. The older adult-specific program included counseling to develop patient self-esteem and peer relationships, reminiscence therapy, and used a more supportive and respectful approach. Those in the older adult-specific treatment were more than twice as likely to report abstinence at one year following treatment. Among patients over 60 years of age, the outcomes were even better.

The Geriatric Evaluation Team: Substance Misuse/Abuse Recognition and Treatment (GET SMART) Program is an age-specific, outpatient program for older veterans with substance abuse problems [48]. GET SMART provided 16 group sessions using a cognitive-behavioral therapy approach. The group sessions begin with an analysis of substance use behavior to determine high-risk situations for substance use. The analysis is followed by a series of modules to teach skills for coping with social pressure, isolation, uncomfortable feelings (i.e., depression, loneliness, anxiety, tension, anger, and frustration), cues for substance use, urges, and slips or relapses. Fifty-five percent of the 49 patients who were contacted at follow-up remained abstinent at 6 months post program completion. An additional 27% were abstinent at the time of follow-up, although they had experienced at least one "slip" since completing the program. Additionally, those who completed treatment were significantly more likely to be abstinent than those who did not.

Concluding Comments

The older population is growing at an unprecedented rate and projections indicate the number of older substance abusers will increase substantially in coming decades. As a result, it can be expected that more and more older patients with substance use problems will present in preoperative settings. Such patients are at heightened risk for negative postoperative outcomes. When considering the addicted geriatric patient, perhaps the first and most important addition to perioperative practice is screening. Screening can be implemented through client intake paper work or through a short conversational screening by a doctor or nurse. As the perioperative physician, and as has been suggested for smoking cessation, Additionally the anesthesiologist is in a position either through a preanesthetic assessment clinic or at postanesthetic follow-up to refer patients to one or more of several screening and interventional programs, either as out patients or through the hospital setting. When substance abusers are identified, brief interventions informed by motivational interviewing and integrated into medical settings can be effective in both reducing substance use and retaining older adults in treatment. Additionally, age-specific substance abuse treatment for older adults has been shown repeatedly to increase retention and improve substance use outcomes among older adults. During preanesthetic assessment, patience and understanding are necessary to obtain the most honest admission of alcohol or drug abuse because of perceived stigma and feelings of guilt associated with clandestine drinking. Intraoperative dosages of benzodiazepines and opioids have to be adjusted according to use and to a more age-appropriate amount. Antibiosis must be considered as infection risks are higher. Postoperatively, the anesthesiologist must have a heightened awareness for the onset of hallucinations and/or withdrawal symptoms. Intravenous and monitoring lines should be well secured lest the patient attempts to disconnect them and/or get out of bed. In fact, at all periods of the perioperative experience, the geriatric abuser is subject to sudden and unexpected changes that deserve attention and prompt treatment.

References

1. US Bureau of the Census. Statistical abstracts of the United States: 2006. Available at: http://www.census.gov/prod/2006pubs/07statab/pop.pdf. Accessed 29 Jun 2007.
2. Gfoerer J, Penne M, Pemberton M, et al. Substance abuse treatment need among older adults in 2020: the impact of the aging baby-boom cohort. Drug Alcohol Depend. 2003;69(2):127–35.
3. National Institute on Alcohol Abuse and Alcoholism. Social work education for the prevention and treatment of alcohol use disorders. Available at: http://pubs.niaaa.nih.gov/publications/Social/Module10COlderAdults/Module10C.pdf. Accessed 27 May 2010.
4. Substance Abuse and Mental Health Services Administration. Results from the 2006 national survey on drug use and health: national findings (Office of Applied Studies, NSDUH Series H-32, DHHS Publication No. SMA 07-4293). Rockville, MD: Substance Abuse and Mental Health Services Administration; 2007.
5. Breslow RA, Faden VB, Smothers B. Alcohol consumption by elderly Americans. J Stud Alcohol. 2003;64(6):884–92.
6. Grant BF, Dawson DA, Stinson FS, Chou SP, Dufour MC, Pickering RP. The 12-month prevalence and trends in DSM-IV alcohol abuse and dependence: United States, 1991–1992 and 2001–2002. Drug Alcohol Depend. 2004;74(3):223–34.
7. Blazer D, Wo L-T. The epidemiology of substance use and disorders among middle aged and elderly community adults: national survey on drug use and health (NSDUH). Am J Geriatr Psychiatry. 2009;17(3):237–45.
8. Han B, Gfroerer JC, Colliver JD, Penne MA. Substance use disorders among older adults in the United States in 2010. Addiction. 2009;104:88–96.

9. Reid MC, Anderson PA. Geriatric substance use disorders. Med Clin North Am. 1997; 81(4):999–1016.
10. Simoni-Wastila L, Zuckerman IH, Singhal PK, Briesacher B, Hsu VD. National estimates of exposure to prescription drugs with addiction potential in community dwelling elders. Subst Abus. 2005;26(1):33–42.
11. Culberston JW, Ziska M. Prescription drug misuse/abuse in the elderly. Geriatrics. 2008;63(9):22–31.
12. Dowling GJ, Weiss S, Condon TP. Drugs of abuse and the aging brain. Neuropsychopharmacology. 2008;33(2):209–18.
13. Simoni-Wastila L, Stuart BC, Sahffer T. Over the counter use by Medicare beneficiaries in nursing homes: implications for policy and practice. J Am Geriatr Soc. 2006;54(10):1543–9.
14. Colliver JD, Compton WM, Gfroerer JC, et al. Projecting drug use among aging baby boomers in 2020. Ann Epidemiol. 2006;16(4):257–65.
15. Drug Topics. 2007;5:24–5.
16. Hanlon JT, Schmader KE, Boult C, Artz MB, Gross CR, Fillenbaum GG, et al. Use of inappropriate prescription drugs by older people Source. J Am Geriatr Soc. 2002;50(1):26–34.
17. National Institute on Alcohol Abuse and Alcoholism. The physician's guide to helping patients with alcohol problems (NIAAA pub. No. 95-3769). Rockville, MD: U.S. Department of Health and Social Services, Public Health Service, National Institutes of Health; 1995.
18. Wang PS, Bohn RL, Glynn RJ, Mogun H, Avorn J. Hazardous benzodiazepine regimens in the elderly: effects of half-life, dosage, and duration on risk of hip fracture. Am J Psychiatry. 2001;158(6):892–8.
19. Fingerhood M. Substance abuse in older people. J Am Geriatr Soc. 2000;48(8):985–95.
20. Schlaerth KR. Addiction: older adults and illegal drugs. Geriatr Aging. 2007;10(6):361–4.
21. Benshoff JJ, Harrawood LK, Koch DS. Substance abuse and the elderly: unique issues and concerns. J Rehabil. 2003;69(2):43–8.
22. Fang A, Hu SS, Endres N, Bradford DS. Risk factors for infection after spinal surgery. Spine. 2005;30(12):1460–5.
23. Galanakis P, Bickel H, Gradinger R, Von Gumppenberg S, Forst H. Acute confusional state in the elderly following hip surgery: incidence, risk factors and complications. Int J Geriatr Psychiatry. 2001;16(4):349–55.
24. Cook DJ, Rooke GA. Priorities in perioperative geriatrics. Anesth Analg. 2003;96(6):1823–36.
25. Bartles SJ, Blow FC, Brockman LM. Substance abuse and mental health among older Americans: the state of knowledge and future directions. Rockville, MD: Older American Substance Abuse and Mental Health Technical Assistance Center, SAMHSA; 2005.
26. Mukamal KJ, Kuller LH, Fitzpatrick A, Longstreth WT, Mittleman MA, Siscovick DS. Prospective study of alcohol consumption and risk of dementia in older adults. JAMA. 2003;289(11):1405–15.
27. Harwood H. Up-dating estimates of the economic costs of alcohol abuse in the United States: estimates, update methods, and data. Rockville, MD: National Institute on Alcohol Abuse and Alcoholism; 2000.
28. Ondus KA, Hujer ME, Mann AE, Mion LC. Substance abuse and hospitalized elderly. Orthop Nurs. 1999;18(4):27–34.
29. Saleh SS, Szebenyi SE. Resource use of elderly emergency department patients with alcohol-related diagnoses. J Subst Abuse Treat. 2005;29(4):313–9.
30. Levin SM, Kruger J, editors. Substance abuse among older adults: a guide for social service providers. Rockville, MD: Substance Abuse and Mental Health Services Administration; 2000.
31. Weintraub E, Weintraub D, Dixon MD, et al. Geriatric patients on a substance abuse consultation service. Am J Geriatr Psychiatry. 2002;10(3):337–42.
32. Alemagno SA, Niles SA, Treiber EA. Using computers to reduce medication misuse of community-based seniors: results of a pilot intervention program. Geriatr Nurs. 2004;25:281–5.
33. Mayfield D, McCleod G, Hall P. The CAGE questionnaire: validation of a new alcohol screening instrument. Am J Psychiatry. 1974;131:1121–3.

34. Moore A, Seeman T, Morgenstern H, Beck JC, Reuben DB. Are there differences between older persons who screen positive on the CAGE questionnaire and the short Michigan Alcoholism Screening Test – Geriatric Version? J Am Geriatr Soc. 2002;50:858–62.
35. Conigliaro J, Kramer K, MacNeil M. Screening and identification of older adults with alcohol problems in primary care. J Geriatr Psychiatry Neurol. 2000;13(3):106–14.
36. Luttrell S, Watkin V, Livingston G, Walker Z, D'Ath P, Patel P, et al. Screening for alcohol misuse in older people. Int J Geriatr Psychiatry. 1997;12(12):1151–4.
37. Bradley KA, Kivlahan DR, Bush KR, McDonell MB, Fihn SD. Variations on the CAGE alcohol screening questionnaire: strengths and limitations in VA general medical patients. Alcohol Clin Exp Res. 2001;25(10):1472–8.
38. Joseph CL, Ganzini L, Atkinson RM. J Am Geriatr Soc. 1995;43(4):368–73.
39. Hinkin CH, Castellon SA, Dickson-Fuhrman E, Daum G, Jaffe J, Jarvik L. Screening for drug and alcohol abuse among older adults using a modified version of the CAGE. Am J Addict. 2001;10(4):319–26.
40. Jones TV, Lindsey BA, Yount P, Soltys R, Farani-Enayat B. Alcoholism screening questionnaires: are they valid in elderly medical outpatients? J Gen Intern Med. 1993;8(12):674–8.
41. Morton JL, Thomas VJ, Manganaro MA. Performance of alcoholism screening questionnaires in elderly veterans. Am J Med. 1996;101(2):153–9.
42. Butler SF, Budman SH, Fernandez KC, Houle B, Benoit C, Katz N, et al. Development and validation of the current opiod misuse measure. Pain. 2007;130(1–2):144–56.
43. de las Cuevas C, Sanz EJ, de la Fuente JA, Padilla J, Berenguer JC. The Severity of Dependence Scale (SDS) as screening test for benzodiazepine dependence: SDS validation study. Addiction. 2000;95(2):245–50.
44. Cummings SM, Bride BE, Cassie KM, Rawlins-Shaw AM. Evidence-based psychosocial treatments for older adults with substance abuse disorders. J Gerontol Soc Work. 2008;50:215–44.
45. Cummings SM, Cooper RL, Cassie KM. Motivational interviewing to affect behavioral change in older adults with chronic and acute illnesses. Res Social Work Pract. 2009;19(2):195–204.
46. PRISM-E Investigators. Improving access to geriatric mental health services: a randomized trial comparing treatment engagement with integrated versus enhanced referral care for depression, anxiety, and at-risk alcohol use. Am J Psychiatry. 2004;161(1):1455–62.
47. Gordon A, Coniigliaro J, Maisto SA, McNeil M, Kraemer K, Kelley ME, et al. Comparison of consumption effects of brief interventions for hazardous drinking elderly. Subst Use Misuse. 2003;38(8):1017–34.
48. Schonfeld L, King-Kallimanis BL, Duchene DM, Etheridge RL, Herrera RL, Barry KL, et al. Screening and brief intervention for substance misuse among older adults: the Florida BRITE Project. Am J Public Health. 2010;100(1):108–14.
49. Kofoed L, Tolson R, Atkinson R, Toth R, Turner J. Treatment compliance of older alcoholics: an elder-specific approach is superior to "mainstreaming". J Stud Alcohol. 1987;48(1):47–51.
50. Kashner M, Rodell DE, Ogden SR, Guggenheim FG, Karson CN. Outcomes and costs of two VA inpatient treatment programs for older alcoholic patients. Hosp Community Psychiatry. 1992;43(1):985–9.

Chapter 15
The Drug-Seeking Health-Care Professional

Dirk Wales and Ethan O. Bryson

Introduction

The potential for addiction among health-care providers, especially anesthesia care providers, represents a significant source of morbidity and mortality and increases the potential for patient harm. Although the incidence of alcoholism and other forms of impairment such as mental illness are similar to other professions, anesthesia personnel have a higher rate of substance use disorders [1]. It is difficult to gather reliable statistics on drug use among health-care providers for reasons of confidentiality, denial, misdiagnosis, or deliberate error. Records can be examined to look for evidence, such as disciplinary actions or mortalities, but there is still no guarantee that all such cases are reported. Because of this, it had been assumed that the true prevalence of addiction in health-care professionals could not be known [2]; however, it is estimated that between 13 and 17% of this population will, at one time or another, be substance abusers [3].

Addiction is a chronic, progressive disease that results in loss of control of one's life. Unless it is recognized and treated skillfully, addiction will result in disability and will often end with death. Physical dependence frequently develops but is not present in all drug addictions. Distinct from drug addiction is drug abuse. Drug abuse involves the inappropriate use of drugs and alcohol but is not accompanied by the uncontrolled compulsion seen with addictions. The addicted health-care professional will continue to divert controlled drugs and use them until he or she either is identified as someone who requires treatment or dies from an overdose, whichever comes first. Denial plays a major role in the individual's response to the relative or associate who is addicted. Following successful treatment, recovering addicts may have lifelong remission; for some, relapses do occur. Return to the practice of medicine is the norm, although each case must be handled individually.

E.O. Bryson (✉)
Department of Anesthesiology and Department of Psychiatry, Mount Sinai School of Medicine, New York, NY, USA
e-mail: ethan.bryson@mountsinai.org

E.O. Bryson and E.A.M. Frost (eds.), *Perioperative Addiction:*
Clinical Management of the Addicted Patient, DOI 10.1007/978-1-4614-0170-4_15,
© Springer Science+Business Media, LLC 2012

253

Background

The history of addiction in medical personnel is a long and pervasive story. In the late 1980s, The American Association of Nurse Anesthetists (AANA) became the first organization to address the issue of addiction formally through the creation of an educational program and a policy shift toward treatment and away from punishment for the addicted anesthesia provider. This effort was led by Diana Quinlan, a certified registered nurse anesthetist (CRNA), who supervised the creation of educational programs designed to provide a safety net for CRNAs who had become addicted to anesthetic agents. With the unfortunate death by self-administered overdose of one of the former AANA presidents in the early 1990s, larger and wider efforts were put into place.

The American Society of Anesthesiologists (ASA) has maintained a Committee on Occupational Health of Operating Room Personnel since 1990, headed at its inception by Dr. William Arnold. During his 6-year tenure, he organized a Task Force on Chemical Dependence in an attempt to provide practical answers to the problem of drug addiction in anesthesia personnel. Bill Arnold and Diana Quinlan can be thought of as the first in anesthesia to learn how to inform their specialties and educate them against substance abuse and its dangers.

The first effective use of media, film, and video in the creation of educational pieces designed to bring the issue of addiction in medical practice to the forefront was initiated by Dr. Tom Hornbein, then Chairman of Anesthesia at the University of Washington. Dr. John Lecky, a self-acknowledged recovering addict who later became a strong voice against substance abuse, worked closely with Dr. Hornbein in the first of the *Wearing Masks* series of educational/informative films warning of the potential for substance abuse in anesthesia providers. This series of educational films was later funded entirely by the AANA. The sad impetus for this funding effort was the death of Jan Stewart, former president of the AANA, who herself died of an overdose in 2002. The *Wearing Masks* series now consists of seven films plus additional features and is distributed by Allanesthesia: The Coalition for the Prevention of Addiction in Anesthesia.[1] It is estimated that 20,000 of these unified programs have been distributed in North America in the past 9 years. Many Canadian institutions have embraced these programs, as well as a scattering of European groups.

During the production of this educational series, research began to hint at the increased role played by chemical changes within the brain of the addict in the addiction process [4]. Evidence began to suggest that chronic opioid abuse leads to physical and chemical changes in the brain that increase drug craving directly. Thus, the addict who continues to use drugs inappropriately does so not because of a conscious psychological choice but due to a physiological urge. These findings underline even more the importance of education in addiction.

Put very simply, medical departments, physician groups, and hospital administrators need to aggressively insure complete drug addiction awareness and instruction

---

[1] www.allanesthesia.com accessed 07/11/2010.

throughout their institutions. An exceptional model for this education was put into place at the Anesthesia Department of the University of Chicago by the then Chair of Anesthesiology, Dr. Michael Roizen, who has conducted an annual series of six sessions promoting awareness of the issue and providing essential information to all members of his department for the past 16 years.

Etiology

Addiction is defined as the overwhelming compulsion to use drugs in spite of the addict experiencing adverse consequences. Drugs of abuse that have the ability to cause addiction activate the reward structures in the brain and in the process induce lasting changes in behavior that reflect changes in neuron physiology and biochemistry [5]. Not everyone who experiments with potentially addictive agents becomes dependent, but there exists a subset of individuals that does. These individuals typically exhibit traits such as novelty-seeking or antisocial behavior, suggesting there is a genetic basis for the susceptibility to dependence [6]. It is this genetic susceptibility that plays a role in the transition from substance use to dependence and from chronic use to addiction.

If proximity to addictive agents increases the risk that a health-care provider may abuse them, it makes sense that the drugs typically abused by anesthesia personnel are those commonly found in the operating room environment: fentanyl, sufentanil, midazolam, and propofol. For other reasons and perhaps due to exposure as well, emergency medicine professionals who abuse drugs are more likely to choose the "street" drugs such as cocaine and marijuana, and psychiatrists are more likely to abuse the benzodiazepines and other sedatives [7].

Personality disorders are commonly diagnosed in substance-abusing health-care professionals admitted to inpatient drug/alcohol-treatment facilities. It has been suggested that one source of motivation for the self-administration of drugs of abuse is the self-medication of symptoms associated with comorbid psychiatric disorders [8]. The observation that individuals with the same personality traits tend to self-administer drugs from the same class, i.e., opioids for anxiety and depression and amphetamines for attention deficit and hyperactivity states, lends credence to this theory. Individuals under evaluation for or treatment for substance abuse should have an evaluation with subsequent management of comorbid psychiatric conditions.

Several theories have been proposed to explain the incidence of drug abuse among health-care professionals. Access to highly addictive drugs may be contributory to the development of addiction in those at risk. Despite strict controls and accounting measures, it remains relatively easy to divert controlled substances for personal use. Some have cited the high stress environment in which today's health-care professionals work as a contributing factor, and others have suggested that exposure to trace quantities to these agents in the workplace sensitizes the reward pathways in the brain and promotes substance abuse. It is important to note that none of the proposed theories has been able to identify a specific cause, but rather merely suggest factors that may increase the risk of developing addiction among health-care professionals.

Some of the factors that contribute to the development of chemical dependence in health-care professionals include:

- *Gender*: The disease is much more commonly seen in men
- *Intelligence*: Correlation between outstanding academic performance and abuse is common
- *Age*: With the exception of alcohol, addiction to drugs usually becomes apparent before the age of 40
- *Denial*: "I can use drugs safely without becoming addicted"
- *Family history* of chemical abuse
- *Availability*: Addiction occurs only to readily obtainable drugs
- *Stress and fatigue factors*

The most important of these factors is probably *availability*. Anesthesiology is unique among medical specialties in that the practitioner administers drugs directly to patients rather than *ordering* others to perform this task. Thus, the drugs are immediately available; they do not have to be stolen from sources not normally available to health-care professionals. Add to this the high potency and rapid onset of drugs commonly used in anesthesia and a deadly situation can result. However, even health-care professionals without easy access to these agents may become addicted. Anyone with access to a prescription pad can easily obtain controlled substances for personal use, and these days it is just as easy to order them over the Internet from an offshore distributor.

While addiction to substances such as alcohol may not become apparent for decades, addiction to agents with shorter half-lives such as fentanyl and sufentanil is clear within weeks of first use. Although some anesthesiologists have become addicted to inhaled anesthetics, abuse of these drugs with the possible exception of nitrous oxide is rare in comparison to drugs taken intravenously.

The Signs and Symptoms of Addiction

The anesthesia care provider who is addicted to anesthetic agents necessarily seeks to maintain a job in close proximity to the drug source. He/she may volunteer for additional evening and weekend assignments or for long cases in which large opioid requirements would be expected. Often, it is the addicted health-care provider who is the last to recognize that a problem exists. It is therefore imperative that the relatives, friends, and co-workers (i.e., those people most likely to observe the signs and symptoms of addiction) gain a clear understanding of the disease and understand what to do if they suspect someone may have a problem. Since early identification of the affected individual can often prevent harm, both to the impaired health-care professional and to his or her patients, it makes sense that all workplace personnel be educated about the signs and symptoms of addiction. Using the University of

Chicago program established by Dr. Roizen as a model, small charts describing the signs and symptoms exhibited by addicted personnel can be posted in anesthesia workrooms, break areas, and on the bulletin board in the operating rooms.

Some of the changes typically observed in the addicted health-care professional include:

- Withdrawal from family, friends, and leisure activities as more time is spent in drug-related activities.
- Mood swings, with periods of depression or bad moods alternating with periods of euphoria or gregariousness, depending upon whether the addicted provider is high or in withdrawal.
- Increasing episodes of anger, irritability, and hostility; increased sensitivity to criticism.
- Spending more time at the hospital, even when off duty, often with odd intentions (in order to obtain and use drugs).
- Volunteering for extra call as an excuse to remain at work.
- Failure to respond to pager, difficult to arouse when on night call.
- Frequent "ampoule breakage" and increased "waste."
- Weight loss and pale skin, as less time and energy are spent taking care of themselves.
- Wearing long sleeves or other clothing designed to hide physical evidence of self-injection.

Changes in behavior are frequently noted with periods of irritability, anger, euphoria, and depression common. When these personality changes are noticed by someone who is educated in the potential for substance abuse in anesthesia providers, an intervention can occur before a critical incident results in patient or provider harm.

The development of *Wearing Masks* and other educational programs has dramatically increased the ability to disseminate this type of crucial information to all hospital personnel, but it is equally important that the family and close personal friends of anyone at risk also be educated. Addiction is frequently first noticed outside the workplace where it is not subject to education, "signs and symptoms" charts, or where it can simply be attributed to the stressful work life of the addict. Friends and family may observe behavioral changes at home that may pass unnoticed by colleagues at work as attributed to stress on the job; therefore it is just as important that these people who are most likely to observe the signs and symptoms of addiction gain a clear understanding of the disease and what to do if they suspect their loved one may have a problem.

The Role of the Family

Commonly, an addict is able to compensate for only so long before a critical incident leads to an investigation. Frequently, this incident leads to an intervention and referral to treatment; occasionally, the critical incident is the death of the addicted anesthesia provider. Chemical dependence in health-care professionals is a disease of loneliness, despair, increasing guilt, and fear. It is not a "social" addiction as seen with marijuana, cocaine, and other drugs. The addicted health-care professional feels trapped, with nowhere to turn, and no way to seek help without losing face, medical license, and career. In spite of progressive difficulty at home, he/she continues to divert and use drugs in what may be viewed as a downward spiral. When the family is notified that an incident has occurred, often there is surprise. Anecdotal reports describe the wife or husband of an addicted anesthesia care provider found dead expressing surprise and disbelief at the news, having not noticed anything odd in spousal behavior. Many express doubts that it would be possible for a person to be addicted to anesthesia drugs and be able to hide this from a spouse or significant other; but denial is a very strong defense mechanism in both the addict and those around them.

Sometimes it is not denial but fear that has allowed the addict to keep the secret. The wife of a young resident who accidentally killed himself with an overdose of fentanyl at the University of Colorado Medical Center in 1992 admitted that she knew of his addiction to fentanyl but did not know what to do about it. Both she and her husband were afraid to report his abuse for fear of recriminations and the loss of a medical license. Fortunately, this was a long time ago, and the specialty has come a long way since then; but it would not be wise to ignore the need of families of anesthesia personnel for education about addiction.

Early detection is often difficult due to the compartmentalized relationships the individual may have with different members of his/her social structure. The spouse of an addict may observe behavioral changes that may pass unnoticed by colleagues at work, and the entire picture is seldom appreciated by any one person. Despite the great strides that have been made, the awareness and educational net needs to be further spread to include spouses and a wider family circle to be effective. Finding ways to inform and educate families of this danger is paramount and possible through meetings, education, and information sent directly to family members.

Intervention

Early identification of addiction before professional impairment occurs is very important; however, this is often difficult. The multiple signs and symptoms of addiction can be subtle and none of them is diagnostic when taken alone. Individual family members and colleagues typically see only a part of the constellation of clues, making it easier for the addicted individual to hide the disease. This is an extremely sensitive situation that must be handled with extreme care to avoid ruining the career of a colleague. Erratic behavior may have many causes and professionals learn to avoid using the term addiction without clear support of such a diagnosis. If a colleague is suspected of having a problem, guidance is available and an individual should not attempt to be the sole source of assistance. Every state medical society in the United States has a program in place to provide help with the identification of the health-care professional in need of care, to refer them to qualified treatment facilities, to monitor them following completion of formal treatment, and to serve as their advocate during the difficult process of returning to work. Not all recovering health-care professionals are able to return to their specialty of choice, but many do so successfully with assistance. ASA serves as an additional source of confidential assistance. Since you will need assistance with confidential investigation, intervention, treatment referral, and aftercare monitoring, a confidential telephone call to the medical society in your state can begin this important process.

Suggestions for how a proper intervention should be conducted include the following:

- Have a trained interventionist present at all times.
- Have a larger group rather than a smaller one.
- Include the individual's spouse, family members, friends, and colleagues.
- Include anyone who is close with the individual so long as they are supportive of the intervention and will not be disruptive.
- Be sensitive to the gender of the impaired health-care professional.
- Bring all of available evidence, including a properly collected drug screen.
- Do not let the person leave the intervention alone.
- Do not let them drive.
- Make arrangements for direct transfer to an inpatient facility prior to the intervention.
- Do not let the addict decide treatment.

It should be made clear that this is not an exhaustive list, nor should someone untrained in the proper way in which to conduct an intervention infer that they would be able to do so by simply reading this.

Legal Issues

When ultimately an addicted health-care professional is referred for treatment or reported to a licensing body, consultation with legal counsel is mandatory for both the reported health-care professional and the institution involved with the reporting, as an individual's license to practice is in jeopardy. Failure to report an impaired colleague has been considered negligence and leaves the individuals and institutions involved open to questions of lability, should harm come to any patient [9]. A good initial source for information in these matters is one of the many diversion programs run by the individual state medical societies. These programs are available to provide consultation concerning intervention strategies, state-specific legal considerations, and reporting requirements. As well, they can be a great resource, providing listings of available self-help groups, therapists, treatment centers, sources of legal advice, and urine monitoring programs.

Limited protection for addicted health-care professionals was offered by the Americans With Disabilities Act of 1992, but it was applied differently to individuals dependent upon alcohol versus illegal drugs. It should be noted that no protection is afforded to the user of substances other than alcohol unless they are currently in a treatment program, and recent case law has further limited protection under this Act [10].

Treatment

Once a health-care provider has been identified as requiring assistance with substance-abuse issues, an addiction psychiatrist should direct diagnosis and treatment. A referral to such a specialist may be obtained from drug treatment centers, the American Society of Addiction Medicine, or any one of the state impaired physician programs mentioned earlier. Addicted health-care providers are commonly sent for residential treatment that may last from 2 months to a year or more. The intention of this initial period is to lay the groundwork for long-term abstinence and recovery. Inpatient treatment is followed by discharge either to a halfway house or directly to the community. A structured halfway house community, with 60–120 h per week of staff contact is often recommended for a 4–8 week period, followed by outpatient therapy as appropriate. Outpatients must be able to function in a normal daily environment and are expected to remain abstinent despite normal availability of alcohol and drugs; therefore this level of treatment may not be appropriate for every patient and the treatment plan is tailored to the needs of the individual.

Under most circumstances, health-care providers are allowed to return to work after inpatient treatment so long as they remain under the supervision of a diversion program sponsored by the state medical society. Part of this supervision includes a monitoring contract which is usually a minimum of 5 years in length and includes regular contact with a caseworker at the monitoring organization, worksite observation, and random urine drug and alcohol screens. The complete abstinence from all mood-altering drugs is typically facilitated through group psychotherapy with other recovering health-care providers and regular attendance and participation in self-help fellowships such as AA or NA.

Risk Management and the True Cost of Addiction

In a medical environment where the newest and most urgent word is "production" with an emphasis placed on increasing the number of patients that can be moved through an operating suite or health-care professional's office in a given day, it is crucially important to take time to educate people on the topic of addiction. The actual cost of not doing this is difficult to quantify, but estimates range from $450,000 to $600,000 for expenses related to the death of an employee from a diversion-related overdose; and if patient harm has occurred and litigation for damages is involved, the cost increases dramatically. To not invest the resources and time required to put in place an educational program because such resources are needed to meet the needs of "production" is, at the very least, shortsighted as the benefits to the institution far outweigh the minimal costs associated with establishing such a program.

Allied to the death of a health-care professional is the stigma and publicity that is generated when the death "goes public" in the media. There is a public fascination with this subject that is fed by aggressive media coverage. The fallout from such an event not only damages the specific institution, but also harms the health-care profession as a whole and contributes to the stigma surrounding the professional use of addictive drugs. Addressing this problem directly from the inside not only results in decreased risk for patient and provider harm but also elevates the health-care profession in the eyes of the layperson. Taking the time to inform, educate, and provide suitable safety nets for those at risk is an effective and inexpensive risk-management strategy.

In addition to education, a holistic approach to risk management must provide for the well-being of health-care professionals at every level in an organization. Historically, residents were a group felt to be most at risk, as new physicians with possibly immature coping skills and with the highest visibility when an incident occurred. Because of the emphasis placed on the evaluation and treatment of the addicted resident, most academic centers have a well-established infrastructure in place. There are, however, no residents in private practice groups, and as such, there is rarely an established department structure in place to provide a "safety net" in these environments. Yet, many private practice groups and hospitals without residents have a physician within the group who sees to the education and management of problems related to addiction, including intervention when necessary. There is such a person in a large private practice anesthesia group in Southern California. This group has created the position of "Director of the Well-being Committee" who is responsible for educating fellow health-care professionals, intervening when necessary, following the course of their treatment, and most importantly, monitoring their re-entry into clinical practice.

Conclusion

Despite the increased awareness of the disease of addiction and the numerous policies and procedures that have been put in place to protect our patients, and ourselves, there is still a significant possibility that a health-care provider will either develop an addiction during their career or have experience with a colleague who does. No matter what the organizational structure of a medical group may be, help, guidance, and assistance can be made available if the group itself understands the need for support of its group members in this crucial area and is willing to back that commitment with resources, both financial and otherwise.

Those who believe that the problems associated with addicted health-care professionals can be addressed with cool clinical solutions will be disappointed. This is a problem mired down in an emotional morass of denial, possible death, and stigma for those who live through it. There are enormous unbudgeted costs to repair loss and damages that directly result from addiction. This issue must be addressed through education and awareness and the willingness to spend the time and energy necessary to develop a group knowledge of the signs and symptoms of addiction. Education must be continual and addressed on a regular basis to ensure the uniform health of staff and to avoid the heartache and guilt that occurs when people realize there was something they could have done to prevent the death of a colleague. This can be done successfully, there are those who have, and there is a solid foundation of educational materials to assist all who will spend the time to educate as well as save lives.

References

1. Bryson EO, Silverstein JH. Addiction and substance abuse in anesthesiology. Anesthesiology. 2008;109:905–17.
2. Brewster JM. Prevalence of alcohol and other drug problems among physicians. JAMA. 1986;255:1913–20.
3. Baldssserri MR. Impaired healthcare professional. Crit Care Med. 2007;35:S106–16.
4. Malison RT, Best SE, Wallace EA, McCance E, Laruelle M, Zoghbi SS, et al. Euphorigenic doses of cocaine reduce [123I]beta-CIT SPECT measures of dopamine transporter availability in human cocaine addicts. Psychopharmacology. 1995;122:358–62.
5. Mohn AR, Yao WD, Caron MG. Genetic and genomic approaches to reward and addiction. Neuropharmacology. 2004;47:101–10.
6. Lesch KP. Alcohol dependence and gene x environment interaction in emotion regulation: is serotonin the link? Eur J Pharmacol. 2005;526:113–24.
7. Berge KH, Seppala MD, Lanier WL. An anesthesiology community's approach to opioid- and anesthetic- abusing personnel. Anesthesiology. 2008;109:762–4.
8. Markou A, Kosten TR, Koob GF. Neurobiological similarities in depression and drug dependence: a self-medication hypothesis. Neuropsychopharmacology. 1998;18:135–74.
9. Kadlec Medical Center v. Lakeview Anesthesia Associates, United States court of Appeals for the Fifth Circuit; 2008.
10. Westreich LM. Addiction and the Americans with disabilities act. J Am Acad Psychiatry Law. 2002;30:355–63.

Chapter 16
Non-narcotic Anesthetic Options for the Patient in Recovery from Substance Abuse

Heather Hamza

Introduction

While there is extensive literature regarding anesthesia for the actively addicted patient, there remains very little to guide the perioperative management of the patient in recovery. Developing a better understanding of the unique needs of the patient presenting for surgery who is in recovery from chemical dependency is essential for those involved in the perioperative care of such patients. Some of the issues that arise in this population are similar to those that confound the management of the chronic pain patient, such as tolerance, opioid-induced hyperalgesia, and withdrawal. In addition, many patients in recovery are maintained on methadone and buprenorphine, which can further complicate their perioperative management. This chapter will discuss pain management strategies involving alternatives to opiates, recommendations for safe use of opiates and other "triggering" agents, and relapse prevention. For the purpose of this discussion, the term "addict" will include persons addicted to alcohol.

Statistics

According to the National Institutes on Drug Abuse (NIDA), in 2008, heavy drinking was reported by 6.9% of the population aged 12 or older, accounting for 17.3 million people.[1] Additionally, an estimated 8% or 20.1 million Americans aged 12 or older

---

[1] National Institute on Drug Abuse (NIDA) 2008 InfoFacts: Nationwide trends. Available online at: http://www.drugabuse.gov/infofacts/nationtrends.html accessed 09-18-2010.

H. Hamza (✉)
Department of Anesthesiology, Los Angeles County Medical Center,
University of Southern California, Los Angeles, CA, USA
e-mail: heather.hamza@gmail.com

E.O. Bryson and E.A.M. Frost (eds.), *Perioperative Addiction:*
Clinical Management of the Addicted Patient, DOI 10.1007/978-1-4614-0170-4_16,
© Springer Science+Business Media, LLC 2012

were current (past month) illicit drug users, meaning they had used an illicit drug during the month preceding the survey interview.

The Substance Abuse and Mental Health Services Administration (SAMHSA) has compiled data specifically on recovery and the use of self-help groups. Combined 2006 and 2007 data from SAMHSA's National Surveys on Drug Use and Health indicate that an annual average of five million persons aged 12 or older attended a self-help group in the past year because of their use of alcohol or illicit drugs. Additionally, 32.7% of persons aged 12 or older who attended a self-help group for their alcohol or illicit drug use in the past year also received special treatment for substance use in the past year.[2]

When considering the millions of people who are either actively using drugs or alcohol and the millions who have reported the use of self-help groups or having received treatment for addiction, there are untold numbers of recovering patients (or patients who would likely benefit from recovery) who present for operative procedures each year.

Definitions

A rational discussion of the issues pertinent to the perioperative management of this population demands consistent definitions of the terms involved. For clarification, the following will apply:

- Tolerance: A naturally occurring phenomenon where, over time, increased doses of a particular drug are needed to elicit the same response (the same dose yields a diminished effect); also known as a right shift of the (opioid) dose-versus-response relationship. This is believed to occur due to desensitization and down-regulation of opioid receptors [1]. After only a few days of abstinence, a left shift (sensitization) of the opioid dose–response curve is noted, demonstrating that tolerance is lost [2].
- Physical dependence: A state of adaptation manifested by withdrawal (defined below). The presence of physical dependence does not automatically imply addiction. Addiction comes with a significant psychological component, and "normal" people do not crave the drug when withdrawing. Physical dependence is commonly accompanied by tolerance [3].
- Withdrawal (or "abstinence syndrome"): Evident when signs and symptoms are experienced after discontinuing the medication, which were not present prior to the initial administration of the medication. Withdrawal might also be precipitated by dose reduction, or by administering an antagonist [4].

[2] Substance Abuse and Mental Health Services Administration (SAMHSA) Office of Applied Studies; participation in self-help groups for alcohol and illicit drug use, 2006–2007. Available online at: http://www.oas.samhsa.gov/2k8/selfHelp/selfHelp.cfm accessed 09-18-2010.

- Addiction: DSM-IV criteria. Manifested by three or more of the following within a 3-month period (APA, 1994):
  - Tolerance (increased amount, or diminished effect with same dose)
  - Withdrawal, or substance use to avoid withdrawal
  - Larger amounts over a longer period than anticipated
  - Unsuccessful effort to cut down use
  - Increased time spent in activities to obtain, use, or recover from the substance
  - Social, occupational, or recreational activities diminish
  - Use continues despite persistent physical or psychological problems
  - Note that tolerance, physical dependence, and withdrawal *do not* automatically determine psychological dependence or addiction
- Pseudoaddiction: People with severe, unrelieved pain may become intensely focused on relief and may appear to be preoccupied with obtaining opiates (drug seeking), but they are actually seeking relief from pain [5].
- Recovery: For the purpose of this chapter, "recovery" will be defined as a person who is no longer self-medicating with alcohol or illicit drugs and who is making a concerted effort to become a productive member of society. This would include the development of effective coping skills and finding pleasure in other activities [6]. It is worthy of note that many experts believe opioid replacement therapy (ORT) is not recovery, since it is not abstinence-based sobriety and distinguish between the patient in a drug-free recovery program and the patient on methadone maintenance. Nevertheless, patients utilizing harm-reduction and damage-control methods, in particular, ORT with methadone or buprenorphine, will be included in this definition of recovery.

Preoperative Assessment

When assessing a patient who may be in recovery, do not stereotype. It is helpful to ask everyone the same questions so that you feel just as comfortable asking a young man in his 20s, covered in tattoos, the same questions regarding illicit drug use as you would a sweet-looking, grandmotherly woman in her 70s. You may find the former has never used illicit drugs while the latter may be currently abusing prescription analgesics. The disease of addiction does not discriminate.

According to Bécheiraz and Thallman, up to 65% of communication is nonverbal [7]. With this in mind, be aware of your body language and volume/tone of voice. All patients deserve privacy, respect, and kindness. When interviewing a minor or a patient with family members present, it is best to ask sensitive questions without visitors.

When questioned inappropriately or incorrectly, patients can very well feel like they are being judged and may answer less than honestly. Historically, the medical profession has not been very kind to this patient population [8]. If the patient appears reluctant to answer, it might be beneficial to say something such as, "I am not the police, I am not here to judge you. I only need to know these things so that I can care for you in a safe and effective manner."

Ask direct questions. For example, some patients might not consider marijuana to be a drug, so it might be helpful to name specific agents when soliciting the history. Additionally, if a patient says "No," be sure to probe further, i.e., "Never?" or, "Have you *ever*?" If the answer is "Absolutely never," or an exact quit date is given, then ask if they are in recovery.

If the patient reveals to you that they are in recovery, or they express the desire to get sober, then congratulate them and give positive reinforcement. It is critical to appreciate that for an addict or alcoholic, achieving sobriety might be the most difficult thing they have ever accomplished, especially if they are newly sober. Assess their feelings regarding opiates, benzodiazepines, and other potential triggering agents. Maybe chat with your patient instead of just giving midazolam (this works for nonaddicted patients too).

Furthermore, be sure to ask what their drug of choice was, how long they used, and how long they are clean. This would also be the perfect opportunity to find out how they are maintaining their sobriety, such as, what kind of support system they have in place (12-step program, sober living, halfway house, family/friends, etc.) [9]. We need to be as comfortable discussing this with our patients as we would any other disease.

These patients may have increased or decreased tolerance, which is highly varied depending on drug of choice, clean time, end-organ function, and individual differences. A sober alcoholic might appear healthier than he/she actually is. Each case is different, but when there is suspicion of organ damage, the healthcare provider should order appropriate tests, i.e., coagulation studies and liver function tests, hepatitis panel, etc. It is also relevant to inquire about the route of administration and assess accordingly. For example, parenteral drug users are at risk for developing skin abscesses and may have been exposed to blood-borne diseases such as the human immunodeficiency virus (HIV) or hepatitis. As well, obtaining peripheral intravenous access is often a challenge in this population. For inhaled drugs (particularly methamphetamine), a thorough airway assessment is warranted as the smoke can be corrosive to the dentition. Chronic marijuana smokers may present clinically with obstructive lung disease. For patients who report nasal administration, such as is common with snorted cocaine or heroin, use extreme caution when inserting a nasogastric tube or nasal endotracheal tube, due to nasal septum atrophy.

Understandably, the sober patient might be terrified of relapse or of receiving inadequate postoperative analgesia, and some investigators have studied nonmedicinal methods of managing preoperative anxiety. Wang and colleagues used music in their randomized, controlled study. They found that the patients in the music intervention group reported significantly lower preoperative anxiety levels [10]. Sjöling et al. assessed the impact of preoperative information in two groups of patients, all receiving a total knee arthroplasty. They found that the intervention (information) group had a more rapid reduction in postoperative pain; their preoperative anxiety state was lower; and they were more satisfied with their postoperative pain management versus the control group [11]. While these studies did not specifically address recovering patients, the principles certainly apply.

Lastly, there are many comorbid conditions to consider in this patient population. Some of the more common ones are smoking, psychiatric conditions (depression, anxiety, post-traumatic stress disorder, and sleeping disturbances), obesity or other eating disorders, and chronic pain.

The "Sober Since Admission" Patient

For many patients, this could be their "bottom" – do not overlook the perfect opportunity to "12th step" them (to suggest recovery). It is extremely common for trauma patients to have coexisting addiction or alcoholism. We perform a tremendous disservice when we treat their stab wounds, gunshot wounds, burns, etc., yet do not address the true underlying cause of their injuries.

Contrary to popular belief, one does not need to be in recovery to effectively suggest sobriety to a patient who would obviously benefit from it. There is always a certain degree of denial, or at least rationalizing/minimizing, that will manifest when the addict or alcoholic is confronted. It might be beneficial to conceptualize separating the patient from the disease. For example, if you feel yourself getting frustrated, do not be upset with the patient; rather be upset with their disease.

Ultimately, addiction is "self-diagnosed," ideally with the individual taking responsibility for their recovery. Many practitioners might not be comfortable or they might not know what to say. Here are some suggestions to open the dialogue and hopefully plant a seed:

- "Have you ever thought that perhaps you are here because of your drinking/drug use?"
- "Have you ever considered getting sober?"
- "Have you ever thought that you do not have to live like this anymore?"
- "Have you ever thought that this could be your bottom – you do not have to keep doing these things?"
- "What are your plans for when you are discharged? Do you have a safe place to go?" (For jail patients, reword it accordingly.)
- When the patient denies that there is a problem, a good comeback is, "I am not necessarily saying that this is *you* – however, we do see a lot of people come through here that have a problem with drugs or alcohol and have sustained injuries exactly like yours. Please think about it."

If the patient tells you that they have tried Alcoholics Anonymous (AA) or Narcotics Anonymous (NA) but that it did not work for them, then encourage them to try it again. It might also be insightful to ascertain why it did not work. Classically, it is because the person did not get a sponsor or work the steps, which are considered integral to successful recovery. It is also beneficial to request discharge planning and social work for appropriate referrals. Due to the "euphoric recall" nature of addiction, the patient might not be interested in sobriety when he/she is feeling better and is about to be discharged, which is why it might be better to get them thinking about it beforehand.

Since not all patients will have access to the Internet, you can go to these web-sites and easily obtain local telephone numbers for the patient to call. It is also important to let your patient know that meetings are free, and in most towns/cities, widely available:

- Alcoholics Anonymous: www.aa.org
- Narcotics Anonymous: www.na.org
- Cocaine Anonymous: www.ca.org

The "sober since admission" patient who has been abusing stimulants presents an additional concern during the perioperative period. Abuse of amphetamines (i.e., methamphetamine, methylphenidate, methyledioxymethamphetamine, and related drugs) can result in complications which persist days after the last ingestion of the drug. The primary mechanism of action of these agents is similar to ephedrine in that indirect sympathetic activation is caused by stimulating the release of norepi-nepherine, dopamine, and serotonin from terminals in the central and autonomic nervous systems. Over time, this leads to catecholamine depletion that is evident even when the person is not actively using these drugs [12]. It is not clear how long this depletion lasts; therefore directing sympathomimetics (i.e., phenylephrine) are recommended in the presence of hypotension. Cocaine, an indirectly direct acting agent, stimulates the sympathetic nervous system by blocking presynaptic uptake of norepinephrine and dopamine, thereby increasing postsynaptic concentrations. Cocaine also has some direct action at dopaminergic receptors, although the cate-cholamine depletion is classically seen with amphetamines. Long-term use of amphetamines and cocaine warrant concern for cardiac dysrhythmias, even when not acutely intoxicated. These patients might benefit from a focused cardiovascular assessment and diagnostics as appropriate (Table 16.1).

Methadone

Commonly used for "methadone maintenance therapy" (MMT), methadone is increasingly being used to manage chronic pain. Although a μ-agonist, methadone has little effect on postoperative or acute pain. Patients on MMT classically exhibit high tolerance for opiates and low threshold for pain (opioid-induced hyperalgesia). It is recommended to not skip doses of methadone preoperatively and also to consider adjuncts/alternatives, discussed in the following section. Another recommendation is to avoid agonist–antagonist medications (i.e., butorphanol and nalbuphine) as they could precipitate acute opiate withdrawal in this population.

Table 16.1 Specific drug–drug interactions between anesthetics and medicines used in the treatment of chemical dependency

	Mechanism of action	Cardiovascular	Respiratory	CNS	Metabolism; miscellaneous
Methadone	Diphenylheptane opiate agonist. Nonopioid activity: NMDA antagonism; also prevents reuptake of serotonin and norepinephrine	Use of positive pressure ventilation may increase postural hypotensive effect of narcotics. Monitor QT interval for patients on higher doses due to increased risk of Torsades de pointes	May be depressed, which may alter rate of onset of inhalational agent delivery	Increased sensitivity to other IV agents due to additive effect of methadone; decreased MAC of inhalational agents	Opioid-induced hyperalgesia. Low threshold for pain; high tolerance for opiates. For all ORT (methadone and buprenorphine), must keep to scheduled dosing, otherwise the patient will have withdrawal
Buprenorphine (Subtex)	Synthetic opiate partial agonist	Potentiation of responses from IV or inhalational anesthetics	Severe respiratory depression when administered with benzodiazepines; respiratory depression with other opiates that is not readily reversed with naloxone	Higher doses of opiate agonists will be required to produce the usual expected response	The systemic or CNS effect of local anesthetics (bupivacaine and mepivacaine) may be potentiated
Buprenorphine and naloxone (Suboxone)	Same anesthetic considerations as plain buprenorphine, unless the patient has crushed the tablets and injected them				The naloxone is *not* bioavailable when taken PO; only when *injected* (in order to discourage IV diversion on the street)

(continued)

Table 16.1 (continued)

	Mechanism of action	Cardiovascular	Respiratory	CNS	Metabolism; miscellaneous
Naltrexone (Revia: PO daily), depo-naltrexone (Vivitrol: injected once a month), also comes in pellet form that lasts 3–4 months	A long-acting synthetic opiate antagonist. Produces a dose-dependent antagonism for as long as 1–3 days after a single dose (in PO Revia). Same anesthetic concerns as naloxone (Narcan), listed here	Rarely seen: hypertension and tachycardia with arrhythmias in patients with preexisting cardiovascular disease who have previously received narcotics	Would need higher than normal doses to reverse opiate-induced respiratory depression	Will need higher doses of opiate agonists (and that is IF they work), while considering the unreliability of antagonism that is present. Consider options and adjuncts	If on daily dose, consider discontinuing 3 days before scheduled surgery
Clonidine (Catapres)	A centrally acting alpha-2 agonist that decreases sympathetic outflow from the CNS. Used to attenuate opiate withdrawal	Only a mild interaction with hypotensive/vasodilating agents. Due to the bradycardia often seen with clonidine, use of beta-blockers may produce an unusually low heart rate		Lowers MAC by 15–50%	Administration of naloxone may precipitate withdrawal hypertension. Also, naloxone has been used for the management of clonidine overdose

Drug	Mechanism	Direct/sympathomimetic effects	Anesthetic implications	Notes
Disulfiram (Antabuse)	Inhibits aldehyde dehydrogenase, causing the accumulation of acetaldehyde from the oxidation of EtOH. This accumulation leads to flushing, vertigo, diaphoresis, nausea, and vomiting after drinking alcohol	Direct-acting sympathomimetics may be more effective due to disulfiram-induced inhibition of dopamine beta-hydroxylase (leading to endogenous catecholamine depletion)	Half-life of barbiturates, benzodiazepines, and phenytoin may be prolonged, therefore prolonging the behavioral effects produced by these drugs	Potential for hepatotoxicity. Recommended to discontinue 10 days before surgery. Miscellaneous: Metronidazole and certain cephalosporins may produce a disulfiram-like reaction with EtOH intake.
Benzodiazepines (chlordiazepoxide, oxazepam, and clonazepam)	Facilitate the actions of GABA		Enhanced respiratory depression produced by IV or inhalational agents	Depressant effects seen with other IV or inhalational anesthetics will be additive to that produced by the benzodiazepine. Or, might see impressive tolerance. May see unusually high plasma levels of bupivacaine due to decreased metabolism. Preoperative administration of cimetidine (Tagamet) may elevate plasma benzodiazepine concentrations and keep them elevated for a longer time

(continued)

Table 16.1 (continued)

	Mechanism of action	Cardiovascular	Respiratory	CNS	Metabolism; miscellaneous
Monoamine oxidase inhibitors: phenelzine (Nardil), tranylcypromine (Parnate)	Inhibition of monamine oxidase, which attenuates oxidative deamination of serotonin, norepinephrine, and dopamine	Indirect-acting sympathomimetics can cause hypertensive crisis. Direct-acting agents appear to be safer		*Potentially fatal interaction* when taken with meperidine. The combination can cause an excitatory response including seizures, arrhythmias, and hyperpyrexia, eventually coma. Meperidine also blocks the neuronal uptake of serotonin.	Propofol and benzodiazepines may result in hypotension and exaggeration of CNS and respiratory depressant effects
Tricyclic antidepressants (amitriptyline, etc.)	Block the uptake of norepinepherine, serotonin, or both	Imipramine and desipramine increase by two- to tenfold the pressor response of injected, direct-acting sympathomimetics		Confusion and delirium postoperatively when centrally acting anticholinergics given preoperatively	
Selective serotonin reuptake inhibitors (example given: fluoxetine or Prozac)	Selectively inhibiting serotonin reuptake causes a potentiation of serotonergic neurotransmission in limbic areas of the brain	Tachycardia and ST segment depression, but only with high doses		Rarely seen: seizures and extrapyramidal rigidity	Half-life of diazepam is increased with fluoxetine. Droperidol may be more likely to produce extrapyramidal effects

Acamprosate (Campral)	The newest FDA-approved medication for maintenance of EtOH abstinence. Inhibits "limbic kindling." No known anesthetic implications at this time.	
Tramadol	Atypical opioid, considered to have low abuse potential. Has centrally acting μ activity; also spinal mechanism of monoamine reuptake inhibition	Possibility for serotonin syndrome when taken with SSRIs or MAOIs

- Methadone undergoes biphasic elimination: α-Elimination (8–12 h) correlates with analgesia (6–8 h), while β-elimination (30–60 h) has plasma levels that are subanalgesic, but high enough to prevent withdrawal symptoms
- Methadone has a cumulative effect: Use extreme caution prior to re-dosing as patients have developed ventricular arrhythmias (Torsades)
- In the opioid naïve, a single dose of >40 mg has been lethal
- Peng et al. recommend a morphine: methadone ratio of 4 or 5:1 (i.e., 30 mg methadone/day is roughly equivalent to 120 mg oral morphine/day),
- Remember that there is NOT a linear relationship when converting from methadone to morphine. Ideally, consult with a chronic pain pharmacist or pain fellow who is very familiar with the complex pharmacology of this drug

Options/Adjuncts to Opiates

There are a large number of techniques described in the literature for managing perioperative and postoperative pain for this patient population. The principles of these techniques could also apply to most, if not all patients. The general consensus seen repeatedly in the literature is:

- To use alternative, nonopiate medications and/or regional anesthesia to minimize opiates
- When opiates are used, adhere to recommended guidelines and prescribing principles
- To consider nonmedical interventions

When selecting alternative agents, it is reasonable to consider their risk to benefit ratio as well as patient comorbidities and type of surgery. White and Kehlet advocate for the use of multimodal, opioid-sparing analgesic techniques but express caution regarding the side effects of the many nonopioid analgesics (acetaminophen, NSAIDs, NMDA antagonists, and gabapentinoids), including those of hepatic and renal toxicity, coagulation, confusion, and oversedation [13]. Furthermore, these effects might be more pronounced when these medications are coadministered with other analgesics and anesthetics.

Regional Techniques, Infiltration of Local by Surgeons, and the "On-Q" System

The benefits of local anesthesia, whether administered by our surgical colleagues or as a regional technique, are obvious, with the need for less supraspinal analgesia (opiates). Regional techniques should be offered to the patient whenever appropriate, especially when there is opiate tolerance, opioid-induced hyperalgesia, and/or the desire to avoid potential triggering agents. Wound-infiltration analgesia as part of a multimodal analgesic regime removes the concern of infection from indwelling catheters or local anesthetic toxicity associated with large volumes.

One study examining the effects of local anesthesia in recovering alcoholics presenting for dental work found that this population is not at increased risk for inadequate analgesia when local anesthesia (mepivicaine) is used [14]. If using large quantities of local, perhaps it would be reasonable to avoid amides if the sober alcoholic has decreased hepatic function. Topically applied local anesthesia has been shown to effectively treat a number of different pain syndromes, including post-thoracotomy, stump neuroma pain, intercostal neuralgia, diabetic polyneuropathy, and postmastectomy pain syndromes [15].

N-Methyl-D-aspartate Antagonists

- Dextromethorphan: Has been recommended by some as an adjunct to reduce opioid requirements [16]. Originally synthesized as an alternative to morphine, it is reported to be practically devoid of symptomatic side effects. When coadministered with morphine, it was mostly effective in the early postoperative period, following spine surgery.
- Amantidine (Symmetrel): Has been recommended for chronic cancer pain [17] but there are still mixed reviews for acute, postoperative pain [18].
- Memantine: The most potent *N*-Methyl-D-aspartate (NMDA) antagonist, it is currently used for a variety of disorders, including Alzheimer's disease, dementia, post-traumatic stress disorder, and others [19].
- Ketamine: When given as a single low-dose bolus (0.15–0.5 mg/kg) with/without a low-dose infusion (2–4 mcg/kg/min) intraoperatively, it has direct analgesic effects, prevents sensitization of nociceptive pathways within the CNS, and reverses or reduces opioid tolerance and opioid-induced hyperalgesia.

Ketamine is commonly used as an adjuvant drug and has been studied extensively. Its efficacy has been shown in bariatric surgery; when used with clonidine it has been shown to improve recovery and reduce postoperative pain when compared to "standard" anesthesia [20]. When administered during induction as a continuous infusion intraoperatively, ketamine has been shown to reduce postoperative opioid consumption [21]. Based on the opioid-induced hyperalgesia literature, including pain management of MMT patients, there is unequivocal recommendation for utilization of an NMDA antagonist; usually it is ketamine that is suggested, although there are other drugs in this class. Furthermore, administration of an NMDA antagonist can attenuate the hyperexcitability or the "wind-up" state that leads to hyperactivity of the nociceptive system.

α-*Adrenergic Agonists*

Clonidine (Catapres) and dexmedetomidine (Precedex) have been shown to be extremely beneficial since they alleviate opioid withdrawal symptoms as well as pain, with proven efficacy as a spinal analgesic [22]. Dexmedetomidine has a $\alpha2/\alpha1$ selectivity ratio that is eight times higher than clonidine and has demonstrated opioid-sparing effects as well as lowered MAC requirements [23]. When clonidine is administered intrathecally, there is a dose-dependent analgesic effect with relative hemodynamic stability, and the nearly immediate analgesic effect argues for spinal versus systemic administration of this drug [22]. Low-dose dexmedetomidine or clonidine, when coadministered with bupivacaine for subarachnoid block, has been shown to produce a significantly shorter onset of motor blockade with a significantly longer sensory and motor block. When used for postoperative sedation, dexmedetomidine has been shown to reduce morphine requirements by 50% and midazolam requirements by 80% [24].

Acetaminophen, NSAIDs, and COX-2 Inhibitors

Nonsteroidal anti-inflammatory drugs (NSAIDs) have been shown to be more effective in the treatment of pain from dental procedures than acetaminophen [25]; however, firm conclusions cannot be made for major/minor orthopedic surgeries due to the limited number of studies. Coadministration of these medications will enhance the pain relief effects, and acetaminophen remains a viable alternative for patients who cannot receive NSAIDs due to their side effects. For patients receiving anticoagulation, acetaminophen should be administered instead of NSAIDs. When multimodal analgesia is performed (acetaminophen, NSAIDs, or selective COX-2 inhibitors) with PCA morphine, there is a significant reduction in morphine consumption as well as a reduced incidence of nausea, vomiting, and oversedation (Table 16.2).

Gabapentin (Neurontin)

Originally developed as an anticonvulsant, gabapentin is now commonly used to treat neuropathic pain, diabetic neuropathy, as well as off-label use for a variety of conditions, such as restless leg syndrome and "dancing eye syndrome" [26]. More recently, it has been trialed for acute surgical pain and has been found to be a reasonable alternative to cyclooxygenase-2 (COX-2) inhibitors, resulting in reduced postoperative opiate use, thus contributing to a more rapid return of bowel function.

The use of a single dose of preoperative gabapentin has been shown to reduce anxiety as well as allowing for more extensive passive and active knee flexion in orthopedic patients and reducing the need for postoperative opioid and NSAID rescue medications [27].

Table 16.2 Should recovering addicts get PCA?

Positive	Negative
Jage and Bey [2] recommend PCA with short-acting opioids; without "background infusion" (? basal rate)	Ziegler [35] does not advocate PCA
Savage et al. [9] recommend PCA with small, incremental doses that are spaced at intervals which do not allow for a rapid rise in serum level of opiate which would produce a big "reward." They also advise caution for the potential of the patient tampering with the PCA system (for the very newly sober or still active addict)	May et al. [6] state that PCA is controversial but that solely dosing on a PRN basis is not good either. They recommend around-the-clock dosing
Peng et al. [33] advocate the use of PCA in MMT patients, especially when they will not be able to resume their usual methadone dose by 48 h	Mehta and Langford [3]: Potentially difficult to optimize due to patient variability; might use PCA for psychological effects versus its intended purpose; PCA must be tamper proof; frequent need of opioid might be viewed as drug seeking or drug craving
Mitra and Sinatra [34] recommend PCA in "selected patients." They advocate starting the infusion in PACU since there might be a delay in dosing upon arrival to the surgical care unit. They also believe that PCA can be supplemented by a basal infusion, but it might not be necessary when the patient has a fentanyl patch. The PCA can also be supplemented with neural blockade and/or nonopioid analgesics. Following their recommendations, the authors give detailed accounts of several individual case reports in which PCA was successful	
Mehta and Langford [3] was the only article reviewed that has an actual table of pros and cons. Highlights: easy to use; is a standard practice; promotes maintenance of stable opioid levels, which avoids sedation at peak levels and pain/anxiety/drug craving at trough levels; patients like being "in control" and possibly reducing any confrontational behavior	

Antidepressants

Many advocate for the use of antidepressants for neuropathic pain, reporting that tricyclic antidepressants and anticonvulsants are the first-line treatment. This also supports the hypothesis that pain and depression share some common biochemical mechanisms. Another interesting find is that antidepressants have an analgesic effect in chronic pain patients who do not have co-occurring depression [28].

Capsaicin

Capsaicin is the lipophilic vanilloid compound that makes hot chili peppers spicy. It is widely available as over-the-counter topical analgesic creams and patches. The agent has a selective action on small peripheral nociceptive fibers; and these effects are mediated by the activation of specific vanilloid receptors, found in nociceptive endings. Capsaicin patches and creams have been recommended for neuropathic/chronic pain, but its opioid-sparing effects need to be investigated further.

Alternative Therapies

Nonconventional methods such as hypnosis, guided imagery, acupuncture, meditation, biofeedback, electrical stimulation, TENS, and physical therapy are reported in the literature, as well as the more commonly employed methods for milder pain such as rest, cold, heat, and elevation.

Mind–body therapies (MBTs) have been shown to be somewhat effective in the treatment of pain resulting from various medical conditions, including postsurgical and chronic pain, but Western medicine has not moved beyond the biomedical model to a biopsychosocial model, for several reasons. These alternative treatment modalities are often overlooked, underutilized, and are underemphasized in medical education. There is also the seeming "lack of evidence" due to the flaws in methodological rigor that are inevitably encountered when testing the effectiveness of MBTs. These interventions cannot be tested with a placebo or in a sham control condition due to the inability of blinding the practitioners to type of treatment, nor blinding the patients to group assignment. Regardless, and in spite of the lack of evidence of effectiveness, many of these treatments have been around for thousands of years and continue to be commonly used in other parts of the world.

Acupuncture

Studies evaluating the efficacy of acupuncture as an analgesic treatment modality are hindered by small sample size, poorly defined/invalidated outcomes, confounding variables, and acupuncturist bias. Studies that have shown its effectiveness report reductions in intravenous supplemental morphine use and postoperative nausea as well as decreased plasma cortisol and epinephrine concentrations. Acupuncture is a viable alternative treatment for pain associated with renal colic and is used effectively in China and Taiwan [29].

Hypnosis

Perhaps the least understood of the alternative therapies, the use of hypnosis in surgery has been implemented for centuries with fascinating, detailed case reports dating back to the early 1800s [30]. As with acupuncture and MBTs, investigation of hypnosis involves small sample sizes and often lacks control groups and statistical evaluations. Several studies have utilized positron emission tomography and functional magnetic resonance imaging to investigate how hypnosis influences neural pain pathways stimulated by evoked potentials. Even if it is not possible to prove effectiveness through studies, hypnosis, emotional support, and positive suggestions are all readily available, safe, and inexpensive and might improve the care of our patients.

Hypnosis has been used in childbirth for over a century to reduce analgesic requirements during labor though it seems to be only effective for stage I labor [31]. Hypnosis, with or without other anesthetic techniques, may offer advantages over conventional analgesic techniques alone. It respects patient autonomy and may be beneficial without significant side effects. Most authors suggest antenatal training could be achieved in as few as four to six sessions, with medical students reading hypnosis scripts to untrained mothers regarding how to facilitate induction of hypnosis to relieve pain and anxiety during labor.

In-Hospital Postoperative Pain Management

Pain is a significant trigger for relapse. Especially for the newly sober, the immediate postoperative period is not the time to quit everything. Stress is also a well-documented trigger for relapse [32], and there are several factors that can cause stress in the postoperative period.

Recovering addicts have a legitimate fear of relapse, as well as a fear of inadequate postoperative pain control due to ineffective dosing. Encourage them to verbalize their concerns. If the patient will have an extended hospital stay, perhaps suggest that they invite their AA or NA sponsor, or other recovering friends to visit. If the patient is newly sober and does not have such contacts yet, it might be worth looking into having a Certified Addictions Counselor (CAC) see them.

During the postoperative period, ascertain if the patient is receiving effective analgesia.

Recovering addicts have pain too, and this is very often is dismissed as "drug seeking." If the prescribed pain regimen is ineffective, this is a good opportunity to be a patient advocate and to educate other healthcare professionals who are more involved in their postoperative care. As well, any patient taking opioids may develop opioid-induced hyperalgesia (increased sensitivity to pain) and this should be considered.

Table 16.3 Guidelines for "self-medicating" after discharge

- Prescriber *must* know history. Only ONE person prescribes; and the prescription is filled at ONE pharmacy
- Have pharmacist divide prescription into 1- or 2-day aliquots, if necessary
- Determine ahead of time what the expected analgesic course should be
- Some recommend drug testing, and also a contract or written agreement
- Agree ahead of time how "lost medications" will be handled; can also do pill counts
- CHECK YOUR MOTIVES! Why am I taking this? Is it physical, mental, or emotional pain? Many addicts cannot differentiate between physical and psychological pain
- Keep accurate track of dosing; perhaps a journal with pain scale ratings. Describe the pain, giving it physical characteristics
- Take it AS DIRECTED. If the pain is refractory, then you must call prescriber. Emergency department visits are highly discouraged, unless previously cleared by primary physician
- Have sponsor, spouse, or other trustworthy person hold prescription if necessary
- Return unused portions to pharmacy – do *not* save for a "rainy day"

Providing recovering patients their postoperative analgesics around the clock instead of on an as-needed (PRN) basis removes the need for the patient to make the decision when to take the medication, and it maintains a therapeutic level of opiate instead of allowing the pain to escalate. Skipping doses can cause anxiety and drug craving; and when the patient asks for medication, it might be misinterpreted as drug-seeking or addictive behavior. It may be helpful to provide the patient a copy of the guidelines for "self-medicating" after discharge (Table 16.3).

Conclusion

There is very little available data regarding the experiences of recovering addicts following surgery, after having received potential triggering agents for relapse. Interestingly, there are two studies that involve recovering anesthesia providers as the sample [36, 37]. The former is unfortunately only published as an abstract, and the latter is unpublished. In the study conducted by Bryson and Hamza, only 10% of the anesthetists surveyed (3/30) subsequently relapsed, and each readily admitted to being in "prelapse" mode prior to receiving a triggering agent. They also reported that they did not have a solid postoperative pain management plan in place. The 90% who did not relapse unequivocally stated that the most significant protecting factor was AA or NA. While this is encouraging, there is much more that needs to be done.

On a personal note, I have countless anecdotal stories of patients where I have taken the time to discuss with them either how they are "working their program of recovery," or strongly suggesting to consider sobriety. I keep photocopies of AA, NA, and Al-Anon literature in my locker, in both English and Spanish, and dole them out as appropriate. I like the patients to have something tangible after I am done talking to them. I have also had so many patients who are already in a 12-step program, who are grateful to have familiar literature to read, for it brings them immense comfort.

I would encourage all perioperative healthcare providers to re-conceptualize addiction and recovery. Addiction is a disease that does not discriminate; and I know of no individual who consciously chose to be addicted. We need to treat all of our patients with dignity and respect and think of what other services we can be offering in addition to perioperative care. If we have patients with a known history of addiction, we are responsible for counseling them and for considering opioid-sparing techniques as appropriate. Patients on ORT should be treated (physically) as active addicts since we know they will have a low pain threshold and a high opiate tolerance.

Directions for future research would certainly involve the efficacy of MBTs and alternative methods in the recovering addict population. Personal accounts of recovering addicts who did not relapse after having legitimately received triggering agents might prove to be helpful as well.

References

1. Alford DP, Compton P, Samet JH. Acute pain management for patients receiving maintenance methadone or buprenorphine therapy. Ann Intern Med. 2006;144:127–34.
2. Jage J, Bey T. Postoperative analgesia in patients with substance use disorders: part I. Acute Pain. 2000;3:141–56.
3. Mehta V, Langford RM. Acute pain management for opioid dependent patients. Anaesthesia. 2006;61:269–76.
4. Prater CD, Zylstra RG, Miller KE. Successful pain management for the recovering addicted patient. J Clin Psychiatry. 2002;4:125–31.
5. Chang G, Chen L, Mao J. Opioid tolerance and hyperalgesia. Med Clin North Am. 2007;91:199–211.
6. May JA, White HC, Leonard-White AL, Warltier DC, Pagel PS. The patient recovering from alcohol or drug addiction: special issues for the anesthesiologist. Anesth Analg. 2001;92:1601–8.
7. Bécheiraz P, Thallman D. A model of nonverbal communication and interpersonal relationship between virtual actors. Computer Animation. 1996;58–68.
8. Scimeca MM, Savage SR, Portenoy R, Lowinson J. Treatment of pain in methadone maintained patients. Mt Sinai J Med. 2000;67:412–22.
9. Savage SR, Kirsh KL, Passik SD. Challenges in using opioids to treat pain in persons with substance use disorders. NIDA Addict Sci Clin Pract. 2008;4:4–25.
10. Wang SM, Kulkarni L, Dolev J, Kain ZN. Music and preoperative anxiety: a randomized, controlled study. Ambulatory Anesth. 2002;94:1489–94.
11. Sjöling M, Nordahl G, Olofsson N, Asplund K. The impact of preoperative information on state anxiety, postoperative pain and satisfaction with pain management. Patient Educ Couns. 2003;51:169–76.
12. Klein M, Kramer F. Rave drugs: pharmacological considerations. AANA J. 2004;72:61–7.
13. White PF, Kehlet H. Improving postoperative pain management: what are the unresolved issues? Anesthesiology. 2010;112:220–5.
14. Fiset L, Leroux B, Rothen M, Prall C, Zhu C, Ramsay DS. Pain control in recovering alcoholics: effects of local anesthesia. J Stud Alcohol Drugs. 1997;58:291–6.
15. Devers A, Galer BS. Topical lidocaine patch relieves a variety of neuropathic pain conditions: an open-label study. Clin J Pain. 2000;16:205–8.
16. Suski M, Bujak-Gizycka B, Madej J, Kacka K, Woron J, Olszanecki R, et al. Co-administration of dextromethorphan and morphine: reduction of post-operative pain and lack of influence on morphine metabolism. Basic Clin Pharmacol Toxicol. 2010;107:680–4.

17. Lussier D, Huskey AG, Portenoy RK. Adjuvant analgesics in cancer pain management. Oncologist. 2004;9:571–91.
18. White PF. The changing role of non-opioid analgesic techniques in the management of postoperative pain. Anesth Analg. 2005;101:S5–22.
19. Suzuki M. Role of N-methyl D-aspartate receptor antagonists in postoperative pain management. Curr Opin Anaesthesiol. 2009;22:618–22.
20. Sollazzi L, Modesti C, Vitale F, Sacco T, Ciocchetti P, Idra AS, et al. Preinductive use of clonidine and ketamine improves recovery and reduces postoperative pain after bariatric surgery. Surg Obes Relat Dis. 2009;5:67–71.
21. Loftus RW, Yeager MP, Clark JA, Brown JR, Abdu WA, Sengupta DK, et al. Intraoperative ketamine reduces perioperative opiate consumption in opiate-dependent patients with chronic back pain undergoing back surgery. Anesthesiology. 2010;113:639–46.
22. Kanazi GE, Aouad MT, Jabbour-Khoury SI, Al Jazzar MD, Alameddine MM, Al-Yaman R, et al. Effect of low-dose dexmedetomidine or clonidine on the characteristics of bupivacaine spinal block. Acta Anasthesiol Scand. 2006;50:222–7.
23. Weinbroum AA, Ben-Abraham R. Dextromethorphan and dexmedetomidine: new agents for the control of perioperative pain. Eur J Surg. 2001;167:563–9.
24. Venn RM, Bradshaw CJ, Spencer R, Brealey D, Caudwell E, Naughton C, et al. Preliminary UK experience of dexmedetomidine, a novel agent for postoperative sedation in the intensive care unit. Anaesthesia. 1999;54:1136–42.
25. Hyllested M, Jones S, Pedersen JL, Kehlet H. Comparative effect of parecetamol, NSAIDs or their combination in postoperative pain management: a qualitative review. Br J Anaesth. 2002;88:199–214.
26. Sirven JI. New uses for older drugs: the tales of aspirin, thalidomine and gabapentin. Mayo Clin Proc. 2010;85:508–11.
27. Srivastava U, Kumar A, Saxena S, Mishra AR, Saraawat N, Mishra S. Effect of preoperative gabapentin on postoperative pain and tramadol consumption after minilap open cholecystectomy: a randomized double-blind, placebo-controlled trial. Eur J Anaesthesiol. 2010;27:331–5.
28. Micó JA, Ardid D, Berrocoso E, Eschalier A. Antidepressants and pain. Trends Pharmacol Sci. 2006;27:348–54.
29. Davenport K, Timoney AG, Keeley FX. Conventional and alternative methods for providing analgesia in renal colic. BJU Int. 2004;95:297–300.
30. Hollander B. Selection of anaesthetics: hypnosis and anaesthesia. Proc R Soc Med. 1932;25:597–610.
31. Wang SM, Kain ZN, White PF. Acupuncture analgesia II: clinical considerations. Anesth Analg. 2008;106:611–21.
32. Sinha R. The role of stress in addiction relapse. Curr Psychiatry Rep. 2007;9:388–95.
33. Peng PWH, Tumber PS, Gourlay D. Review article: Perioperative pain management of patients on methadone therapy. Canadian Journal of Anaesthesiology. 2005;(52) 5:513–523.
34. Mitra S, Sinatra RS. Perioperative management of acute pain in the opioid-dependent patient. Anesthesiology. 2004;101 (1):212–227.
35. Ziegler PP. Addiction and the treatment of pain. Substance Use & Misuse. 2005;40:1945–1954.
36. Williams MJ, Tinnell C, Gibbs CP. Adverse Experiences of Recovering Physician Addicts/Alcoholics in the Perioperative Period: Exposure of anesthesia providers in recovery from substance abuse to potential triggering agents. Anesthesiology, September 1992;77(3A):A1113.
37. Bryson EO, Hamza H. Exposure of anesthesia providers in recovery from substance abuse to potential triggering agents. Journal of Clinical Anesthesia, In-press.

Index

E.O. Bryson and E.A.M. Frost (eds.), *Perioperative Addiction:*
Clinical Management of the Addicted Patient, DOI 10.1007/978-1-4614-0170-4,
© Springer Science+Business Media, LLC 2012